CHINESE MEDICINE
IN CONTEMPORARY CHINA

SCIENCE AND CULTURAL THEORY

A Series Edited by Barbara Herrnstein Smith

and E. Roy Weintraub

CHINESE MEDICINE

IN CONTEMPORARY CHINA

Plurality and Synthesis · VOLKER SCHEID

DUKE UNIVERSITY PRESS   Durham & London 2002

2nd printing, 2005

© 2002 Duke University Press

All rights reserved

Printed in the United States of America on acid-free paper ⊗

Typeset in Trump Mediaeval by Tseng Information Systems, Inc.

Library of Congress Cataloging-in-Publication Data appear

on the last printed page of this book.

Portions of chapter 5 were originally published in "Shaping
Chinese Medicine: Two Case Studies from Contemporary China,"
in *Innovation in Chinese Medicine*, ed. Elisabeth Hsu (Cambridge:
Cambridge University Press, 2001), pp. 370–404.
Portions of chapters 6 and 8 were originally published in "Kexue
and Guanxixue: Contemporary Chinese Medicine and the Origins
of Plurality," in *Medical Pluralism*, ed. Waltraud Ernst (London:
Routledge, 2001).

This book is dedicated to my parents

CONTENTS

LIST OF FIGURES AND TABLES

Figures

Tables

ACKNOWLEDGMENTS

I gratefully acknowledge the help and support of many individuals and institutions who supported me through various stages of writing this book. Their kindness, criticism, and encouragement not only helped to make the entire process an exciting intellectual adventure but also created many new relationships while deepening others.

To Gilbert Lewis, my doctoral supervisor at the University of Cambridge, I give my most grateful thanks. He provided me with many of the tools of anthropological inquiry and guided me in their use. He showed great patience in dealing with ideas sometimes quite different from his own and supported me through the various difficulties encountered in preparing the dissertation on which this book is based. Judith Farquhar, from the Department of Social Anthropology at the University of North Carolina, has been an inspiration, mentor, and friend without whose help and guidance I would have lost my way on more than one occasion. I hope that through the writing of this book I can justify some of the trust she has placed in me over the years. My friend and colleague Dan Bensky was an ever-present source of support without whose manifold inputs—too numerous to list in detail—this book would never have been realized.

At the Department of Social Anthropology in Cambridge, where I wrote the Ph.D. dissertation that eventually matured into this book, I was guided toward a more profound familiarity with anthropology and enabled to formulate my interests in such a way as to make them worthy of inquiry. Particular thanks go to Françoise Barbira-Freedman, who supervised me for one term; to Esther Goody for making me so welcome during my first year at the department; to Marilyn Strathern for supporting me after my return from the field; and to Caroline Humphrey for her valuable criticisms.

My fieldwork was possible only with the help of Xu Shaoying, who went to considerable trouble to organize my stay at Beijing University of Chinese Medicine. After I arrived in Beijing, Mrs. Xu provided many of the introductions that later enabled me to carry out my fieldwork. At the University of Chinese Medicine the staff of the Foreign Training Institute arranged for me to study with the teachers I selected, as did the administrative offices of the Dongzhimen Hospital, the China-Japan Friendship Hospitals, and the Guoyitang Clinic. Their help is greatly appreciated. Ren Tinge, of the Basic Theory Research Institute of the university, helped me find books that even libraries did not carry.

During a different phase of my research the staff of the library at the Academy of Chinese Medicine in Beijing was helpful in accommodating my requests. Particular thanks go to the director of the library, Qiu Jian, who made each of my three stays at the library a most enjoyable experience, and to Yang Kangwei, the senior librarian. The same warm welcome was extended to me at the library of the Shanghai University of Chinese Medicine. I am most grateful to librarians Ma Ruren, Deng Lijuan, and Wang Ronggen for assisting me with various tasks.

The openness, support, and warm hospitality afforded to me by my teachers, fellow students, patients, and all the other people I met during my visits to China deeply touched me. The many individuals who helped me are too numerous to list. I wish to express my particular gratitude, however, to a small number of teachers and friends who went out of their way to help me see and understand and to make me feel comfortable. Their patience, warmth, and humanity made my time in China rewarding and pleasurable. I thank Professor Xu Zhu for taking me under her wing and for helping me whenever I needed it. Professor Lu Tianxin and his wife, Professor Qian Zhenhuai, welcomed me with warmth and affection and taught me much. To Wang Jun, my research assistant, friend, and sister, I owe thanks for support, encouragement, and just being herself. Zhao Baixiao had the openness of mind to engage with my strange ideas and the patience to help with the practical side of things: from finding accommodation to lending me his bike. As a result, he became a very special friend. Professor Wu Boping tirelessly provided me with information and introductions, taught me the subtleties of prescribing, and took time to comment on parts of my manuscript. Professor Wu helped me to understand what I value most deeply in Chinese medicine. Last, I owe more than just gratitude to Professor Shi Zaixiang, who accepted me as his student and, together with his wife, Professor Huang Liuhua, made their family my family. His consistent inspiration as a clinician, teacher, and scholar has touched me deeply.

I also wish to express thanks to Professors Dong Changhong, Guo Zhi-qiang, Huang Yunliang, Liu Jingyuan, Wang Mianzhi, Wang Ziyu, Xu Runsan, Yang Weiyi, and Zhang Shijie. In their own particular ways each of them profoundly deepened my understanding of Chinese medicine. Others who helped me in various ways during my visits to Beijing and whom I remember with affection include Laura Caretto; Echo and her brother, Yu Mingzhe; Eric Hagt; Hao Zhen and her husband, Cai Zhiwei; Brenda Hood; Fan Yongping; Jia Hai-zhong; Li Ge; Li Jing; Wang Hao; Xiao Yi; Xu Chunhong; and Zhang Shunan.

Several friends and colleagues commented on drafts of my manuscript at various stages of its transition from thesis into book. I am grateful to all of them for their patience and for sharing their knowledge with me. Professor Nathan Sivin not only took the time to read through my entire dissertation but returned it to me with useful annotations on almost every page. I am deeply indebted to his scholarship and support, which helped me to express my ideas much more clearly than might otherwise have been the case. Professor Geoffrey Lloyd also read my dissertation and pointed me in the right direction on many points. Francesca Diebschlag, Waltraud Ernst, Eric Karch-mer, Hugh McPherson, Andrew Pickering, Kim Taylor, and the participants of the Agora Conference on "Travelling Facts" at the Wissenschaftkolleg in Berlin read through various parts of my manuscript and aided my understanding of many issues, enabling me to amend inadequate points and passages. Whatever deficiencies remain are entirely attributable to my own limited understanding.

Grants from the Richards Fund, the Ling Roth Fund, and the Wyse Fund supported the writing of my dissertation. Norma Beak paid for my travel to China. I am much indebted to her generosity and kindness. I also gratefully acknowledge support from the Wellcome Trust in the form of a research fellowship during the final stages of drafting this book. The formulation of my initial research proposal, the composition of my thesis, and the writing of this book benefited from the help and criticism of colleagues, scholars, and friends not yet mentioned: Christine Bodenschatz, Steve Clavey, Keith Hart, T. J. Hinrichs, Elisabeth Hsu, Stephen Hugh-Jones, Mohammed Tabishat, Paul Unschuld, Franz Zehentmayer, and the participants of the writing-up seminars at the Department of Social Anthropology in Cambridge.

One of the many things I have learned is that writing a book is exciting but producing it can be hard work. My grateful thanks go to everyone at Duke University Press for their generous help and support. I am obliged in particular to J. Reynolds Smith and Sharon P. Torian for guiding me through the entire process with great patience; to my editor Pam Morrison and my copy editor Mindy Conner, who are responsible for turning my manuscript into this book; and to Mary Mendell for taking care of the design and artwork.

I apologize to Matteo for having to endure the many disadvantages that my attempts at becoming a scholar-physician have brought to his life. Most of all I want to express my gratitude to my wife, Cinzia, for her enduring love and support.

TIMELINE ON CHINESE HISTORY

Zhou dynasty 周   c. 1030–c. 221 B.C.
   Spring and Autumn (Chun qiu 春秋) period   c. 722–480 B.C.
   Warring States (Zhan guo 战国) period   480 B.C.–221 B.C.
Qin dynasty 秦   221 B.C.–207 B.C.
Han dynasty 汉   202 B.C.–220
Three Kingdoms period 三国   221–280
Jin dynasty 晋   265–479
Northern and Southern dynasties   479–581
Sui dynasty 隋   581–618
Tang dynasty 唐   618–906
Five Dynasty period 五代   907–960
Song dynasty 宋   960–1179
Jin dynasty 金   1115–1234
Yuan (Mongol) dynasty 元   1260–1368
Ming dynasty 明   1368–1644
Qing (Manchu) dynasty 清   1644–1911
Republican period 民国   1912–1949
   1927–1949   Nationalist Party (Guomindang 国民党) rule
   1946–1949   Civil War between Guomindang and Communists
People's Republic 中华人民共和国   1949–present
   1956   China declared socialist
   1957   Great Leap Forward
   1966–1976   Cultural Revolution
   1978 onward   Period of economic reform and opening up to the West

In this world, things are complicated and decided by many factors. We should look at problems from different aspects, not from just one. —Mao Zedong, "On the Chungking Negotiations"

Basing oneself on the affirmation of past experience, yet feeling one's way through to how one might employ dead methods in order to treat living people [truly] is to synthesize the old and the new, is to consider and deliberate both the foreign and the Chinese. —Yue Meizhong, "Without Persevering It Is Difficult to Become a Physician"

I deeply believe that the theories and treatment methods of Chinese medicine and Western medicine are not alike. The objects of research in both cases, however, are diseases and the results that can be obtained by treatment. —Qin Bowei, "Survey of Famous Shanghai Physicians: Foreword"

CHINESE MEDICINE
IN CONTEMPORARY CHINA

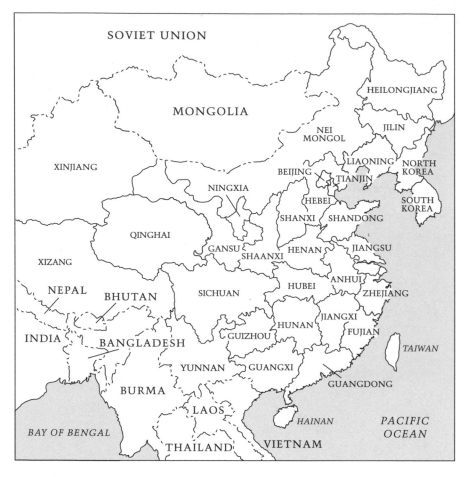

Geographical Map of China (Provinces)

INTRODUCTION

As a traditional healing art that is establishing a global presence in the post-modern world, Chinese medicine defies many of the conventional categories that order our lives. If Chinese medicine is indeed traditional, why has it not disappeared by now together with the rest of traditional Chinese society? If it is a science, what does that imply for our views of science at large? If the key to Chinese medicine lies in an intimate familiarity with Chinese culture and its concepts, how can it be used by increasing numbers of non-Asians who possess at best a very superficial understanding of that culture? If, on the other hand, Chinese medicine is—like biomedicine—not tied to time or place, why do we refer to it as Chinese? And what, finally, is the secret of Chinese medicine's remarkable adaptability that has allowed it to prosper for more than two thousand years?

Suggestions for Reading This Book

Engaging with a complex and complicated phenomenon such as Chinese medicine requires patience and a willingness to abstain from easy generalizations if questions such as those above are to be answered. Hence, in writing this book I have consciously embraced an interdisciplinary attitude that refuses to be constrained by the boundaries of any one academic discipline or tradition of inquiry. My ethnographic approach is that of a medical anthropologist, even though I rarely refer to culture or society. I draw for theory on models developed in the sociology of scientific knowledge, but I do not engage in much discussion regarding the nature of science and technology. I frequently and unapologetically take the perspective of an insider, though I am sure physicians of Chinese medicine in China and the West will find my views regarding the essential plurality and plasticity of their tradition challenging.

I write not for one particular audience but for anyone with an interest in contemporary Chinese medicine. Different people may benefit, however, from reading this book in different ways. For this purpose I have constructed each chapter as a self-contained unit and grouped these into three main parts. Each chapter explores a distinctive problem, and each of the three parts draws a loose boundary around a particular topic of inquiry.

Part 1 foregrounds theoretical and methodological problems encountered in our explorations of Chinese medicine. Chapter 1 locates my own position within this encounter and defines the precise goals of my inquiry. It is within this context that plurality emerges as the main thesis of the book. Chapter 2 expands the theme by means of a brief historical overview and an ethnographic case study that allow me to define plurality as being characterized by an essential heterogeneity and multiplicity of elements conjoined in the practice of Chinese medicine, as well as the simultaneous emerging and disappearing of these elements in practice.

Part 2 constitutes the ethnographic core of the book. Here I examine from six different perspectives a plurality of agencies and processes involved in the shaping of contemporary Chinese medicine. These include: politicians and the state (chapter 3); patients and physicians (chapter 4); the practice and transformation of Chinese medicine in the coming together of modern institutions of health care and classical scholarship (chapter 5); the institutions, networks, and kinds of knowledge involved in becoming a physician (chapter 6); and the emergence of knowledge and practice at the intersection of ideological, clinical, institutional, historical, and personal struggles (chapters 7 and 8). Each chapter can be read on its own. Read together they furnish an understanding of Chinese medicine in contemporary China as a network of intersecting processes and structures that do not have any single center to which they could be reduced.

Part 3 moves from description to intervention. The manner in which we define Chinese medicine as an object of inquiry impinges on debates regarding its position in our lives. At present, these debates tend to be constrained by hegemonic biomedical models of efficacy even where positions are developed as alternatives to these models. Chapter 9 defines all medical practice as fundamentally experimental, with each practice embodying in its construction differential evaluations of risk and desire for control. I suggest that it is the task of anthropology and other social sciences to make transparent these alignments and thereby facilitate decision-making processes that touch all our lives.

Given the different background knowledge and interests different readers will bring to this book I suggest two different reading strategies. Anthropologists, sociologists of science, historians of medicine, and others with some background knowledge in any of the above disciplines, who are likely to be interested in the theoretical debates that guide my inquiry, should read the book from front to back. Practitioners of Chinese medicine, physicians, and others without background knowledge in any of the disciplines mentioned above, who are likely to be interested in Chinese medicine as a medical practice rather than as a sociocultural phenomenon, might first want to read the ethnographies of part 2 and the conclusion in part 3 before approaching the more demanding theoretical discussions of part 1.

Notes on Terminology

Given that this book addresses a very diverse audience, many of whom will have little prior knowledge of Chinese medicine, I provide brief explanations of medical terms and concepts wherever necessary. For a more thorough explication I refer readers to accounts of Chinese medical thinking and practice and of Chinese medical history that are by now available in English and all other major European languages.[1]

Throughout this book I use the term "Chinese medicine" to refer to the medicine of the scholarly elite during the imperial era and also to the subsequent transformations of this medicine in the course of the Republican, Maoist, and post-Maoist periods. This is the literal translation of the Chinese term zhongyi 中医, which is used in the People's Republic of China (PRC) to refer to both of these uses.

I explicitly avoid the term "traditional Chinese medicine" (TCM), which is commonly employed by both scholars and practitioners of Chinese medicine in the West to refer to the post-1949 official, state-sanctioned practice of Chinese medicine, for a number of reasons. First, the term "traditional" is not widely used in China itself when referring to Chinese medicine. The term "TCM" was created in the mid-1950s for use in foreign-language publications only with the explicit aim of generating a certain perception of Chinese medicine in the West. Second, the term "traditional" invokes the inappropriate sense that Chinese medicine is unchanged or unchanging, neither of which is true. Third, opposing pre-1949 Chinese medicine with post-1949 TCM generates perceptions of discontinuity that, although true in one sense are false in many others. It suggests that post-1949 changes within Chinese medicine are of an altogether different order than changes during previous periods. The only reason I can see for subscribing to such a view is that we perceive the times in which we live as somehow more important than others. Fourth, practitioners of Chinese medicine in the West commonly employ "TCM" to designate specific forms of Chinese medical practice (most often those based on pattern differentiation according to the eight rubrics, or *ba gang* 八刚) in order to juxtapose these with other forms of Chinese or Oriental medicine. This use of "TCM" has become so entrenched that it depletes the acronym of any value for the purposes of academic discourse.

"Western medicine" is the literal translation of the term *xiyi* 西医 that is used in the PRC to refer (1) generically to the practice of Western-origin medicine rooted in the biosciences (biomedicine), and (2) to the post-1949 official, state-sanctioned practice of that medicine in China including its institutional and ideological separation from Chinese medicine. Throughout this book I use the term "Western medicine" when emphasizing etic Chinese perspectives (or myself as their ethnographer). I use "biomedicine" when emphasizing emic Western perspectives (or myself as interventionist anthropologist) because of the widespread use of this term throughout the academic literature, despite the fact that it invokes an inappropriate sense of objectivity as integral to that medicine. I have not always succeeded, however, in being as strict (or schizoid) as this opposition implies and requires.

As in all areas of sinology, translation of Chinese medical terms is a sensitive and hotly disputed issue.[2] I am not a sinologist and have considered it wisest not to embark on an extensive program of novel translations. Wherever possible I have followed Wiseman's *Dictionary of Chinese Medicine* and other authoritative texts.[3] Only where I do not agree with available translations do I offer my own suggestions. Only where available terms appeared to me especially controversial are my choices discussed explicitly. Some terms have been left untranslated. These include widely known medical concepts such as *yin/yang* 阴阳 and *qi* 气 because these have already been assimilated into the English language. They also include terms for which an English-language translation is suggested but then abandoned in favor of the original Chinese, such as *guanxi* 关系 (social networks), in order to preserve the polysemy of the Chinese term or to avoid the use of cumbersome descriptive translations.

Throughout the book all specialist Chinese terms have been transcribed using the pinyin system. Simplified Chinese characters are given at least on the first occurrence of such terms in a chapter. The exceptions are, once more, *yin/yang* and *qi*, as well as proper names, place-names, and the names of historical periods. Such terms occur regularly in English-language texts without special designations, and the use of italics would be confusing. In order to protect my informants' privacy all names of living persons with the exception of public figures are fictitious.[4]

All monetary values are given in yuan renminbi (RMB) or their US $ or £ sterling equivalents. During the period of my fieldwork £1 equaled approximately 13 RMB or $1.50.

PART I
CHINESE MEDICINE
AND THE PROBLEM
OF PLURALITY

1. ORIENTATIONS

With few exceptions, modern textbooks and physicians of Chinese medicine view their tradition as having unfolded in the course of an unbroken development that stretches back over two thousand years. Many Western historians, on the other hand, perceive the same development as a history of ruptures and ongoing adjustment to social change, of the continuous assimilation of extraneous knowledge and a never-ending struggle for identity. Chinese medicine, then, can be conceived of as being shaped by processes internal to itself but also by the desires and resistance of other peoples and things. Consequently, at any point in its long evolution Chinese medicine has been characterized by a diversity that encompasses every aspect of its organization and practice, from theory and diagnosis to prognosis, therapeutics, and the social organization of health care.[1]

The concrete realities of such diversity are rendered visible by even the most fleeting visit to any hospital or outpatient clinic of traditional medicine in contemporary China. No two doctors diagnose, prescribe, or treat in quite the same way. It would be most unusual, for instance, if after consulting ten senior physicians for the same complaint one did not walk away with ten different prescriptions.[2] Chinese physicians and their patients seem little perturbed by this. Both view personal experience, accumulated through years of study and clinical practice and by definition diverse, as a cornerstone of Chinese medicine. Doctors pride themselves on their individual styles of prescribing or needling. They define their identity by emphasizing their place within a medical lineage, but also by demonstrating that they are engaged in reshaping Chinese medicine through the use of biomedical knowledge and technology. Senior doctors state that no good physician ever writes out the same prescription twice, yet they actively collaborate in the formulation and marketing of patent remedies (*chengyao* 成药). Western, Chinese, shamanist, and religious forms of healing not only exist side-by-side, they are also integrated in many different ways. Patients move easily from one doctor, clinic, or hospital to the next if the present one does not deliver the expected results. In time-honored tradition (especially if they can afford the expense), they may consult several doctors and compare their prescriptions before deciding which one's treatment to follow.

There is nothing unusual about such diversity and contradiction. They are documented for other medical traditions undergoing modernization, but also for biomedicine and for Western science at large. Wherever we look, syncretism and ambiguity abound.[3] Nevertheless, diversity is often experienced as problematic by both insiders and outsiders to a particular health care system in the context of first- and second-order inquiries. First-order inquiries are defined here as arising in immediate relation to clinical practice (i.e., as having to do with choosing between different therapeutic possibilities, the ordering of experience, etc.); second-order inquiries analyze first-order processes.[4] Given an environment in which a plurality of possible diagnostic and treatment strategies is imagined possible, physicians and their patients must devise methods to select from the array of available options those considered most useful or appropriate. Such choices may be left to individuals and their families, but there may also be institutionalized procedures or practices that prescribe, enable, or restrict choice.

For physicians in imperial China such methods and institutions included memorization and rote learning, apprenticeship involving the acquisition of tacit knowledge, and the continued interpretation of canonical texts in the light of personal experience. Without a state-controlled teaching system that had the authority to effectively define and police the form and content of medical practice, each doctor was, as Nathan Sivin notes, "expected to arrive at his own synthesis through the interaction of deep book learning and practice. The goal was to be fully responsible for his very limited power over life and death, not to become a technician manipulating bodies."[5] In contemporary China efforts are being made to replace reliance on subjective experience with objective knowledge according to perceived universal scientific standards; older practices, however, endure.

Chinese patients have always been well versed in accommodating to the wide variety of health care choices available to them. In imperial China it was considered one of the duties of a filial son to care for his parents medically. This was taken to mean that a gentleman or scholar should be conversant with the works of the medical canon. He might prescribe medicines himself, but more usually he would decide on the appropriate treatment based on his medical knowledge. If a family member fell ill, several physicians might be invited to the house to make a diagnosis and submit a prescription. The household would then select from among these diagnoses and prescriptions the one they felt was most appropriate or convincing. This practice still exists. I observed it during my fieldwork in Beijing, as in the case of a rich businessman from Taiwan who was searching for treatment for his terminally ill daughter. He consulted several famous physicians before making a choice. Less well off patients choose between practitioners by considering their reputation, the fees they charge, the service they offer, and the institution at which they practice. Chapter 4 describes in detail several cases of such health seeking and the complex choices it involves.

Descriptions of how individual physicians and patients confront the pluralities of a given health care system can be distinguished from investigations that take these first-order inquiries as their topic.[6] Such second-order inquiries may be intrinsic to a medical tradition, as in the contemporary Chinese medical subdisciplines of *zhongyi ge jia xueshuo* 中医各家学说 (doctrines of schools of Chinese medicine) and *zhongguo yixue shi* 中国医学史 (history of Chinese medicine).[7] Or they may be extrinsic, as in the case of medical anthropology or Chinese studies. Confronted with a diversity of health care practices and health-seeking behaviors on the descriptive (first-order) level, second-order inquiries strive to explain how and why the diversities discovered arise, how they are structured and relate to each other, and how they compare across different contexts of health care delivery. This book is one such inquiry.

In medical anthropology the concept of medical pluralism is widely employed to flag research into health care systems in which different medical traditions coexist in a cooperative or competitive relation with each other.[8] Conventionally, the most commonly adopted methodology for this purpose is to sort the diverse forms of medical practice encountered in a given context into different medical systems and then to explore how patients and their families choose from them on the basis of distinct cultural knowledge and belief systems.[9]

There are many problems, however, with this kind of analysis. First, contemporary ethnographies demonstrate that patients and their families do not simply make rational choices from the array of therapies available to them. Rather, health-seeking behavior is a dynamic, discontinuous, and fragmentary process involving complex negotiations of social identity and morality, in the course of which people draw simultaneously on local and global perspectives.[10] Second, medical traditions, including biomedicine itself, have been revealed to be far less systematic than had originally been imagined. Rather than possessing clearly definable boundaries, medical systems are permeable to all kinds of technological and ideological influences effecting systemic change and local adaptations. The establishment of biomedicine in non-Western societies, for instance, is not merely a transfer of knowledge, practices, and institutions but involves important accommodations of that which is transferred. So-called traditional practices, on the other hand, can frequently be uncovered as inventions of twentieth-century modernizers profoundly influenced by Western knowledge and thought.[11]

Discourse on medical pluralism has never been able to resolve the ensuing tension between expectation and reality. With regard to Asian medical systems, for instance, researchers have found it inordinately difficult to reconcile assumptions about the systematic nature of these traditions with the observation that, in practice, they are characterized by frequent inconsistencies and low levels of actual systematization.[12] Should this tension be interpreted as a sign of disorganization and, by implication, of the inferiority of Asian medical systems vis-à-vis biomedicine?[13] Or is it instead an essential dimension of these systems, turning them into flexible tools in the hands of skilled practitioners?[14] Is inconsistency a sign that modern physicians no longer understand the theories on which their medicines are based?[15] Are traditions such as Chinese medicine useful but no longer really alive, comparable to the function of Latin during the Middle Ages?[16] Or perhaps consistency is not to be found in medical theories at all, but rather in the "practical logic of the clinical encounter," which in the case of Chinese medicine may be revealed as a "coordinated use of 'logically inconsistent' methods to produce a nuanced specificity."[17]

Plurality thus continues to be an unresolved problem in all second-order accounts of Chinese medicine. Diversity, readily admitted on the level of description, is all too often reduced to some form of monism on the level of explanation, whether in the form of enduring cultural practices or essences or in teleological narratives of gain or loss. Such search for deeper unities is not merely an attempt at explanation, however. It is also a construction (disguised as representation) of Chinese medicine as a commonsense object. The most important purpose of such construction is comparison, so that attributes of one object can be contrasted with those of apparently similar objects: Western medicine versus Chinese medicine, Chinese medicine in the imperial era versus modern TCM,[18] scholar-physicians versus shamans, science versus traditional knowledge, medicine versus art, and so on. In particular, indigenous, traditional or folk medicines continue to be constituted in anthropological, historical, and professional discourse as the "other" or opposite of biomedicine, even when such constructions are motivated by a critique (often romanticized) of biomedicine itself. Whether Chinese medicine is seen to be an "integrated system" or an assemblage of empirically useful theories and practices, whether it is imagined to be closed or open, whether it is described as holistic or reductionist—all these are not objective aspects of Chinese medicine itself, but indexes as to where, by whom, and for which purposes Chinese medicine has been constituted as an object of description and analysis.

My own encounters with Chinese medicine have shown these dichotomies and the desires motivating their construction—their "logics of equivalence and panics of reduction"[19]—to be flawed. In most cases, for each discontinuity described other continuities can be found that break asunder carefully constructed categorizations. And what appears disconnected from one perspective often connects from another. Epistemologically, their frequently unstated a priori assumptions construct distinctly Orientalist knowledge (even in the most charitable sense of the term)—a charge to which any ethnography of Chinese medicine written at the end of the twentieth century must be extremely sensitive.[20] For even when such constructions and comparisons are not a reflection of latent Western imperialisms, they reveal a tendency to construct Chinese medicine in terms of specifically Western discursive categories when a willingness to adapt these categories to the realities of Chinese medicine would perhaps be more rewarding.

In this book I will write a different ethnography of Chinese medicine, an ethnography that accepts plurality as an intrinsic and nonreducible aspect of all medical practice. For this purpose I relate ethnographic descriptions from my fieldwork in Beijing, China, to models about the interrelation between knowledge, technology, society, and self that have been developed in medical anthropology and the interdisciplinary field of science and technology studies (STS).[21] As a result of this dialogue I advance two propositions. The first is negative. It states that Chinese medicine in contemporary China is not a totality. By this I mean that the visible pluralities of Chinese medicine I describe are not reducible to a singular cultural logic or process of cultural production. The second proposition is positive. It argues that Chinese medicine in contemporary China can be modeled as a dynamic process of simultaneous emergence and disappearance. By this I mean that Chinese medicine and the multiple and heterogeneous elements that constitute it are best described as emergent global states, or *syntheses,* that are produced by local interactions of human and nonhuman elements, or *infrastructures.* Accounting for and describing the plural and often dispersed interactions at local levels that create, support, destabilize, and tear apart global coherences that are never more than temporarily stable thereby emerges as the new task of any anthropology of medicine.

Ethnographic Orientations

The ethnographic fieldwork on which this book is based was carried out predominantly in Beijing, where I stayed for a total of sixteen months between 1994 and 1999. The final writing up was carried out in Shanghai, where I was able to collect valuable information at local libraries. During my fieldwork in Beijing I observed more than four thousand treatment episodes while working with venerated senior physicians (*laozhongyi* 老中医); senior consultants (*zhuren yishi* 主任医师); attending physicians (*zhuzhi yishi* 主治医师); undergraduate (*benkesheng* 本科生), master's (*shuoshisheng* 硕士生), and doctoral students (*boshisheng* 硕士生); as well as doctors undertaking further training (*jinxiusheng* 进修生). I attended institutions that ranged from large university teaching hospitals to pharmacies, from prestigious clinics employing only famous physicians to a clinic operated in the evenings from a one-bedroom apartment.

My status as a practitioner of Chinese medicine provided me with numerous opportunities to engage directly with patients. For a while I was the physician-in-residence for the staff of the guesthouse at which I lived. I was invited to conduct many impromptu consultations with perfect strangers in shops and markets and also during one memorable thirty-six-hour bus journey. I developed close relationships with several physicians and their families, with students and laypeople. All of these facilitated my access to contemporary Chinese medicine by a number of routes: from daily discussions with fellow students to semistructured interviews with ten Beijing households concerning specific illness episodes; from a longitudinal observation of a doctoral research project to a quasi apprenticeship with one of my teachers.[22]

The professionalized elite Chinese medicine with which I deal in this ethnography continuously refers us to an ever-expanding archive of canonical texts and commentaries that reach back at least two millennia. My teachers in China never failed to impress on me that reading, writing, and memorizing are intrinsic aspects of medical practice. No ethnography of Chinese medicine can, therefore, ignore the significance of written sources. Given the sheer size of the material this is a formidable task. No practicing physicians, even those with the desire to do so, have studied all the classics, and I cannot profess more than an eclectic familiarity with this vast literature. My readings have been, of necessity, selective and often lacking in the intimate familiarity with all those other classical sources (literary and philosophical) that would properly be required for their understanding but which demand time and resources far beyond the scope of this study. Nevertheless, written texts inform my entire ethnography, and in particular chapters 3, 7, and 8. They are intended, inter alia, to provide a counterpoint to the observational data on which my other case studies are based.

A number of factors specific to Beijing as a fieldwork site and to myself as a fieldworker must be mentioned. From the 1980s onward the influence of private enterprise in the development of the health care sector has steadily accelerated. Unlike many other parts of China, however, Beijing has maintained a relatively well developed state health care sector.[23] As the national capital, Beijing is also the country's premier research and administrative center. Beijing hospitals and research institutes of Chinese medicine are staffed by the nation's most eminent scholars and attract some of its brightest students. This is reflected in the fact that Beijing physicians have made extraordinarily influential contributions to the shaping of contemporary Chinese medicine. Beijing is also, of course, a center of international exchange. A considerable number of foreigners (mainly from other East Asian countries but increasingly from the West) study there for degrees in Chinese medicine. In addition, international training centers at universities, colleges, and major hospitals offer courses of varying duration and sophistication for an ever-expanding market of physicians and lay practitioners from abroad.

For the most part I received no support, financial or institutional, from local Chinese or overseas organizations during my fieldwork. It was logistically impossible, therefore, to carry out large-scale surveys or clinical follow-ups, or to employ any other method of research dependent on such assistance. I was forced, instead, to rely entirely on that essential skill required for survival in modern China—the cultivation of extensive networks of personal relations (see chapter 6). To a significant degree this task was facilitated by the fact that I encountered most of my informants as a student not only of anthropology but also of Chinese medicine. I have studied Chinese medicine since 1980, and by the time I arrived in Beijing I had worked already for more than ten years in private practice. During my fieldwork my knowledge of Chinese medicine was constantly tested by fellow students and teachers, and passing these tests opened many doors to me that might otherwise have remained closed.[24]

Certain implications that arise from the above must be addressed at this point. First, my account is biased toward an elite stratum of Chinese medical physicians and their clientele within the state health care sector dominant in Beijing.[25] Second, it is impossible to separate the complex subjectivities I carried into the field. Being simultaneously a physician and a student of Chinese medicine, an anthropologist and a European, impinged on the issues I explored, the relationships I formed, and the data I collected. I contend, however, that these factors did not preclude me from carrying out anthropologically meaningful research. Their relevance to my project is of no different order than being a biomedical physician *and* an anthropologist or Asian (and by implication exposed to and involved in ongoing redefinition of postcolonial national identity) would be to anthropological analyses of non-Western modes of modernization.[26] In fact, I would argue that only someone intimately familiar with Chinese medicine can undertake a meaningful investigation of that tradition. Meaningful in this context points to an investigation that does not rely on the separation between internal (i.e., implicit and explicit doctrinal knowledge and skills) and extraneous factors (i.e., social, cultural, and historical agencies) in the construction of a practice. This requires of the ethnographer more than a fleeting acquaintance with Chinese medical theory and practice and of readers the same willingness to follow complex arguments and descriptions that is demanded and accepted by the ethnography of nuclear physics or mathematics.

Conceptual Orientations

Throughout this book I follow contemporary Chinese usage in the labeling of health care practices. Modern Chinese apply the term "Chinese medicine" (*zhongyi* 中医) to a seemingly well defined aspect of the official health care system with its own educational institutions, hospitals and outpatient clinics, professional organizations, and journals. In both lay and professional discourse Chinese medicine is distinguished, on the one hand, from Western medicine (*xiyi* 西医), and, on the other, from various officially recognized folk medicines (*minjian yixue* 民间医学) and "unofficial" popular therapeutic practices such as divination (*suanming* 算命), witchcraft (*wushu* 巫术), and physiognomy (*xiangmian* 相面). Official and professional discourse makes the further distinction, in certain contexts, between Chinese medicine and integrated or combined Chinese and Western medicine (*zhongxiyi jiehe* 中西医结合). "Folk medicine" implies both the empirical use of drugs and the medical systems of non-Han minority cultures (*minzu yixue* 民族医学). Like Chinese medicine, the latter are taught at state colleges and are supported by an infrastructure of special hospitals. Unofficial healing practices are not supported by the state.[27]

In official and private discourse healing practices are delineated by means of variously intersecting oppositions. Western medicine is more modern and scientific, and therefore more naturally associated with progress and development than either Chinese or minority medicines. However, all three are characterized by the possession of theoretical knowledge (*lilun* 理论) and an evolutionary history of progressive transformations. Chinese medicine may be ancient (*gulao* 古老), but it is not necessarily old and backward (*jiu* 旧).[28] Hence, it can be modernized (*xiandaihua* 现代化) and developed into a science (*kexuehua* 科学化). This is in stark contrast to unofficial healing practices, which are often associated with "feudal superstitions" (*fengjian mixin* 封建迷信) and either ignored or discouraged by the state. The backward character of empirical and unofficial medicines is reflected, too, in the view that they do not possess a theory.

Moving from discourse to actual healing practice blurs even further the boundaries between apparently distinct medical systems. Physicians who refer to themselves and are referred to by their patients as "doctors of Chinese medicine" (*zhongyi yishi* 中医医师) routinely make biomedical diagnoses, prescribe biomedical drugs, and even perform surgery. Many of their Western medical colleagues, on the other hand, use drugs from the Chinese materia medica (*zhongyao* 中药), though not always on the basis of a Chinese medical diagnosis. Many doctors, with the explicit support of the state, attempt to integrate Chinese and Western medicines, but there exist no clear guidelines about how such an integration might be advanced or what its end product should look like. Some of my teachers had studied Western medicine before becoming Chinese medical physicians or had undertaken extensive postgraduate training in biomedical specialties. One had studied Kampo, the Japanese variation of Chinese medicine; another Uigur medical practices. Some regularly practiced meditation or other body techniques to strengthen their *qi* and enhance their healing powers. One doctor took me to his spiritual master, a senior monk at a Beijing Buddhist temple, who writes out prescriptions under the telepathic guidance of Hua Tuo 华佗 (?–203), a famous physician of the Three Kingdoms period. Another asked me to accompany him to make offerings to Sun Simiao 孙思邈 (c. 581–682), a Tang dynasty physician who is venerated as the "King of Medicine" (*yaowang* 药王) at the White Cloud Temple (*Baiyunsi* 白云寺) in the south of Beijing.[29]

Outside the official state sector such border crossings multiply. Historically, elite physicians, who tended to be pharmacologists, also included symbolic techniques in their repertoire and exorcized demons while folk healers drew on the herbal prescriptions formulated by the elite. In contemporary China the visible reemergence of unofficial healing practices is closely linked to the privatization and commodification of medicine; in other Chinese cultural contexts they never disappeared. The integration of "unofficial" divination into "official" traditional medicine, small entrepreneurial clinics peddling secret prescriptions and treatment techniques, exorcism by means of acupuncture, and the flowering of qigong 气功 movements are examples that I observed personally or were recounted to me by informants and are documented in the literature.[30]

Chinese medicine, furthermore, is no longer a purely "Chinese" phenomenon. Actively supported by the World Health Organization (WHO), promoted by the Chinese state, dispersed by Chinese physicians for whom it has become a passport to fame and fortune abroad, studied by conventional and alternative medicine practitioners throughout the world, sought after by an international clientele of patients—Chinese medicine in the 1990s was a global phenomenon and big business, too. In 1987 the World Federation of Acupuncture and Moxibustion Societies was established in Beijing with a total membership of more than fifty thousand physicians from more than one hundred participating countries. Beijing University of Chinese Medicine, where I resided during my fieldwork recently accredited a five-year degree program in England organized cooperatively with Middlesex University. Similar joint ventures have been set up in Spain, France, the United States, and Australia. A hospital staffed by physicians from the Dongzhimen Hospital of Chinese Medicine in Beijing has been operating in Germany for more than a decade. Most of my teachers in Beijing had lectured or worked abroad: in Malaysia, the United States, Japan, Singapore, Denmark, Mexico, France, Great Britain, Switzerland, Spain. At least two told me their closest disciples were non-Chinese. Students of Chinese medicine make up the second largest contingent of foreign students at Chinese universities, and by the end of 1998 more than seventeen thousand foreigners had participated in official courses of Chinese medicine in China. In 1993 the foreign exchange revenue obtained by exporting Chinese medicine drugs amounted to more than $500 million, which was expected to increase to over $800 million by the turn of the century.[31]

Historically, Chinese medicine has never been purely "Chinese" in any case. Throughout its long history it has been receptive to foreign imports—of ideas, of technologies, of drugs.[32] Most recently, biomedical concepts and practices have constituted a crucial though by no means singular influence in the development of Chinese medicine.[33] As it traveled to other parts of the world Chinese medicine was integrated into or forced to compete with existing health care practices. Some of the resultant reinterpretations of the original product have found their way back to China, where they have contributed to the ongoing transformation of traditional medicine.[34]

In the light of these observations "Chinese medicine in contemporary China" becomes a thoroughly problematic category, a vain attempt to contain an essence that has long since seeped through the cracks between whatever fragile articulations bind "Chinese" to "medicine," and further to "contemporary" and "China."[35] Thus, not merely because of actual or perceived crises of representation in the Western academy but also in response to empirically tangible complexities and complications, the question arises as to whether a localized exploration of Chinese medicine is still desirable. Would it not be more realistic to produce an ethnography that reflects the global restructuring and mobilization that are creating everywhere new hybrid cultures, new ruptures, new fragmentations, new dislocations? Is it not necessary, at least, to widen the purview from Beijing to include Shanghai, from the north to the south, from the city to the rural hinterland?

Such problematic articulations and disassociations between the local and the global are not properties merely of contemporary Chinese medicine. In a world that is simultaneously moving closer together and farther apart, they have moved to the forefront of debate in many different arenas and disciplines. As some ethnographies diagnose the emergence of an increasingly homogeneous global culture or even of a world system, others reveal the global to be itself provincial in the face of ever-multiplying expansions of fragile localities.[36] Likewise, anthropologists' claims to a privileged understanding of the local through viewing it from a global perspective have been shattered as just another Enlightenment illusion and tool of imperialism.[37] Contemporary anthropologists accept that the boundaries between home and elsewhere, between self and other, are real only inasmuch as they are constructed through intersubjective processes. If I insist on writing an ethnography of "Chinese medicine in contemporary China," this does not, therefore, indicate a return to outdated concepts of bounded cultures or a shying away from problematic definitions. On the contrary, it marks an explicit desire to contribute to debates that take my ethnography out of a narrowly defined concern for "medicine" or "China."

Sahlins has argued that the boundary permeability of culture is not necessarily reflective of its inherent fragility but that it can be read, inversely, as a sign of culture's power to include by assimilating alien objects and persons.[38] From this vantage point, the local always encompasses the global while globalization reveals itself as nothing more than the assimilatory practices of particularly localized imperialisms.[39] "Global" and "local" cease to be differences of quality and become mere differences of scale.[40] Nevertheless, global and local also indicate a tension and a dynamic, whether conceived of as between a self-referential nonreducible macrocosm and specifying limiting microcosms, the one extracted from the other, or as between the concrete spaces where relations are enacted and where they can be observed and the larger contexts against which they can be imagined and which make them possible.[41]

It is crucial, therefore, to define Chinese medicine in contemporary China from the outset as something locally constructed and capable of assimilating many different elements (Chinese and non-Chinese, ancient and contemporary, medical and nonmedical), yet also as a global reference that makes local agency possible. This will require me to describe the emergence of Chinese medicine in contemporary China in terms of interrelated performances and not as being the result of a system of representations or stable cultural practices. It means that I cannot base my ethnography on a priori assumptions about the existence of bounded communities, networks, traditions of knowledge, styles of reasoning, or even person and self that could somehow ground my investigation. Thus, while I rely on categories such as "Chinese medicine" and "Western medicine" to establish the objects of my study, I do not thereby accept their actual existence. Rather, they are concepts both for and against which my argument works, a position and methodology reflected also in the complementarity propositions outlined in the first section of this chapter.[42]

Disciplinary Orientations

Contemporary Chinese scholar-physicians see Chinese medicine as being many things at once and as being influenced by many forces at the same time. As one reference manual for university lecturers states: "Chinese medicine relates to both natural and social science, it is the product of their mutual overlapping" (*Zhongyixue sheji ziran he shehui kexue, shi liangzhe xianghu jiaocha de chanwu* 中医学涉及自然和社会科学, 是两者相互交叉的产物). The same text also calls it "the product of an osmotic exchange between many disciplines" (*duo xueke jiaohu shentou de chanwu* 多学科交互渗透的产物), a craft and art (*jiyi* 技艺), and the ethically charged enterprise of "practiced benevolence" (*ren ren zhi shu* 仁人之术). It is thus seen as the organic unity of a scientific striving for truth (*zhen* 真), a humanist concern for efficacy (*shan* 善), and an aesthetic desire for the beautiful (*mei* 美).[43] And it is precisely this heterogeneous constitution that—for these scholar-physicians at least—makes plurality not only inevitable but also nonproblematic.

I am not alone, then, in challenging the reification of medical systems into stable conceptual categories. The self-reflective discourse by contemporary Chinese scholar-physicians regarding the nature of their medicine does much the same thing. There is, nevertheless, an important difference of perspective between their stance and mine. Almost without exception contemporary scholar-physicians refract Chinese medicine through the lens of modernism, even if that modernism is reflected through Maoism, Deng Xiaoping thought, and other particularly Chinese prisms. Imported Enlightenment models of the concurrent progress of knowledge and time dominate their internal histories of medicine.[44] The same models inform the standardization (*guifanhua* 规范化) and sifting of the national medical heritage (*zhengli zuguo yixue yichan* 整理祖国医学遗产) in progress since the 1920s.[45] Most practicing physicians with whom I discussed the issue were convinced that the contending voices (*zhengming* 争鸣) of past and present would merge in the course of Chinese medicine's development; what was taken for granted for society at large naturally applied to medicine as well.[46]

As an ethnographer who in the course of his training has learned to employ the tools of critical theory and postmodern anthropology, I find it difficult to accept this perspective. On the other hand, I have found very few Chinese physicians who view the plurality of their tradition as an intellectual problem. Faced with the task of portraying Chinese medicine through the reifying categories of Western scholarship, I have experienced considerably more difficulty in this respect. This dilemma—my inability, as anthropologist, to accept "native" discourse on its own terms, yet an equally acute awareness of the ever-present danger of Orientalist modes of *re*-presentation—is not easily resolved.[47]

I suggest that any escape from this dilemma must begin with the acknowledgment that anthropologists never stand above their subjects; that differences between first- and second-order inquiries are constructed rather than essential. All second-order inquiries always and of necessity intervene in ongoing struggles and thus participate in the first-order processes they describe and analyze—whether by distinguishing between objective "facts" and subjective "beliefs" or by "speaking for" their subjects as self-appointed representatives.[48] Only when this role of the objective outsider is relinquished does a more honest participatory stance become possible. Such a stance still aspires to produce critical knowledge, though a knowledge that is "knowledge for" rather than "knowledge of" or "knowledge about."

Such a participatory stance can be developed through the pursuit of two interrelated questions. First, what can we (as Westerners, as anthropologists, as social scientists) learn from the engagement with Chinese medicine? Second, what can we (as Westerners, as anthropologists, as social scientists) contribute to Chinese medicine's understanding of itself? For at least three reasons, addressing these questions is significantly enabled by adopting a broad interdisciplinary perspective. First, because the Chinese themselves describe the emergence of their tradition as a multidisciplinary event; second, because only a plurality of perspectives can be adequate in the pursuit of plurality itself; and, third, because it represents a way out for anthropologists whose own tradition is encumbered by a tenacious bias toward monist explanation.

Archer demonstrates that the anthropological notion of culture has since its inception been based on the "*a priori* assumption that there always was a discoverable coherence in culture" and that this produced "a mental closure against the discovery of cultural inconsistencies."[49] Intracultural diversity, a phenomenon described ethnographically at least since the 1930s, remained for a considerable time associated in the minds of anthropologists with pathology and decay.[50] Even anthropologists who readily accepted the pervasiveness of such diversity did not thereby escape completely from the monistic doxa of their profession. Distributive models of culture were intended to produce a sociology of knowledge that could map cultural systems on social systems. As Hannerz remarks, an implicit assumption of these models was that "the somehow non-cultural creates differentiation, and often threatens with conflict and disintegration, while shared culture, whether through consensus or hegemony, unites."[51]

Tracing in detail the roots of anthropology's holistic habitus is not the goal of the present discussion.[52] That habitus is, however, closely intertwined with the problematic demarcation of the modern from the traditional. As Schwartz demonstrates, one finds in much of modern Western discourse on culture an opposition between closed, static, and therefore unchanging traditional cultures and the dynamic heterogeneous cultures of modernity.[53] This explains why until quite recently anthropologists avoided paying attention to complex non-Western societies. According to Appadurai, "a kind of reverse Orientalism" is involved in this avoidance, "whereby complexity, literacy, historical depth, and structural messiness operate as disqualifications in the struggle of places for a voice in metropolitan theory."[54] Yet, an inverse opposition is as easily invoked, and many writers have contrasted the boundedness, coherence, and universality of science as a superior form of cognition from the fragmented and often incoherent nature of unequally efficacious local belief systems.[55]

Such ideas have their proximal roots in turn-of-the-century social theory and its implications in the Western imperialist project. Culture, for instance, became an important analytic category in Western thought precisely at that historical moment when "Atlantic nations began to establish their domination over much of the rest of the world," which involved a "process of self-definition through contrast with characteristics imputed to colonized others."[56] Theories of social practice, frequently presenting themselves as alternatives to culture theory, emerged around the same time in debates among German neo-Kantians on the role of social norms (Sitten) and among British political theorists on the tension between custom and nature in the regulation of behavior, and thus share with culture theories a common heritage.[57]

This heritage can be traced back even further to Enlightenment perceptions of knowledge and subject formation, and in particular to the philosophy of Immanuel Kant. We may recall that Kant took plurality in the form of sensory data as given and argued that unity had to be synthesized from these by a newly constituted entity, the universal subject. As Luhmann notes, it was precisely this separation of unity and plurality that defined the subject as subject (namely, the subject of the connection between unity and plurality) and marked complexity as the definitive problem of modernity.[58] Anthropologists accepted Kant's intuitions but, following Montesquieu, also allowed for the mind to be shaped by different societal environments. Human subjects were defined as possessing universal cognitive capacities, yet also as acting in accord with locally defined modes of practical reason. Anthropology's task accordingly became to deduce from outward complexities of behavior for each society or social group the underlying unity of rules, norms, and representations that constitute its specific form of practical reason.[59]

This search for unity has been challenged dramatically over recent decades by the discovery everywhere of syncretism, hybridity, and heteroglossia. Yet, in anthropology—as in postmodernist writings—disclosures of plurality all too often remain parasitic on prevalent monist orthodoxies. They are easily criticized, therefore, for contributing to understanding in a negative manner only, or credited, at best, with showing up the dilemmas, paradoxes, and ambivalences generated by established systems of order.[60] On the one hand, this is due to a tendency in postmodern writing to emphasize resistance to rather than transformation of current systems of power; on the other, it is grounded in the inherent ambivalence of concepts such as "hybridity" and "syncretism" that underpin such discourse. Is hybridity the "space betwixt and between two zones of purity," or is it "the ongoing condition of all human cultures, which contain no zones of purity because they undergo continuous processes of transculturation"?[61]

Two conclusions can be drawn from this discussion. First, grasping Chinese medicine through a framework that does not insist on the a priori reduction of its intrinsic plurality necessitates the redefinition—perhaps even the abandonment—of concepts such as culture, practice, system, and tradition by means of which medicines of all kinds are conventionally comprehended. Second, in order to transcend anthropology's pertinacious commitment to these concepts (and the monistic bias they imply), a radically pluralist ethnography of Chinese medicine may need inspiration from other disciplines such as cognitive studies, systems theory, or cultural psychology that are less mired in postmodern passivity and self-reflection yet equally critical of modernist discourses and social arrangements.

STS rather than traditional anthropology has provided me with many of the most immediately useful tools, models, and inspirations for this endeavor. Like anthropology, STS is interested in understanding fields of human practice. Unlike anthropology, however, whose holistic bias and search for cultural constants render encounters with plurality intrinsically problematic, the disciplinary history of STS is a critique of such unity.[62] Placing themselves against neopositivist philosophy and a Whiggish history of science, the various research traditions within STS show that scientific knowledge is constructed rather than discovered. Such construction can be visualized as the alignment of human and material agencies within historically specific microworlds. STS thereby emphasizes the intrinsically local character of all such knowledge, the global impact of which depends on its ability to re-create microworlds that share essential elements—elements whose dominance within a microworld forces accommodations from other elements—in many different locations.

More recently, STS researchers have moved away from a concern mainly with undermining traditional accounts of science toward a critical but positive engagement with scientific practice. This shift is mirrored (not surprisingly) in a changed relationship between STS and anthropology. Initially, the sociology of scientific knowledge (SSK), the dominant research tradition within STS, had borrowed from anthropologists their ethnographic method, but ended up calling for an anthropology of science "without anthropologists."[63] Anthropologists, on the other hand, complained that they could find in laboratory ethnographies and the anthropology of science much theory but "little if any culture." They argued that the microsocial orientation of STS fails to explain how macrosocial factors such as race, class, and gender not only shape science but are themselves in-formed and trans-formed through science.[64] This led to the emergence of an entire new subdiscipline referred to by its creators variously as the cultural studies of science and technology (CSS) or as "critical STS." More self-consciously political and interventionist, writers in this tradition draw attention to how science is built (or builds itself) into local and global constellations of power and exclusion/inclusion. The result is a much richer understanding of how similar microworlds differ even if they share many of the same elements in their construction.[65]

Locating an ethnography of Chinese medicine with specific reference to STS and CSS constitutes an intervention in these debates. It is, on the one hand, an expression of appreciation for the vistas this interdisciplinary field has opened up for me. Here, it is precisely the contradirectedness of STS as opposed to anthropology—tracing global coherences back to local interactions rather than looking for enduring deep structures as generators of local agencies—that makes its theoretical perspectives so attractive for my purposes. On the other hand, it also presents an anthropologically informed challenge to STS and that field's conception of science as a largely Western and modern enterprise. I thus take from anthropology a concern for the thick description of local complexities and contradictions while I look to STS for its theoretically more evolved analyses of local processes of knowledge construction. I also intend to play off the pull toward synthesis that informs anthropology's search for pattern against the primacy of plurality and heterogeneity rooted in the constructivist foundations of STS.[66] A concrete framework and methodology for this enterprise is developed in chapter 2.

Having emphasized the potential of this approach, I will conclude this introduction by drawing attention to some of its shortcomings. At least two potential problems can be identified. The first concerns the danger of placing oneself at the borders of established research traditions. Positions at the margin can open up new horizons and enable decisive action, but they also carry the risk of marginalization and of speaking to no one but oneself. Traditions, as MacIntyre has shown, are debates to which one can contribute only if one has been admitted beforehand as someone entitled to speak.[67] In a narrow professional sense, I consider myself neither an anthropologist nor a sociologist of science and technology, but rather a scholar-physician who uses these disciplines to make sense of what he does. To clinicians suspicious of academics dealing in mere "theory" and to those academics who view my direct involvement with the clinical as equally polluting I can only profess the sincerity of my intentions and the hope that what I bring back to their disciplines makes me a worthwhile recipient of the tools I have borrowed.

The second danger is political. Practitioners of Chinese medicine in both China and the West may be extremely suspicious of what I have to say. Having to defend their tradition in a day-to-day struggle against a dominant biomedical-industrial complex, they are proud of what they perceive to be its holistic and systematic nature, its intrinsic difference from biomedicine, and its continued existence for over two thousand years. They may therefore see me as applying—in an apparently corrosive manner—tools crafted to eliminate the separation of nature and culture in science to a medical practice which itself does not know of this separation. They may see me as deconstructing the fragile unity of contemporary Chinese medicine that has been carefully established during a century of struggle with Western medicine. Why, indeed, should they not be suspicious? My answer to them is simple and straightforward. First, I am a practitioner of Chinese medicine who loves what he does. Second, I have a track record of speaking for the independence of Chinese medicine as an alternative to biomedicine. Third, I perceive the dominant strategies currently employed by proponents of Chinese medicine—strategies that imply that Chinese medicine must live up to the standards of objectivity and systematicity set by biomedicine even though biomedical practice consistently fails to do so itself—as Trojan horses that will smuggle the power of the biomedical-industrial complex into the very heart of the tradition. Most concepts by which Chinese medicine at present seeks to define itself—paradigm, system, science, progress—are terms taken from a modernist discourse that intrinsically supports biomedicine. If Chinese medicine wishes to escape from the stranglehold of this discourse, it can do so only by creating a new and autonomous discourse, a discourse that honors tradition and succeeds in taking Chinese medicine into the postmodern world. In this endeavor practitioners of Chinese medicine may find powerful allies in anthropologists, sociologists of science, and others committed to an understanding of medicine that does not grant implicit rights to some practices while denying them to others.

2. PLURALITY AND SYNTHESIS
Toward a Multisited Ethnography of Chinese Medicine

The immediate task that arises from the reflections of chapter 1 is to translate its programmatic objectives into a viable framework for ethnographic description and analysis. Such a framework should form a bridge between the debates regarding modernization; globalization; and the nature of science, tradition, culture, and self that constitute the invariable background to our engagement with Chinese medicine and the concrete realities of medical practice as observed from different points of view. I begin this effort with a historical overview of diversity in Chinese medicine. Besides providing essential information for readers not intimately familiar with the Chinese medical tradition, this survey documents how plurality is woven into the very fabric of Chinese medicine, extending from perceptions of the body to the social relations embodied in learning, teaching, and practice; from the canonical texts of the Han dynasty to present-day research in urban hospitals.

Analytically this diversity can be grasped by means of two interrelated concepts: heterogeneity and multiplicity. After introducing these concepts I will draw on debates regarding the modernization of Chinese medicine to explore different possible strategies for examining them. This discussion leads me to suggest that Andrew Pickering's "mangle of practice" may function as a useful model for an ethnography of contemporary Chinese medicine that captures its plurality without undue distortion.

The Diversity of Chinese Medicine Past and Present

Plurality in Chinese medicine commences at the most fundamental level, that of the description and organization of body structure and function. No single term in classical Chinese corresponds to the English "body," with its implicit meaning (shared with other Indo-European languages) of a vat or container and its categorical opposition to "mind." Different terms such as *shen* 身 (the lived body), *hsing* 形 (the bodily form or shape), and *ti* 体 (embodiment of any number of things, including spiritual, cosmic, and moral states) were used, instead, to evoke various aspects of the "shape or disposition of human process." Inasmuch as such shapes and dispositions are always emergent, they are context bound and therefore plural.[1]

The body in Chinese medicine, then, is not an aggregate of discrete morphological substances linked to each other anatomically by means of mechanical structures and physiologically by way of interactive functional systems. Rather, it is a complex unit of functions and a site of regular transformations. While these transformations have discernible patterns, the body itself is always becoming. Classically, it was described by means of organic metaphors that related it to the functioning of the imperial government, the waterways that were essential to transportation and communication in China, the climate and seasons, and the other myriad interactions between heaven and earth. In general, such descriptions were perspectival and therefore incomplete, couched in language that valued evocation, metaphor, and allegory. Many aspects of body, therefore, remained provisionally defined and always open to revision.[2]

Debates concerning the exact nature and function of various visceral systems of function, for instance, have flared up repeatedly in the history of Chinese medicine. The concept of the *sanjiao* 三焦 provides a good example of such polemics. The *sanjiao* is one of the eleven regular visceral systems of function (*zangfu* 脏腑) of Chinese medicine and is recognized as such in early medical writings. Less equivocal have been precise descriptions of its functions, structure, or associations. In the *Huangdi neijing* 黄帝内经 (*The Inner Classic of the Yellow Lord*), the oldest canonical text of the Chinese medical tradition, the three *jiao* 焦 which together make up the *sanjiao* are visualized as distinct entities in space comparable to an irrigation system for the distribution of various types of *qi* and fluid.[3] The *Nanjing* 难经 (*Classic of Difficult Issues*), a first- or early second-century A.D. commentary on the *Neijing* that later became a canonical text in its own right, no longer links these functions to concrete anatomical structures. It stipulates that the *sanjiao* "has a name, but no bodily shape" (*you ming er wu xing* 有名而无形).[4] The contradiction between these opposing views has never been resolved in a satisfactory manner.[5] It was exacerbated with the arrival of Western anatomy. While rough correspondences could be established between Western anatomy and other visceral systems of function of Chinese medicine, no anatomical substratum resembling the *sanjiao* has ever been established.[6]

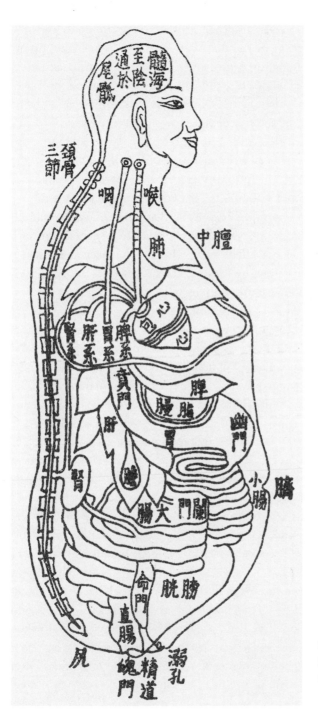

FIGURE I. Ming dynasty illustration of the internal organs of the body

Disagreement exists, too, about other attributes of the *sanjiao*. Some authors emphasize its function in the distribution of water and fluid, others that of generating and distributing various types of *qi*.[7] On some occasions it is paired with the heart governor (*xinzhu* 心主) or pericardium in an external/internal (*biao/li* 表里) relationship. Other texts pair it, instead, with the bladder (*pangguang* 膀胱) and the kidneys (*shen* 肾). In some texts the *sanjiao*'s distribution of defensive (*wei* 卫) *qi* is linked to the upper *jiao* and the lungs (*fei* 肺). Others view defensive *qi* as emanating from the lower *jiao* and the gate of life (*mingmen* 命门). This plurality is further exacerbated by the fact that seemingly contradictory statements can be found in the same text.[8]

Moving from conceptions of the healthy body to those of disease and illness one encounters a similar diversity. Physicians of Chinese medicine have not one but several languages available with which to diagnose and describe dysfunction.[9] In 1992 a report by the Xinhua News Agency stated that physicians of Chinese medicine currently employ more than one hundred different diagnostic systems.[10] At least seven methods of pattern differentiation are taught in today's universities and colleges.[11] To these might be added a large number of other widely used methods, including biomedical diagnostics and methods derived from biomedicine but assimilated into Chinese medicine.[12] There is no agreement between physicians about which method should be applied to a particular case, nor are there any established mechanisms to bring about convergence.[13]

Even at the most basic level one can distinguish at least three disease models and treatment strategies in contemporaneous use: (1) the empiricist use of specific treatment technologies; (2) an ontological disease nosology leading to specific treatments for defined diseases or, at least, locally limited interventions designed to deal with specific causes; and (3) an individually based functional disease model giving rise to the medicine of systematic correspondence. None of these strategies, according to Unschuld, can be said to be exclusively Chinese.[14]

Diagnostic technologies are usually summarized in classical and "modern" texts as the four methods of diagnosis (*sizhen* 四诊). These are inspection (*wang* 望), listening and smelling (*wen* 闻), questioning (*wen* 问), and palpation (*qie* 切) especially of the pulse (*mai* 脉). No unanimity exists, however, regarding the details of specific diagnostic techniques, the interpretation of diagnostic data thus obtained, or the relative value of various types of diagnosis. One can find, for instance, several different systems of pulse diagnosis practiced on various sites of the body. Even within particular systems there is little unanimity. Correspondences between different sections of the radial pulse and various visceral systems of function have been debated throughout the history of Chinese medicine, but differences of opinion continue up to the present day.[15]

Treatment practices are equally varied, and the history of Chinese medicine is characterized by polemics between advocates of different schools of thought.[16] Such polemics might concern theoretical issues or the correct interpretation of textual sources as much as the diagnostic and treatment techniques appropriate to a given case.[17] During my fieldwork, for example, I observed that the same acumoxa point was located differently by different physicians, and that points were selected on the basis of personal experience and stimulated by means of highly individualized needle techniques (*shoufa* 手法). Practitioners may use the same stylized terms taken from the canonical literature to describe a therapeutic intervention, but in practice they apply to it their own interpretations.[18]

If we turn to the social organization of medical practice, we find considerable diversity between types of practitioners and modes of transmission of knowledge. Throughout the history of Chinese medicine no group of practitioners ever succeeded in establishing itself as a profession in the sociological sense of the term.[19] Medical knowledge, whether transmitted orally or through written texts, was available to diverse groups of people. While the state did at times attempt to control medical practice, it never succeeded in disciplining the activities of practitioners at large. As Unschuld comments, "the Chinese physician as a definable entity did not exist." Instead, medical resources were widely distributed among "shamans, Buddhist priests, Daoist hermits, Confucian scholars, itinerant physicians, established physicians, 'laymen' with medical knowledge . . . , midwives, and many others."[20]

Lacking external disciplines that created and maintained standards of knowledge and practice, distinct streams of medicine, designated by the term *pai* 派, emerged as foci of interdisciplinary organization. The conventional translation given to *pai* is "school," such as in *piwei xuepai* 脾胃学派 (the spleen and stomach school) or *Hejian xuepai* 河间学派 (the Hejian school). If one examines the emergence of such groups, however, one finds that the various doctors who assigned themselves to a particular stream did not necessarily subscribe to a common theory directing their research as the term "school" would imply. Nor were they bounded by real or fictive kinship relations. Wu thus argues that it is more appropriate to speak of *pai* as designating a "group of people sharing some ideas or principles or at least claiming to do so." (We shall see in chapter 6 that such claims cannot be dissociated from a wide range of practices whose goal it is to establish and secure a person's position in society by means of various networks of social relations.) Within any *pai* various types of relations between student and teacher and various modes of transmission of knowledge could coexist, from secretly guarded transmission of secret recipes and texts within a family, to explicit teacher-student bonds with formal instruction, to the autodidactic study of certain key texts.[21]

Three factors have to some extent bridged the rifts between previously contending factions, schools, and streams in contemporary China: (1) attempts at professional unification in the face of threats posed to the existence of Chinese medicine by proponents of Western science from the 1920s onward; (2) moves to standardize Chinese medicine (*guifanhua* 规范化) that originated within Chinese medical circles as a strategy in their struggle for autonomy during the Republican era but were significantly accelerated and extended following the introduction of state-controlled education in the late 1950s; and (3) the regulation of Chinese medical practice and its integration into a nationwide health care system following the establishment of the communist regime in 1949.[22] In the late 1970s, for example, the Chongqing Chinese Medical Research Institute organized a series of seminars to discuss theoretical and clinical aspects of the *sanjiao* problem and proclaimed these to be resolved.[23] However, not all of my teachers in Beijing seemed to have been convinced, as not all shared the same opinions. Individual patterns of practice, family traditions, secret formulas, conceptual diversity, contending interpretations of classical texts, and struggles about the goal and meaning of Chinese medicine never disappeared. There are many indications that in the current climate of economic competition and relative decline of central political control they are, in fact, resurfacing more openly again.

Politically motivated convergence among contending factions within the Chinese medical community was one aspect of its encounter with Western medicine; another was the emergence of additional diversity. Western medical knowledge had stimulated debates within Chinese medical circles ever since its introduction into China in the sixteenth century. Initially these were limited to a small number of persons and to controversies that had been unresolved for centuries but were rekindled by newly arrived ideas from the West. More profound changes began to take shape only from the beginning of the twentieth century, when China's turn toward science and technology ushered in a new era.[24] "Mr. Science" (*sai xiansheng* 赛先生), adopted as a culture hero by the May Fourth movement, personified the belief in modernization that has been the enduring credo of all variants of scientism in post-imperial China.[25] If it wanted to survive, Chinese medicine could not afford to isolate itself from this movement.[26] Today, continuation of tradition and its simultaneous development under the joint guidance of biomedical science and the Communist Party—summarized in the slogan "inheriting and carrying forward" (*jicheng fayang* 继承发扬)—are accepted as equally important goals shaping Chinese medicine.[27] Yet, how precisely they might be synchronized so as to bring about the modernization of tradition is a question still unanswered.

The emergence of a stream working toward the integration and convergence of Chinese and Western medicine (*huitong xuepai* 汇通学派) at the turn of the twentieth century, the search for a new medicine (*xinyi* 新医) in the 1950s and again during the Cultural Revolution, and the contemporary state-supported combination and integration of Chinese and Western medicine (*zhongxiyi jiehe* 中西医结合) are labels attached to successive stages of this process.[28] None of these succeeded in providing models of inquiry or practice that were acceptable to all the physicians and politicians involved. Polemics between traditionalists and modernizers continue unabated to this day, and various interpretations of Chinese medicine are known under different names. Thus, "classical" (*gudaide* 古代的), "traditional" (*chuantongde* 传统的), "modern" (*xiandaide* 现代的), "scientific" (*kexuede* 科学的), and "new" (*xin* 新) are terms applied to Chinese medicine by different authors to signify their different perceptions of what "Chinese medicine" stands for.[29] Whatever else the interaction between Chinese and Western medicine may signify, it has added to the diversity of Chinese medicine without resolving its inner tensions.[30]

Tradition and Modernity in Contemporary Chinese Medicine

Moving from description to analysis, we can capture the plurality of Chinese medicine outlined above by means of two interrelated concepts: "multiplicity" and "heterogeneity." Heterogeneity implies that the Chinese medical tradition, its practitioners, and practices are open to and constituted by influences from a variety of domains and from various periods in time. Biomedical knowledge, technology, and research are infiltrating contemporary Chinese medicine around the world even as poetry, painting, and calligraphy continue to exert powerful forces on Chinese physicians.[31] In Europe and the United States Chinese medicine is reshaped by its association with peculiarly Western understandings of concepts such as holism, energy, and spirit,[32] while in China (as discussed above) it is redefined through particularly Chinese perceptions of science and modernization. New practices such as auricular acumoxa continually emerge in the ongoing commerce of ideas and technologies between East and West and are soon added to the tool bag of "traditional" medicine.[33] Apparently immutable core concepts of Chinese medicine such as *qi* are continually up for discussion as social, cultural, technological, and economic factors penetrate into the medical domain.[34] And as in any other medical system, what constitutes an illness and what does not is never a purely medical decision but is subject as well to political power and cultural trends.[35]

Multiplicity is a consequence of heterogeneity. Due to the permeability of medicine to outside influences—technological as well as ideological—we usually find at any one place and time a variety of ways of thinking about the body and of diagnosing and treating illness, and of ideas regarding the nature of good medical practice. We observe various types of practitioners, various ways of transmitting knowledge, and ongoing competition for status, influence, and power between individuals and groups. As we shall see in subsequent chapters, such multiplicity exists at every level of description, within as well as between medical traditions, and even with respect to individual physicians, who reveal themselves to be far more complex than conventional images of the subject and medical practice have previously imagined.

Although multiplicity and heterogeneity are now widely accepted as characteristic aspects of Chinese medicine, such plurality stubbornly resists all attempts to reduce it to the conventional categories of scholarly Western discourse. This is revealed in exemplary fashion in the analysis of modernization in Chinese medicine.[36]

China embraced modernity as a consequence first of the realization of military weakness and later of actual defeat at the hands of both Japan and the Western colonial powers. Within the context of the Self-Strengthening movement (*Yangwu yundong* 洋务运动) lasting from 1860 to 1895, the New Culture movement (*xin wenhua yundong* 新文化运动) of about 1915–28, and the May Fourth movement (*Wu si yundong* 五四运动) starting in 1919, intellectuals and politicians set out to transform China into a "modern" country. Science and technology in particular were seen as crucial for effecting this transformation. As a consequence, technicism and the valorization of scientific knowledge (some authors speak of a "Chinese obsession with science") were constant guides on China's tortuous path toward modernization throughout the twentieth century.[37]

During the first half of the century Chinese medicine was widely perceived as a symbol of the old society for which the modernizers, many of whom had studied Western medicine abroad, could envisage no further use. Controversies and polemics between proponents of Chinese and Western medicine culminated in 1929 in an ultimately unsuccessful attempt to legally abolish the practice of Chinese medicine. One of the outcomes of these confrontations was a significant reorientation within the Chinese medicine community itself toward embracing reforms that encompassed the scientization and standardization of medical knowledge and practice, the supplementation of apprentice-based learning with professional schools and colleges, and the organization of physicians within professional organizations rather than clan- or native place–based local networks.

The institutional status of Chinese medicine changed radically after the establishment of the People's Republic in 1949 leading to its progressive integration into the state-controlled health care system. Inasmuch as the various facets of socialist revolution and reform from 1949 to the present were governed by ideologies of progress similar to those that guided earlier reformers, the ongoing modernization of Chinese medicine was, if anything, accelerated. For almost all observers—Western historians, anthropologists, and practitioners of Chinese medicine as well as Chinese politicians, physicians, and most patients with whom I spoke—contemporary Chinese medicine therefore constitutes an entity categorically different from the medicine of the imperial era.[38]

This perception raises important scholarly questions that take us back to the problematic differentiation between tradition and modernity and its conjoining with the problem of plurality discussed in chapter 1. If contemporary Chinese medicine, or TCM, is really different from the medicine of the previous periods, where precisely (historically, conceptually, practically) runs the boundary between the two? If Chinese medicine is no longer "traditional" (or old, or ancient, or prescientific), what does this imply for the claims of biomedicine to be the only truly "modern" (or scientific) medicine? If several forms of "modern" medicine (Chinese medicine and Western medicine in China, or Chinese medicine in China and the United States, Britain, or Germany, all which are clearly different from each other) can exist contemporaneously, what implications does this have for our perceptions of modernity?

How we approach these questions—let alone how we answer them—clearly depends on how we define modernity and mark it off from tradition. Contemporary writers employ three broadly different strategies for this purpose. The first defines the "modern" by means of universal attributes such as the disjunction between science and tradition, knowledge and belief, nature and culture. Modernization then becomes the process by means of which these disjunctions are established and maintained. Standardization and regularization of knowledge and practice, professionalization, a belief in progress and the ability to improve the human condition by means of science and technology, emphasis on the global and universal coupled with a disregard for the local and specific, and the emergence of bureaucracies in the service of nation-states are some of the criteria often used to measure whether or not a given society or culture is "modern."[39] The distinction between "modern" and ancient ("traditional," old, etc.) Chinese medicine outlined above, for instance, is established precisely through this mode of analysis.

On the plus side, this perspective allows us to tie transformations in Chinese medicine to similar changes in other social domains such as education or the policing of civilian populations, and, by implication, to global theories of historical and social development.[40] It is less suitable, however, for teasing out the actual complexities and contradictions of specific historical transformations such as the conjunction between modernist and nationalist ideologies in the development of "modern" Chinese medicine both before and after 1949.[41] Its linear narrative furthermore fails to account for the fact that historical time does not move with the same speed in all regions of a culture or society. As a consequence, there is little agreement among scholars regarding the point at which the transition between "traditional" and "modern" Chinese medicine occurred. While for some historians it is an ongoing and incomplete process leading to the coexistence of traditional and modern elements that can nevertheless be clearly demarcated, others feel able to specify a distinct epistemological event that marks this transition.[42]

At this point I shall interject into the discussion a brief case study drawn from my fieldwork in Beijing in 1994. This study exemplifies within the space of a single event that in contemporary Chinese medicine the "modern" and "traditional," the old and the new, the Western and Chinese, are connected by multiple strands and conjoined into complex hybrids that not only obscure what is actually transforming what but challenge the very reality of these oppositions.

CASE 2.1. *Dr. He Acquires a New Needle Technique (I).* Dr. He is a Ph.D. student in the acumoxa department of Beijing University of Chinese Medicine (*Beijing zhongyiyao daxue* 北京中医药大学). He comes from Shanxi Province, where he completed his bachelor's and master's degrees. His supervisor in Beijing is Professor Xia, one of China's most famous and influential acupuncturists. One evening Dr. He asked me to show him my needle technique (*shoufa* 手法). The term *shoufa* refers to the method by which the needle is inserted and manipulated in acumoxa therapy.[43] Through needling, acumoxa practitioners enter into a direct relationship with their patients' *qi*. "Grasping the *qi*" (*deqi* 得气), for instance, indicates that the needle has made contact with a patient's *qi*. This is experienced by the physician through sensations such as pulling or firmness at the tip of the needle, and by the patient through sensations of pain, numbness, cold, or heat. Once the *qi* has been grasped in this way it can be further moved around a patient's body (*yun qi* 运气) by means of needle manipulations that may or may not involve projections of the physician's own *qi*.

Throughout the history of acumoxa therapy many different needle techniques have been promoted. "Modern" technology has increased the scope for developing new methods by allowing for better sterilization, deeper needling, and longer retention of needles.[44] Simultaneously, it also has engendered different relations between physicians and their patients and physicians and their own bodies, as electronic needle stimulators remove the necessity to cultivate complex body practices designed to attune the *qi* of physicians with that of their patients. Nevertheless, today as throughout the history of acumoxa therapy, individual acupuncturists recommend different styles of needling and manipulation. For many, one's personal needle technique still represents a skill honed during years of training and application. And even experienced acupuncturists can be observed cultivating their *shoufa* through daily practice on tangerines or cotton cushions.

Dr. He's curiosity about my needle technique was thus a way of finding out more about me. It was also, as it turned out, an offer to deepen our relationship. He explained that for nine years he had used a technique taught at the Shanxi College (fig. 2), but recently he had adopted the needle technique of his supervisor, Professor Xia (fig. 3). Although he had used this needle technique for only six months, Dr. He considered it far superior to that of his previous teacher. After all, Professor Xia was renowned throughout China. Efficacy alone, however, did not exhaust the reasons that had convinced Dr. He to change his style. He explained that if he wished to benefit from Professor Xia's experience to the maximum extent, he had to come as close as possible to thinking and feeling like him. How could that be done without needling like him? Furthermore, if he stubbornly stuck to his old needle technique Dr. He would not be showing respect to his famous teacher. How could he then expect him to share his knowledge?

Thus, for the last six months Dr. He had practiced Professor Xia's needle technique every evening for half an hour. Now he was sharing it with me. In doing so he assumed the role of my teacher, but also that of a

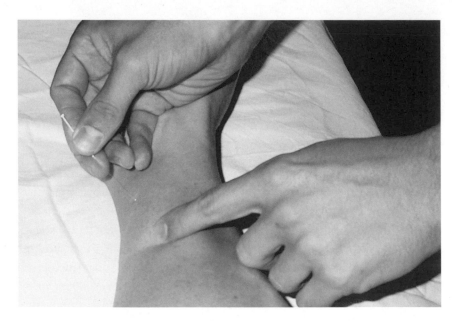

FIGURE 2. Dr. He's previous needle technique

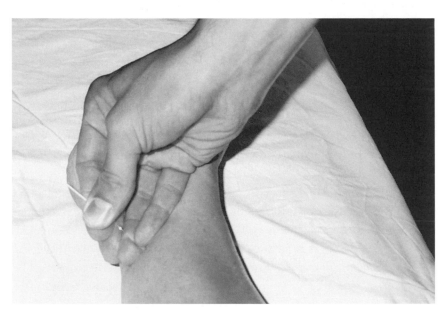

FIGURE 3. Dr. He's current needle technique

friend, with all the reciprocal obligations this involved. In my relationship to Dr. He, just as in Dr. He's relation to Professor Xia, there was no alternative but to accept the gift and change my style.

Modernization as Local Process

My short case study succinctly demonstrates how apparently "modern" and "traditional" elements of practice are conjoined in contemporary Chinese medicine. Dr. He, practicing in a hospital and studying for a doctoral degree at a state university, inherits a personalized needle technique within a relationship that is at once structured by what Dr. He himself perceives of as "traditional" morality and a bureaucratic process that is "modern" in the Weberian sense. In actual practice, Dr. He uses this needle technique to treat patterns on the basis of a method of diagnosis synthesized and imported into acumoxa in the 1950s and 1960s. In addition, he often combines it with electro-acupuncture, a product of "modern" technoscience, or auricular acupuncture, a Western invention that is now considered part of "traditional" Chinese medicine.[45]

A second strategy for distinguishing modernity from tradition increasingly employed by anthropologists and historians seeking to accommodate to this plurality therefore has been to treat modernity as an essentially local phenomenon. Their writings use universal features of modernization to link inquiries across disciplines, historical periods, and geographical areas, while understanding the dynamics of modernization as possible only in relation to concrete contexts of practice.[46] From this perspective, the modernization of Chinese medicine in Republican China can be interpreted as having emerged through a historically specific dialectic between scientism and nationalism that shaped not only Chinese medicine but also Chinese perceptions of science at the time. Modernization of Chinese medicine in post-Mao China, instead, can be made intelligible as structured by different contradictions: Chinese medicine's status as a national treasure decreed by Mao Zedong, the imperatives of social development that unfolded from Deng Xiaoping's theory of four modernizations, and the hospitalization of Chinese medicine as an aspect of state-controlled health care. This conjunction of forces made the utilization of science and technology as primary tools for the development of Chinese medicine imperative while at the same time its institutionalization removed state-controlled Chinese medicine from the target list of more radical modernizers.

Without surrendering the benefits that accrue from a comparative point of view, perceiving of modernization in terms of different processes related by family resemblance rather than uniform characteristics enables an understanding of modernity and its constitutive practices as locally configured and implicitly plural. It allows the investigator to tease out of a particular constellation of events those forces that are specific and unique to it, yet always relates such singularity to more general principles of social transformation. From such a vantage point, the "traditional" and "modern" elements in Dr. He's practice cease to be contradictory and become the key to apprehending its local construction. That various aspects of modernization should progress at different paces or penetrate into some domains of practice but not into others ceases to be a problem and becomes a reflection of the particular local constellations of power, and hence of resistance and accommodation.

This mode of analysis thus allows for the persistence of local differences without surrendering the notion of modernization as a more encompassing global event. The authority of Professor Xia that styles itself according to Confucian models of social relations, for instance, is merely inserted locally into an institutional system modeled on Western exemplars that it does not thereby transform. Likewise, Dr. He's needle technique as an example of body-centered practice made meaningful by ancient notions of qi transformation does not exhaust his therapeutic repertoire but merely constitutes one among many different clinical tools. Increasingly, as in the case of electronic point-location devices, electro-acupuncture apparatuses, and national or international standards for acumoxa point locations, these tools are produced through technological and bureaucratic processes rather than individual experience and personally transmitted craft. The standardization intrinsic to these processes of production necessarily configures local contexts of practice, even if individual skill still adapts their specific local usage. Dr. He's inclusion of electro-acupuncture, which disallows bodily centered idiosyncratic needle techniques, into his treatments is one example. Another is his use of pattern differentiation (bianzheng 辨证), which has dominated acumoxa practice only since it was manufactured as the pivot of Chinese medicine in a process stretching over several decades from the early 1950s to the 1980s.[47]

The problem of what precisely is meant by "modern" and "traditional," however, still is not decisively resolved here. Professor Xia's manual needle technique might seem traditional because it is person-centered, transmitted within kinship-like master disciple networks, and refers itself to the manipulation of qi and thereby to a traditional canon of medical concepts, texts, and practices. It may be contrasted to technoscientific forms of electro-acupuncture that discipline physicians' bodies by uniting them with industrially produced electronic stimulating devices and severely curtail the space for local variation and personal adaptation. Classical forms of needle manipulation may also be compared with modern forms of insertion that do not refer to *qi* but concern themselves only with muscles, blood vessels, and nerves as viewed from a biomedical perspective and thus subsume acupuncture as a mere technique to the global networks of biomedicine.

Examined more closely, however, these apparently clear distinctions are immediately rendered opaque once more. Historically, both Professor Xia's needle technique and the one Dr. He learned from his previous teacher can have emerged only after the introduction of stainless steel needles in the late 1940s and early 1950s. Previously, acupuncture needles manufactured from soft steel, silver, or gold did not allow for quick penetration of the skin but virtually had to be "screwed" into it. Do innovations in the domain of needle technique that occurred as a result of introducing stainless steel needles imply the assimilation of a modern technology to traditional physiology or the transformation of traditional body practice by modern instruments? Physicians who have made major contributions to mapping the classical body of channels and collaterals (*jingluo* 经络) onto the modern body of muscles and nerves consider themselves simultaneously modernizers, traditionalists, and a bridge between tradition and modernity.[48] And what kind of body is the one presented on modern acupuncture charts, a body that renders nerves and channels of *qi* as equally visible and real? Is it a "modern" innovation? A distortion of anatomical facts by "traditional" fantasies? Or a hybrid that partakes in equal measure of tradition and modernity?

Such questions draw our attention to the fact that categories of thought such as tradition/modernity, science/ethnoscience, nature/culture, and fact/fetish are themselves local productions and therefore in some sense traditional even where they present themselves as modern. Furthermore, inasmuch as such oppositions become meaningful only within the discourse of modernity itself—the attempt to label certain phenomena and practices "modern" and thereby mark them off from others—these categories do not function as neutral signifiers. Rather, they invoke implicit evaluations that limit understanding and constrain adaptability. Two examples relevant to the ethnography of contemporary Chinese medicine will demonstrate these effects.

Inquiries into local processes of modernization are most often organized within the framework of a world system's perspective. Contemporary ethnographies and postcolonial writings thus focus on the encounter of local groups and persons with the forces of globalization and the macroprocesses

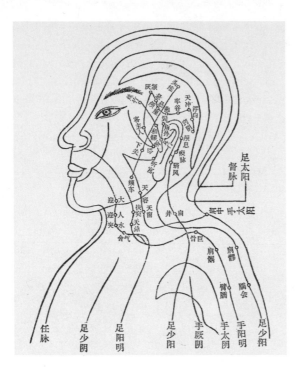

FIGURE 4. Qing dynasty illustration of the acupuncture channels of the head

associated with capitalist political economy in its many forms. Relationships between tradition and modernity are therefore interpreted as being marked by distinctive qualitative differences that construct modernity as naturally dominant. As a consequence, relationships between the "modern" and the "traditional" are most often viewed through a framework of resistance and accommodation in which tactical resistance and subversive deferral constitute resources by which nonmodern forms of life can undermine—but never actually overcome—the hegemony of the "modern."[49] Consequently, academic investigations of Chinese medicine in the West often focus on the loss of "traditional" skills and concepts and view its future with considerable apprehension.[50]

However, Dr. He's needle techniques demonstrate that the apparently "traditional" is often merely the "modern" in disguise. Furthermore, as we shall see throughout my ethnography, that which we choose to label "traditional" is not merely inventive in its own right but is also capable of assimilating and thereby transforming the "modern" into an aspect of tradition.

Second, even when modernity is conceived of as locally emergent, its opposition to traditional forms of practice invariably impinges on judgments regarding the desirability of these local transformations. Thus, in contempo-

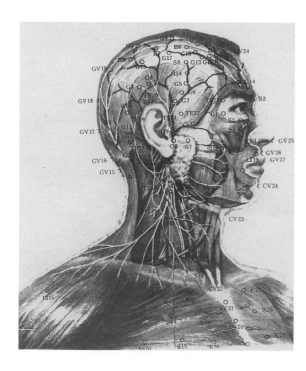

FIGURE 5. Modern illustration of the acupuncture channels of the head

rary China, where scientism is state sponsored, hardly any of the physicians and patients I met did not countenance the modernization of Chinese medicine as absolutely necessary. This attitude has led to a pressure for "developing" (*fazhan* 发展) Chinese medicine with little discussion regarding the actual need for or consequences of such development. In the West, on the other hand, where the popularity of Chinese medicine is intimately associated with romanticist critiques of modernity, its associations with tradition are consciously emphasized. Hence, Westerners do not practice "Chinese medicine" but rather "traditional Chinese medicine" (TCM). This makes it very difficult for Western advocates of modernization to view Chinese medicine as anything other than a return to outdated modes of thought and practice, while on the other side its supporters easily lose sight of the transformative potential implicit within Chinese medicine itself. The result, in China as in the West, is a foreclosing of multiple other options of engagement with Chinese medicine—options that may be less easily recruited to conventional oppositions between "tradition" and "modernity" but that may enable less prejudicial judgments regarding the benefits of different medical practices in the plural health care systems arising everywhere as a consequence of globalization.

Escaping from this impasse requires recognition of the processes whereby distinctions between "tradition" and "modernity" are locally configured within the context of historically specific endeavor and struggle. This can be achieved only if Western medicine and modernization lose their status as singular points of reference in the analysis of non-Western medical practices. I therefore turn to a third perspective regarding modernity that has evolved in the field of science and technology studies.[51] This perspective resolves the various dilemmas we have discussed by denying modernity any distinctive qualitative characteristics by which we could mark it off from tradition. Rather, knowledge and society, nature and culture, the old and the new, are seen as always co-constructing each other through practices of the present in which both their past and future are continuously at stake.

Dissolving the essence of previous conceptions of modernity in this way empowers my ethnography of Chinese medicine in three ways at once. First, by drawing attention to the implications of the rhetorical construction of modernity it enables the kind of interventionist anthropology advocated in chapter 1. Second, the theoretical models made available by this research tradition provide conceptual tools that explain how and why the "modern" and "traditional," kept apart in thought, align without difficulty in practice. Third, by disabling the reductionist pressures implicit in all teleology, plurality can be transformed from a mere surface phenomenon in constant need of explanation to an object of research that deserves to be taken seriously in its own right. In the next section I introduce Andrew Pickering's "mangle of practice," a model of network construction that explicitly relates itself to the above perspective, as particularly fitting for the ethnography of contemporary Chinese medicine.

Practice and Practices

Pickering's "mangle of practice" is a model for thinking about the construction of practices that conjoin nature and culture in real time.[52] For this purpose Pickering distinguishes between culture, or *practices*, on the one hand, and the work of *practice*, by which such cultures or practices are constructed, on the other hand. "Culture" here describes the "transverse connections across multiple and heterogeneous fields" whereby diverse entities such as skills and social relations, machines and instruments, and beliefs and knowledge are aligned with each other *in* practice at a given place and time.[53] In Pickering's view, irrespective of whether one speaks of culture or practice or whether one uses some other related designation such as "form of life," "episteme," "disciplinary regime," "actor-network," or "cyborg," and irrespective of what style of description and analysis a particular author might favor, cultural studies (of which anthropology is a prime example) implicitly tend to focus on the mapping and exploration of such synchronous structure.

Pickering therefore distinguishes a second dimension of analysis aligned orthogonally to that of cultural studies. In this dimension one examines how cultures change through and *in practice*. This is the dimension in which Pickering's "mangle of practice" (or "mangle," for short) is located. The concrete mode of operation of this mangle is the "interactive stabilization" of "disciplined human agency" and "captured material agency." Interactive stabilization refers to the idea that none of the elements belonging to a particular culture or practice are pregiven or ready-made for assemblage. Rather, they emerge in the very process through which a practice constructs itself. Put another way, the mangle that produces culture at the macrolevel operates simultaneously in constructing all the various constitutive elements of a culture at the microlevel. This implies that no culture or practice can be reduced to a deeper level—whether of meaning, agency, habitus, or environmental context—that would provide us with privileged access to its mode of (re-)production. Rather, culture is always and forever self-generating within practices that extend from the formation of individual selves and social units to the construction of technical apparatus and machines, and beyond to their integration into emergent nature-cultures and also, of course, to our models of such nature-cultures themselves.

Human agency—the beliefs and knowledge that inform it, the desires that motivate it, and the skills that express it—arises and is transformed in the course of concrete practical interactions with other agencies both human and nonhuman. Such agency is disciplined because it does not arise spontaneously; it is always already part of practices sustained by ongoing interactions between participating elements. Human agency can, however, be aligned to new and other elements in the course of practice, at which point it opens itself up to adaptive transformation. The same is true for nonhuman, or "captured," material agency. Pickering uses the term "captured" to denote that what precisely a machine, quark, amoeba, or phenomenon of nature will do, or is capable of doing, at a particular place and point in time can never be known by human agents other than through the insertion of such material agency into human practices of knowing and doing.

Human agency and culture, in this view, are neither imposed onto the world by meaning-giving human subjects nor are they mere reflections of objectively existing social or natural environments that constrain human autonomy. Constraints, in fact, do not exist other than as the resistance they offer to human agency, and they emerge only in the course of humans' attempts to transform the world they inhabit. The mangle—that is, the processes through and in which culture, subjectivity, and history are constructed and transformed—is therefore likened by Pickering to a "dance of agency" between humans and nonhumans. From the perspective of participating humans this dance can be described as a dialectic of *resistance* and *accommodation* in which "resistance denotes the failure to achieve an intended capture of agency in practice, and accommodation an active human strategy of response to resistance."[54] How the dance looks from the side of nonhumans we cannot know. All we can do is formulate models of such agency in the course of practical engagement with it.

Pickering's model of the mangle emerged in the context of his science and technology studies. Its author explicitly states, however, that he intends it to be used as a "theory of everything." He claims that the mangle provides us with a model for thinking about all practice and that it is applicable equally to microlevel analyses of how science works, to macrolevel studies of cultural and historical change, and even to the understanding of human engagement with "nonstandard agency" (Pickering's term for agencies outside disciplined human and captured material agency such as spirits, shamans, and witches). Pickering thus presents us with a model of the world in which the way the world is and how we know this world mutually construct and support each other.[55]

The mangle is a particularly attractive model for the kind of ethnography I have in mind for three reasons. First, it furnishes a nonreductive account of practice that can easily accommodate to the diversity of Chinese medicine. Second, as a general theory of *practice* (and not merely of *cultural* practices) it cuts through the science/tradition distinction that characterizes modernist analyses of Chinese medicine. Third, its posthumanist account of agency and view of the world as continually emergent resonates by way of elective affinity with important tenets of thought within the Chinese medical tradition itself. Not having to process Chinese medicine through entirely alien categories of understanding yet allowing for sufficient critical distance to it, Pickering's model thus enables (though by no means guarantees) a more profound understanding of Chinese medical practice than do attempts to ground such practice in stable configurations of history, knowledge, culture, or practice.

Rethinking Agency

Before proceeding any further a brief discussion of the conflation of human and nonhuman agency that underpins Pickering's model and related post-humanist studies of science is necessary. Granting agency to humans and nonhumans alike is primarily a strategy for getting around enduring questions in social explanation and their relation to the problem of plurality discussed in chapter 1. If social and natural environments are shared, what makes individual agency possible? And what is the locus of such agency? Is it determined and collective so that each act represents a deeper order and habitus, or is it spontaneous and individual? If it is both, how do the two levels of activity relate to one another?

Critics of such conflation argue that human agency, though crucially configured by external constraints as well as disciplinary regimes and articulations of power, clearly differs from nonhuman agency in its possession of unique characteristics such as intentionality. These characteristics should be reflected in meaningful accounts of human practice. Rather than attributing agency to nonhumans and thereby dragging social scientific analysis onto the level of primitive fetishism, these critics suggest that it would be more profitable to explore the mechanisms by which humans variously accord agency to people and things through processes of delegation and representation. A traffic light, for instance, clearly has agency only inasmuch as it is inserted into specific human practices.[56]

Posthumanists reject these arguments, viewing them as an attempt to return to a language of human subjectivity engaging with objectively existing constraints and the problematic dialectic between structure and agency that such thinking entails. Rouse, for instance, poignantly demonstrates how talk of intentionality reintroduces a vestigial sense of meaning as something uniquely bestowed to a situation by humans into the analysis of practices. His solution is to argue that "the role of active subjects in configuring practices is not the bestowal or imposition of meaning but a responsiveness to the solicitations of their situation." Subjects thus become agents only inasmuch as they respond to the givens of a context of action using their skills of comportment, intellectual as well as practical. While such skills encompass the engagement with both physical objects and social meanings present in a situation, they do not require thinking of such engagement as having meanings categorically different from other forms of engagement with the world.[57]

Accounts of agency in Chinese medicine and philosophy resonate with the views of Pickering, Latour, Rouse, and others. Chinese medicine certainly

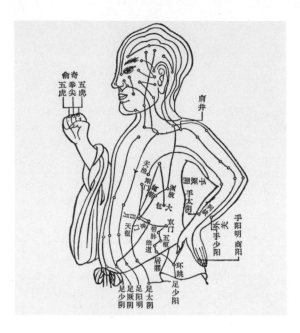

FIGURE 6. Qing dynasty illustration of the acupuncture channels of the abdomen

allows for heterogeneous agencies and a multiplicity of entities, both human and nonhuman, to contribute to the transformations of the world. These conceptions challenge humanist/antihumanist accounts of agency from a different angle than the perspectives developed in science and technology studies, even if (or perhaps especially because) discourse on agency in Chinese medicine is today conducted in politically correct materialist terms.[58] He Yumin writes that "according to Chinese medicine the origin of the world, its material [makeup], that which fills out the entire universe, the finest matter whose movement does not cease—these [all] are generated by the interactive transformations of *qi*. All things in the world are the results of these material movements and transformations of *qi*."[59]

At the basis of all agency in Chinese medicine thus stands *qi*. In early Chinese writings about nature *qi* simultaneously refers to that which "makes things happen in stuff" and "stuff in which things happen."[60] According to Porkert, *qi* is both an "energetic configuration" and a "configuration of energy," while Unschuld translates the term as "(finest matter) influences," "emanations," or "vapours."[61] Different types of *qi* such as *xue* 血 (blood), *jing* 精 (essence), *jinye* 津液 (body fluids), *zangfu zhi qi* 脏腑之气 (visceral *qi*), *yuanqi* 元气 (original *qi*), *zongqi* 宗气 (gathering *qi*), and *daqi* 大气 (great *qi*) can be distinguished, each with its own presence in space and function in time. *Weiqi* 卫气 warms the body and secures its external boundaries; *yingqi*

营气 nourishes skin, muscles, bones, sinews, and visceral systems of function (*zangfu* 脏腑). Different types of *qi* are derived from and transformed into each other. The visceral systems of function in Chinese medicine directly express this physiology of *qi* transformation: "liver stores blood" (*gan zang xue* 肝臟血), "lung directs *qi* downward" (*fei jiang qi* 肺降气), "spleen controls blood" (*pi tong xue* 脾统血), and so on.[62]

Chinese accounts of *qi* transformation thus provide us with a model of the world that implicitly accepts nonhuman agency. Just as important, these accounts also undermine conventional Western notions regarding the unitary agency of human subjects. A famous passage in *Suwen*, chapter 8, which compares visceral systems of function to court officials, is still memorized today by students at Chinese medical colleges. Thus, in a seminar in London in 1996, a Chinese professor began his lecture on the liver by reciting: "Liver holds the office of general, whence strategies emanate" (*Ganzhe, jiangjun zhi guan, moulu chu yan* 肝者, 将军之官, 谋虑出焉).[63] In other (con)texts visceral systems of functions are predicated by the verb *zhu* 主. *Zhu* is commonly translated as "rules," "dominates," or "governs," though its semantic range is

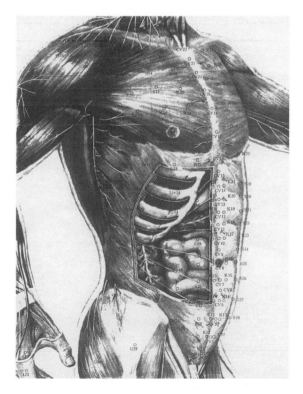

FIGURE 7. Modern illustration of the acupuncture channels of the abdomen

far more complex. According to Hay it refers to relations among the visceral systems of function that are not exhausted by cause and effect.[64] Farquhar suggests rendering *zhu* as "to unfold," to convey an image of visceral systems of function as constituting, like persons, "points of centrality that organize radiating and shifting fields around themselves," though in the context of the *Neijing* it is more correctly translated as "is responsible for."[65]

Visceral systems of function are responsible for agency in heterogeneous domains. Thus, we learn that "liver is responsible for the sinews" (*gan zhu jin* 肝主筋), "liver is responsible for fright" (*gan zhu jing* 肝主惊), "liver is responsible for the making of strategies" (*gan zhu moulu* 肝主谋虑), "liver is responsible for ascending and effusion" (*gan zhu sheng fa* 肝主升发), "liver is responsible for free coursing" (*gan zhu shuxie* 肝主疏泄), "liver is responsible for the sea of blood" (*gan zhu xuehai* 肝主血海), and "liver is responsible for physical movement" (*gan zhu yundong* 肝主运动). The agency of visceral systems of function, like that of the persons they constitute, is interactive rather than reactive. Visceral systems of function initiate, sustain, and support the activities of body/mind but are also subject to the power of agencies that affect body/mind from within and without. Liver, for instance, "forms tears" (*wei lei* 为泪), is "averse to wind" (*wu feng* 恶风), and "lives on the left" (*sheng yu zuo* 生于左). It pathologically "attacks the spleen" (*cheng pi* 乘脾), while physiologically "liver and kidney are of the same source" (*gan shen tong yuan* 肝肾同源). "Anger damages liver" (*nu shang gan* 怒伤肝), but when "liver *qi* is depleted there is fear" (*ganqi xu ze kong* 肝气虚则恐).[66] Disorders of liver function are reflected in a wide range of problems that impinge not only on body/mind but also on morality and the ordering of social space. *Lingshu*, chapter 8, gives a flavor of these processes: "When the liver is [affected by] being disheartened and grief that perturb the middle this injures the etheral soul [*hun* 魂]. When the etheral soul is injured the person runs amok disregarding [conventions] and is not pure. One who is not pure will not be an upstanding person. The genitals will shrink and the sinews spasm. The two rib cages will not rise. The heart is withered and the complexion perished. They will die during autumn."[67]

Chinese medicine's ideas about the making of strategies carried out by the liver challenge core aspects not only of humanist accounts of "agency" but also of "self," "person," or "subject" with whom the former is interlocked. This does not imply, however, that Chinese physicians, ancient and contemporary, were or are unable to distinguish between human and nonhuman agencies. Rather, all things are made up of and connected by matter-influences such as *qi*. Hence, they can interpenetrate and influence each other organically within processes of transformation and organization. In Chinese medicine, too, thought and affect constitute a different dimension of being than the movement of food through the bowels. But inasmuch as both are types of *qi* transformation they are not categorically different. Thought and affect may influence bowel movements, but bowel movements or the weather may also influence affect. Therefore, while many physicians suggest that it is best to treat emotional disorders by regulating affect, they see no reason why it should not also be done with drugs or needles. And while they suggest that intentions crucially affect how medicine becomes efficacious, they also accord to needle manipulations and drugs an efficacy all of their own.[68]

Different physicians, schools, and streams of transmission interpret these interactions through their own particular modes of understanding. While this is not the place to follow up any of these in detail, we can note, nevertheless, that the interpenetration of human and nonhuman agencies permitted by Chinese thought led some of its key thinkers to formulate ideas that resonate with contemporary posthumanism in striking ways. The neo-Confucian philosopher Zhu Xi 朱熹 (1130–1200), whom Fung refers to as "probably the greatest synthesizer in Chinese thought," presents an intriguing example. Zhu Xi orders all phenomena in the universe into groups according to a hierarchy at the apex of which stands humanity.[69] Interactions between these phenomena are orderly and intelligible. There is, however, no single agency (human, natural, or superhuman) that determines how the universe comes to be the way it is. Rather, the universe and all phenomena in it are as they are because at each given moment they fit together in the only way they can fit together. Chen Chun 陈淳, an immediate pupil of Zhu Xi, explains: "*Li* [pattern] is a natural and unescapable law of affairs and things. . . . The meaning of 'natural and unescapable' is that [human] affairs, and [natural] things, are made just exactly to fit into place. The meaning of 'law' is that the fitting into place occurs without the slightest excess or deficiency."[70] Needham argues that for neo-Confucianists in the tradition of Zhu Xi this fitting together—a fitting together that is "living and dynamic to the highest extent" and is designated by the technical term *li* 理, or "pattern"—is the ultimate ground of being. Hence, for Zhu Xi—much as for Pickering eight centuries later—"all things [are] 'dancers' in a universal pattern."[71]

The Past and Future Orientation of Practices

"*Li* permeating things is the natural unescapableness of them," Needham insists. "Righteousness [*yi* 义] is how to handle this *li*."[72] State-sponsored neo-

Confucianism came to perceive of engagement with the world ultimately in terms of accepting and adapting to the given order in nature and society. For contemporary anthropologists and sociologists of science, on the other hand, it is precisely the constructed nature of what is given that is always at stake. Nevertheless, I will not surrender so easily the affinity between the two traditions. For it seems to me that the notion of *li* can help us to address certain problems of Pickering's model of the mangle, such as the tenacious persistence of the structure/agency dichotomy implicit in the distinction between *practice* and *practices*. Pickering insinuates that we must choose whether we want to investigate *practice* (defined as the temporal extension of culture) or *practices* (defined as the structural alignment of heterogeneous elements in culture). Zhu Xi's notion of *li*, which Needham translates as both "pattern" and "organization," effectively undercuts this dichotomy because *li* designates both how things are and the reason why they are "just so."

The present is "just so" because each thing, each element of a practice or culture as well as that practice or culture at large, is continually emergent at the intersection of its own past and future. Structurally, that with which we engage is always already at hand through the historical positioning we take up in the environment in which we live and work or in relation to the tools we use. It is given temporally, inasmuch as situated agency is a response to the "specific configuration of meaningful possibilities of action which emerges from past practice."[73] Yet, all practice is simultaneously also future oriented even when it intends to maintain a status quo or re-create a status quo ante. This effect can be grasped structurally by observing that elements of a practice—but also entire practices themselves—are constitutive elements of other practices. Practicing acumoxa, for instance, requires not only a coming together of patients, physicians, ideas about the body, needles, and other tools in the context of particular institutions; it is simultaneously tied to practices of knowledge transmission, professional organization, manufacturing and commerce, health insurance, the circulation of money, and so on. The ongoing development of any one practice is therefore fundamentally influenced by that of other practices. Inasmuch as there exists only one way in which different practices can be articulated into an overarching pattern so that it is "just so," we can speak of future states determining the present.[74]

The mechanisms of this relation—the manner in which the past intrudes into the present but simultaneously in which the present rewrites the past by means of its own future orientation—are what constitute practice and practices as spatiotemporally extended.[75] Furthermore, such emergence is not merely a coming into being; it is simultaneously also always a disappearing.

Attention is thereby drawn to the fact that conceptually as well as method-ologically Pickering's mangle focuses only on those agencies that contribute positively to the emergence of a particular practice. There exist many pro-cesses in life and nature, however, that do not produce definitive end-products that can then serve post hoc as handles on the elucidation of practice. Beside the stories of the victors stand the stories of the victims, the excluded, and the vanquished, the stories of those agencies for which there is no place in the practices of the present. These stories and their traces are much more difficult to hear, however, from Pickering's perspective. Yet for political as much as for epistemological reasons, their inclusion into the bigger pattern is important to anthropologists.[76]

Elements that are no longer articulated with other elements *in practice* do not simply disappear but may persist, more or less visible, for long periods, constantly threatening to interrupt present alignments and offering different futures. One reason, certainly, why contemporary Chinese medicine appears more immediately plural than some other traditions (such as biomedicine but also the timeless traditions of a certain type of ethnography) is that its past is too much of a presence—a past not merely of fragments, ruins, and memories but of entire libraries, living commentatorial traditions, and embodied lines of descent.[77]

Infrastructural Synthesis

In chapter 1 I identified the Kantian conception of synthesis as the point of origin for the monistic bias that characterizes anthropological theories of cul-ture. An anthropology open to the idea that plurality may be a fundamen-tal rather than a derivative aspect of social life must therefore exchange the Kantian vision of synthesis as grounded in the synthesizing capacities of a universal subject for one that views synthesis (as a state) as an emergent prop-erty of synthesis (as a process), and vice versa.[78]

The emergence of multisited ethnography—the juxtaposition of different perspectives in the examination of an object of research—during the last de-cade indicates that such a shift is already well under way. Multisited ethnogra-phy indicates not merely a change of methodology from conventional single-site locations to a set of shifting contexts and positions but also a changed understanding of how culture and the world are made up. Whereas the conven-tional anthropological focus on local situations and peoples, intimately asso-ciated with the established dichotomy between local life-worlds and a global (world) system easily fits into the categories inherited from Kant via Montesquieu, multisited ethnography can posit no given entity to be examined and no a priori ground to which it may be reduced. Rather, says Marcus, comparison emerges from putting questions to an emergent object of study whose contours, sites, and relationships are not known beforehand."[79]

I believe that Andrew Pickering's mangle of practice constitutes a workable model through which such an approach to Chinese medicine can be developed. The mangle and its subsidiary concepts such as agency, accommodation, and resistance furnish tools that can easily be translated into anthropological analysis. For the reasons outlined above, I consider it necessary, however, to extend Pickering's model in three directions. First, we need to resist as much as possible its latent structure/agency dichotomy. Instead, an ethnography of synthesis should emphasize at all times the interrelation and mutual determination of *practice* and *practices*.[80] Second, synthesis should be conceived of not merely as an emergence but as a simultaneous emerging and disappearing. Third, an anthropology of synthesis needs to pay attention not only to what is aligned in practice but also to what is actively excluded and suppressed.

I therefore suggest locating the operation of Pickering's mangle in spatiotemporally extended fields of practice (i.e., patterns of interconnected practices). The inclusion in and exclusion of agencies from practices structure fields of practice via patterns of connectivity that are continually emerging and disappearing. Which agencies are available for inclusion into given practices and which others must be excluded to guarantee the cohesion of distinct patterns of practice are functions of the nature of given fields. This differentiates the notion of a field of practice from naturalistic conceptions of "the world" in which some things are objectively given and others are mere figments of the mind, but also from perceptions of cultural practices as tied to specific social groups. A bacteria, a wind evil, or a physician of Chinese medicine exists only if connected (whether positively by inclusion or negatively by exclusion) to at least some other agent within a given field of practice. Agencies can continually be added to a field of practice by recruiting them from other fields. They can be marginalized within a field but also vanquished by physical extermination or the redefinition of field boundaries.

My definition implies that individual agencies within a given field are not necessarily all related to each other, nor is each single local interaction connected to the field as a whole. Fields of practice, in which agencies compete with each other for inclusion into given practices, can thus be conceived of as balancing on a dynamic center that need not correspond to a concrete or real center. This allows us to make global descriptions or analyses of the field—

that is, of networks, practices, institutions, and so on—without reducing local events to effects of global determinants, or vice versa. Evidence of such partial connections and dispersed agency will be found throughout my ethnography.[81] For the moment it is more important to appreciate the theoretical point that plurality is an intrinsic effect of this overdetermination of global fields by the local unfolding of focal agencies. Put another way, although a field of practice has a distinct shape and history—a shape and history that we can describe—it is not necessary to posit a single agency or practice that determines it or to which it could be reduced.

For the sake of clarity I shall from now on employ the term "infrastructures"—borrowed from the philosopher and literary critic Rodolphe Gasché—to refer collectively to the various elements that can be integrated into a given *synthesis* at any moment. Gasché defines synthesis with respect to infrastructures as involving "a complicity and complication that maintain together an undetermined number of possibilities, which need not necessarily be in relation of antithetical contrast with one another, as is the case in the classical concept of synthesis."[82] The term "infrastructures" thus retains the idea that social life is constructed and that this construction is intelligible without insisting that such intelligibility must be monistically biased.

Chinese medicine can now be conceived of as a field (even better, a number of fields) of emergence and disappearance of infrastructural syntheses, noting that all infrastructures as well as the larger field(s) of emergence and disappearance are also conceptualized as syntheses. Synthesis signifies process and product, event and result. On the outside syntheses appear stable, while on the inside they are always potentially falling apart, threatened by the intrinsic insecurity of infrastructural alignments. Syntheses can extend across analytical domains (accommodating both heterogeneity and multiplicity) by relating to each other various kinds of infrastructures: bodies (organic, inorganic, technological, social, institutional, political), selves (social, psychological), and signifiers (concepts, texts, signs). They can simultaneously reach back to the Yellow Lord and project themselves forward into the future as Chinese physicians proclaim self-confidently that "the twenty-first century will be the century of Chinese medicine."[83] Syntheses can link up physicians in Beijing trained in the 1930s, diagnostic tests from the United States, herbal medicines imported from Arabia since the Ming, and the newly emergent interests of multinational drug companies without the need to posit bounded systems or historical periods. Synthesis, finally, is a scalable process applicable to and connecting micro- and macrolevel events. As infrastructures syntheses make themselves available for participation in emergent syntheses on a higher scale, while as coherent patterns they impose constraints on the alignment of their own infrastructures.[84]

This vision of the mutual determination and structuring of infrastructures within wider fields of practice accommodates each of the three constitutional aspects of plurality—multiplicity, heterogeneity, and simultaneous emergence and disappearance—previously defined. It furthermore accords with the way many Chinese physicians think about their work—a work in which the synthesis (*zonghe* 综合) of tradition and modernity and the understanding of dynamic patterns developing through an unfolding of internal contradictions (*maodun* 矛盾) and their consequences constitute recurring reference points.[85] Plurality thus is both a reflection and a consequence of the multiple ways in which infrastructures at various levels of organization interact, determine, and constitute each other in the formation of syntheses. And because this interactive co-determination produces patterns that are always "just so," plurality as a reflection of infrastructural synthesis implies neither a relativist nor an antirealist position, nor does it privilege plurality or process above synthesis or structure.[86]

Before translating this model into a method for ethnographic research, I will show its ability to facilitate the thick description of local practice while at the same time integrating such description into a nonreductionist understanding of plurality. For this purpose I shall return once more to my case study of Dr. He.

Dr. He Acquires a New Needle Technique (II). My case study demonstrates in an immediately accessible manner that medical practices are not reflections of beliefs or knowledge alone. They are not determined by social structures, nor do they reflect distinct types of social agency. And they never exhaust themselves in the merely clinical or in narrow definitions of efficacy. Assumptions about the relationship between needle techniques, movements of *qi* in the body, and therapeutic results constitute only one input into Dr. He's style of practice. Dr. He adopts the new needle technique because he assumes that it is clinically useful (after all, Professor Xia is more famous than his previous teachers), but simultaneously because it is a tool in the construction of social relationships. Likewise, while Dr. He himself believes in theories of *qi*, many of his colleagues do not, although to most observers both groups will appear to practice acumoxa in the same way. Dr. He's assumptions regarding the efficacy of the two needle techniques between which he has to choose are furthermore determined by his current status vis-à-vis his teachers, their hierarchical rank in the Chinese medical teaching establishment, and his own future expectations for advancement within the system.

These various factors (in my terminology, infrastructures)—all of them syntheses in their own right—do not contribute to the synthesis of Dr. He's needle technique in an additive manner that could be represented in terms of a simple algorithm. Rather, the various infrastructures we observe influence and modify one another in the unfolding of a real-time process that can be made visible as a pattern. On one level, adopting a needle technique is a tool through which Dr. He constructs and maintains social relations. It is also a process whereby his own person and self are being formed: physically, through adaptations of bodily comportment; clinically, via a changed mode of interaction with his patients and their qi; socially, as he surrenders a relationship with one teacher in favor of establishing one with another. Dr. He affirms established moral codes by submitting to what he refers to as "traditional" models of filiality, yet he simultaneously undermines these codes as he manipulates them to his own advantage, a contradiction of which he was all too aware. In certain contexts, Dr. He could become extremely critical of the patriarchal system of values embodied in his relationship with Professor Xia. He compared it unfavorably with the less authoritarian and, in his perception, "Western"-style relationships between teachers and students in science departments of Chinese universities. Yet, Dr. He was also very proud to be the student of Professor Xia, whose authority he admired and hoped one day to emulate.

In the context of his relationship with me, Dr. He used the needle technique as a gift. Such gift giving is central to Chinese perceptions of self-definition, social status, and propriety.[87] By presenting me, a Westerner, with a gift from the treasure-house of Chinese medicine, Dr. He made me more Chinese in two ways at once: he turned me into a more accomplished practitioner of Chinese medicine and he inserted me into a distinct network of social relations. Yet, in doing so he also (and for the most part inadvertently) opened up his own self to change. In the course of constructing a relationship with me he was confronted with ideas and actions that were sometimes inspirational to him, yet at other times uncomfortable and even painful.

Something as basic as the holding, inserting, and twisting of a needle is thus revealed as a synthesis constituted by a multitude of heterogeneous infrastructures. Once in place, the needle technique itself becomes a polyphonous instrument that can be integrated into different kinds of actions operating at various levels of efficacy. Such integration requires many skills: skill in the rotation, lifting, and thrusting of acumoxa needles; skill in the shaping of bodily practice; and skill in the manipulation of social roles and moralities. Dr. He has a visible agency in the emergence of these syntheses, yet he is equally visibly shaped by them and is therefore himself continuously emerging. Neither can these various levels of efficacy be neatly separated from one another. An acumoxa needle is an instrument that can be manipulated in different ways, yet its materiality does not allow for just any kind of handling: it can bend or break and will fail to grasp the *qi* if not manipulated correctly.

Many Chinese, finally, believe that people—including physicians and their patients—are brought together by a kind of predestination (*yuan* 缘). We do not have to accept the metaphysics behind this belief for it to remind us of the connections, at once clinical and social, that via a needle technique link Dr. He's patients to him, to Professor Xia and his medical ancestors, and beyond to the entire infrastructure of Chinese medicine's past and present.

In terms of the model of synthesis previously outlined we find in this case study numerous examples of multiplicity and heterogeneity. Multiple possibilities of manipulating needles and of relating to one another exist and are connected in heterogeneous alignments traversing different fields of practice. Synthesis describes these as simultaneously emerging and disappearing connections between infrastructural agencies into distinctive patterns. Adopting one needle technique implies to Dr. He that another will be rejected. This other needle technique does not thereby disappear, however, from the field of practice of Chinese medicine. It is maintained in the context of other social relations but also exists within Dr. He as a bodily memory which he may resurrect in other contexts. As a mature practitioner he might want to experiment with different needle techniques, though how well his body remembers will be affected by what else it is and has been doing, and with what other infrastructures it is and has been aligned.

Choosing or conforming to one kind of social relation negates others. Dr. He has to adapt his subjectivity to forms of etiquette commonly found between teacher and student in Chinese medicine circles. He and his teacher are thereby aligned with one another in a distinctive pattern that structures social relations within their field of practice. Yet, Dr. He also seeks to modify this relationship by limiting its powers to specific contexts of instruction. In the triangulation between his teacher, himself, and the code of conduct according to which both parties relate, nothing is therefore predetermined. Professor Yang might come to find that his students respect him more if he adopts the less paternalistic stance of his colleagues at Western medical schools. Dr. He might adjust to older, Confucianist-inflected models of studentship and—as other students have informed me—find that he becomes a "better" because less selfish person in the process, for Confucianism values not only patriarchal authority but also benevolence. Or he might flexibly accommodate his agency to one kind of relation in one context and to another in a second.

With regard to the definition of the infrastructural field in which these syntheses take place, we can note that it is populated by tools (such as needles and instruments for electro-acupuncture), people (patients, physicians), and ideas (about *qi*, acumoxa, etiquette). We can see how the import of new tools or ideas (such as electro-acupuncture) changes the field and the connections between infrastructures within the field (wiring up a needle to a machine is a less personal skill than manipulating needles by hand and, by implication, more resistant to being recruited to the regulation of interpersonal relationships). We can also see how the field itself, on the other hand, is constituted by the syntheses that constitute it. Whether or not machines for electro-acupuncture persist in the field will depend not only on their clinical effects but also on their integration into or exclusion from the social relations in which acumoxa practice is daily (re-)produced.

Translations: From Anthropological Model to Ethnographic Practice

On the basis of ethnographic and historical evidence I have argued that social life must be accepted as irreducibly plural but that this plurality negates neither coherence or pattern nor meaningful analysis. In this view plurality is characterized by three interrelated features: heterogeneity, multiplicity, and synthesis. Heterogeneity and multiplicity are primarily descriptive concepts emphasizing the plural constitution of fields of practice. Synthesis is an analytical concept employed to capture the constitution of such fields as a process of simultaneous emergence and disappearance. Synthesis and syntheses can thus be qualified by four attributes.

1. *Locality:* Syntheses are by definition local, taking place at a particular place and a particular time. They can, however, connect infrastructures across conventional spatiotemporal boundaries such as geographical regions, political states, or historical periods.

2. *Connectivity:* Syntheses interconnect with one another into larger and smaller patterns. In this manner the global frames the local while the local simultaneously constitutes the global without one being reducible to the other. Global and local are thus defined along different scales of order rather than according to different qualities of existence.

3. *Agency:* Syntheses are simultaneously viewed as processes of interactive stabilization between interrelating infrastructures, both human and nonhuman, and as processes of inclusion and exclusion. The interaction between infrastructures in the process of synthesis can be captured via concepts such as accommodation, resistance, and struggle without implying the existence of invariable relations of domination or the dichotomies between local life-worlds and global (world) systems.[88]

4. *Topography and Topology:* Syntheses take place in and reciprocally create fields of practice. Fields of practice are envisaged as presentations of infrastructures currently included in or excluded from actual syntheses. Such inclusion/exclusion structures fields of practice via patterns of dynamic connectivity that can be observed and described.[89]

Given the vastness of the field that is contemporary Chinese medicine and the multitude of syntheses that take place in it, which of these are included and excluded from any given ethnography will be a subjective and political choice. The implications of this were discussed in chapter 1 and do not need reiteration here. Suffice it to say that a self-consciously interventionist ethnography such as the one presented in this book aims to engage with its topic in a manner that opens new vistas and facilitates new possibilities of action. George Marcus has shown that such an epistemological position emerges from (or, as in the present case, leads back to) a methodology that eschews the conventional anthropological focus on single fieldwork sites in favor of a more complex form of tracking through observation and participation at and within multiple research sites.[90]

I believe that in the present case this can best be achieved by focusing on the role of a small number of key infrastructures participating in the transformations of contemporary Chinese medicine: the state, patients, physicians, and Chinese medical knowledge. Each of the chapters in part 2 is centered on one or more of these infrastructures, exploring their input into contemporary

Chinese medical practice as well as their own transmutation in the process of the ensuing interactions. Methodologically, I have chosen a case study approach as the most suitable vehicle for this purpose. Case studies allow detailed descriptions but do not necessitate reductionism. They allow for the testing and explication of general models, yet do not verify them and thereby appear to manufacture truth. Case studies acquire meaning only in relation to specific theoretical models and thus will highlight reflectively the performative production of my own ethnography.

One last question: Will the translation of my case studies into the model of synthesis add anything new to conventional thick description in anthropology? If we define as the purpose of ethnography the tracing of subtle relations between infrastructures related to one another in the course of practice, perhaps not. Anthropology, however, also seeks to relate ethnography to general models of social life, and these models invariably influence what we pay attention to. In this respect, I do believe that my model directs us toward a less reductionist and more fluid understanding not merely of Chinese medicine but of medicine in society, and perhaps even further than that. Read together, the case studies will provide readers with a sense of Chinese medicine in contemporary China as a pattern that has no single shape and has not one but many histories but that is, nevertheless, real and intelligible. Disappearing as it emerges, this pattern tells us something about how health, illness, culture, medicine, and society constitute each other in a rapidly transforming China. If we pay close attention it also tells us something about ourselves.

PART II
CONTEMPORARY
CHINESE MEDICINE:
SIX PERSPECTIVES

3. HEGEMONIC PLURALISM
Chinese Medicine in a Socialist State

In the concluding section of chapter 2 I decided on a strategy of multisited ethnography as the most suitable methodology for analyzing plurality in contemporary Chinese medicine. I argued that this strategy allows the systematic examination of processes of emergence and disappearing and the patterns to which these processes give rise without the need for suitable master narratives (such as modernization) or deep structures (culture, practice, or system) to tie these patterns and processes together. In the present chapter I embark on this project by examining the involvement of the Chinese state in the transformations of Chinese medicine. I begin with a brief historical overview of the development of Chinese medicine since 1949.[1] The choice of this starting date is as sensible as it is arbitrary. After the establishment of the People's Republic, and particularly from 1954 onward when it won active support from the Chinese Communist Party (CCP), the development of Chinese medicine became inseparably intertwined with the establishment of the new China. Chinese medicine, previously practiced in private clinics and hospitals and transmitted through apprenticeships or private schools, was transformed into the "traditional Chinese medicine" (TCM) now taught in state-controlled institutions.

Many authors thus draw a line between Chinese medicine before and after 1949 or between Chinese medicine and TCM. On closer inspection it quickly becomes clear that the development of Chinese medicine in Maoist and post-Maoist China has been guided by a plurality of different and sometimes contradictory political imperatives. Nationalism, Maoism, the valorization of science and technology, market economics, the desire to project to the outside an image of China as a country with a profound and unbroken cultural heritage—yet also, conversely, a deeply felt pressure to emulate Western models of rationality—and many other factors have shaped this development.

It would therefore be difficult to single out one influence that dominated this period. Likewise, in spite of many ostensible differences, in many respects the transformation of Chinese medicine in Maoist and post-Maoist China merely continues various and by no means homogeneous processes of transformation initiated during the Republican period, which in turn were facilitated by earlier transformations during the late imperial era. Many physicians actively involved in the National Medicine (*guoyi* 国医) movement of the 1920s and 1930s, for instance, became key players in the shaping of Chinese medicine after 1954. And many of the ideological cornerstones of modern TCM—such as the resonance between dialectical materialism and the natural philosophy of the Chinese medical classics or the scientization and systematization of Chinese medicine—have a history that long predates Mao.[2]

Hence, our decision to focus on continuities or ruptures, on what stays the same or on what changes, is influenced by our position and what we want to explain as much as by what actually happened. Narrowing this introduction to the history of Chinese medicine after 1949 does not imply that I see this date as a watershed. Some things changed after 1949 because the state redefined (several times, in fact) the function of Chinese medicine within its larger project of social transformation. Some things changed because they were already changing. And many things, lest we forget, remained the same. Presenting a short and by no means comprehensive overview of the development of Chinese medicine after 1949 allows me, however, to keep my narrative brief and still to argue one essential point: that the role of the state in shaping contemporary Chinese medicine is that of a powerful, but not all-powerful, agent. While the state decisively frames the ongoing transformation of Chinese medicine, it by no means controls it, and the state itself, therefore, is also reshaped in its engagement with Chinese medicine.

For the sake of convenience I have divided the period under discussion into three sections: (1) the period from 1949 to 1965, which corresponds to the formal institutionalization of Chinese medicine; (2) the period of the Cultural Revolution from 1966 to 1976; and (3) the post-Maoist period from 1977 to the present. This tripartite division is conventionally employed by modern Chinese authors and politicians.[3] In oral discourse my informants also tended toward this division. I have therefore adopted it throughout this and subsequent chapters, even if it does not match the sophistication of historically more detailed analyses.[4]

During the first half of the twentieth century the debates between proponents of Chinese medicine and Western medicine gradually turned into open
confrontation. In the ensuing exchange of polemics Chinese medicine came
under increasing attack from modernizers of every political persuasion, including prominent CCP scholars such as Guo Moruo 郭沫若 and even Mao Zedong himself, for being outdated and unscientific.[5] To counteract such threats
Chinese medicine physicians responded by creating a tactically useful association between their medicine and a presumed national essence. Simultaneously, they also began to modernize their tradition by importing Western
models of teaching, organization, and practice. These strategies proved successful in defeating a law proposed in 1929 by Western medicine physicians
and their allies within the Guomindang government to outlaw Chinese medicine outright. They did not, however, manage to significantly alter the balance of power within the domain of the state between the two medicines or
the association prevalent among large sections of the elite between Chinese
medicine and the old China. During the last years of the Republican period
most schools and colleges of Chinese medicine were closed. In spite of its
continued popularity among the populace Chinese medicine clearly lacked
political power. If there was any future for it at all, it lay in a fundamental
transformation by means of Western science and technology.[6]

Following the establishment of the new China in 1949, state support
for Chinese medicine emerged gradually in a series of stages. As Taylor has
shown, this emergence was "the product of an undetermined and piecemeal
process" that owed more to "a careful manipulation of [Chinese medicine's]
value as a 'cultural legacy'" than to "any consideration of its actual therapeutic value."[7]

During the time of the Civil War (1945–49) CCP policy regarding Chinese
medicine had been guided by encouraging the "cooperation of Chinese and
Western medicine" (zhongxiyi hezuo 中西医合作). This strategy reflected a
pragmatic utilization of medical resources in the context of revolutionary activity based predominantly in the countryside but still influenced by Soviet
(i.e., metropolitan) ideologies and models of modernization.[8] Once in power,
CCP policy makers undertook a critical appraisal of available resources in the
health care sector. On the basis of this review "four great guiding principles"
(si da fangzhen 四大方针) of health care policy were formulated and implemented following the First and Second National Health Conferences in 1950
and 1951. These principles can be summarized as follows: (1) medicine had to

serve the working people; (2) preventive medicine programs were to be given priority over curative ones; (3) Chinese medicine was to be united with Western medicine; and (4) health programs were to be integrated with mass movements.[9]

Implementation of policy in the health sector was the joint responsibility of the Ministry of Health (MOH, Weishengbu 卫生部) and the Chinese Communist Party, whose bureaucratic organizations paralleled each other. Broadly speaking, while the MOH, dominated by biomedical physicians, favored modernization following Western models of professional health care, the CCP under the leadership of Mao Zedong, for political as well as ideological reasons, favored preventive care, mass campaigns, and the subservience of professional knowledge to revolutionary goals.

Regarding the relation between Chinese and Western medicine the four principles of health care policy noted above are significant in two respects. First, the development of medical knowledge and practice was, initially in principle but increasingly also in practice, taken out of the hands of physicians and made subservient to political aspirations. Second, cooperation between Chinese and Western medicine was replaced by the goal of creating a single "new medicine" (xinyi 新医) that would embody the unique spirit of the Chinese revolution. Under the slogan "unify Chinese and Western medicine" (zhongxiyi tuanjie 中西医团结) this vision guided policy roughly until 1956, albeit from two distinctly different directions. These emerged from complex power struggles among political factions in the CCP and the MOH but also through a process of "learning from experience" by Mao Zedong and other politicians.[10]

Initially, modernizers within the MOH aligned to Western medicine succeeded in imposing their views on the intended unification. Communist policy regarding Chinese medicine during the early 1950s thus accorded Chinese medicine an inferior place within government policy but did not significantly alter the political desire to do away with it altogether at the earliest possible moment. In the words of Crozier, early MOH policies meant nothing other than "the road to oblivion for Chinese medicine."[11] In my opinion, therefore, this period is one of transition marked by continuity with the policies of the Guomindang government, which had systematically kept Chinese medicine out of state health care. One pertinent example is the fact that Yu Yunxiu 余云岫 (1879–1954), notorious for having proposed the law forbidding the practice of Chinese medicine in 1929, was invited to the First National Health Conference in Beijing in 1950 and apparently maintained considerable influence over leading MOH bureaucrats at the time.[12]

Like many other prominent modernizers and reformers, Yu Yunxiu had studied Western medicine in Japan. He had been influenced by Japanese models of modernization and Darwinist ideas of social evolution prevalent in both China and Japan at the time, which accorded health care and hygiene an important position in national self-strengthening. Yu's opposition to Chinese medicine, perceived as an emblem as well as a cause of China's inferior position vis-à-vis the West, thus was nationalist in origin and motivation. Yu's ideas of "medical revolution" (*yixue geming* 医学革命) and his perception of Chinese medicine as effective only in "consoling the spirit" (*jingshenshang zhi weijiede* 精神上之慰藉的) resonated with MOH designations of Chinese medicine. During the early 1950s Chinese medicine was viewed as a "feudal society's feudal medicine" (*fengjian shehui fengjian yi* 封建社会封建医) that, like other aspects of the old society, needed to be transformed through strict controls on medical practice and reeducation of its practitioners. It was deemed "not too late to train large numbers of new physicians possessing both adequate levels of scientific training and experience as replacements" (*shang laibuji peiyang dapi you kexue shuiping yu jingyan de xin yisheng qu zhihuan* 尚来不及培养大批有科学水平与经验的新医生去制换).[13]

Accordingly, licensing of Chinese medicine practitioners was introduced in 1952 by way of state-controlled examinations. These required extensive knowledge of Western medicine, and many Chinese medicine physicians who lacked such knowledge lost their entitlement to practice. Simultaneously, starting in 1951, Chinese medicine improvement schools (*zhongyi jinxiu xuexiao* 中医进修学校) were established throughout the country, and even older and well established physicians were required to attend. Twenty of these institutions had been set up by 1955 teaching a total of 143 classes.[14] These schools were intended to raise levels of theoretical and practical knowledge (particularly that of Western medicine) among physicians of Chinese medicine as well as to inculcate ideologically correct thinking.

In addition, a number of young but already established physicians were selected on the basis of competitive examinations to study Western medicine for five years.[15] It is important to note that the intended unification of Chinese and Western medicine at this time already had political as well as clinical functions inasmuch as Western medicine was thought of as a tool by means of which perceived ideological shortcomings of Chinese medicine, in particular its plurality, could be remedied. Mao Zedong, for instance, stated during a meeting of the CCP Central Committee in 1953 that in the course of uniting the two medicines "Western medicine definitely must smash the sectarianism [of Chinese medicine]" (*xiyi yiding yao dapo zongpaizhuyi* 西医一定要打

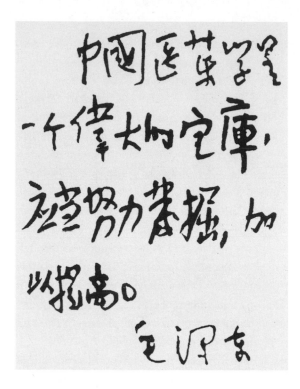

FIGURE 8. Calligraphy by Mao Zedong: "Chinese medicine is a great treasure-house and should be diligently explored and improved upon" (1958)

破宗派主义). Inasmuch as the Chinese medicine improvement schools played a key role in preparing the way for the establishment of new orthodoxies in Chinese medicine, this estimation may be perceived as a correct judgment (see chapter 7).[16]

The direction of the initial phase of bringing about a new medicine through "Chinese medicine studying Western medicine" (*zhongyi xuexi xiyi* 中医学习西医) was suddenly reversed in late 1953. The policy reversal culminated in a succession of official pronouncements regarding the value of Chinese medicine throughout the following year. Following severe criticism of the MOH's policy toward Chinese medicine by Mao Zedong himself, two ministers of health were forced to resign. The reasons for the change are not entirely clear but definitely included the following (not necessarily in order of importance): attempts toward greater utilization of all possible resources in health care in a country where everything was in short supply; efforts to avoid excessive dependency on imported technology and drugs; increased efforts to control and rectify "the undesirable ideological tendencies of the Western-trained doctors" by counterbalancing these with a profession more easily dominated precisely because its dependence on tradition made it vulnerable in a society in the grip of modernization; Mao Zedong's personal concern for social stability (*shehui anding* 社会安定); and, finally, an increasing sense of national pride that wanted to creatively inherit some aspects of the old culture and that perceived of China as capable of making a unique contribution to the world.[17]

Indeed, by September 1954 Liu Shaoqi 刘少奇 went as far as pronouncing that "despising Chinese medicine is servile and subservient bourgeois thinking" (*kanbuqi zhongyi shi nuyan bixi nucaishi de zichanjieji sixiang* 看不起中医是奴颜婢膝奴才式的资产阶级思想).[18] As a consequence, Chinese medicine was increasingly accorded value in its own right. It was accepted into the national insurance scheme, and in October 1954 the Culture Department of the CCP Central Committee made recommendations regarding the improvement and strengthening of Chinese medicine that included the establishment of the Academy of Chinese Medicine (Zhongyi yanjiuyuan 中医研究院), the integration of Chinese medicine into the larger hospitals, as well as a general expansion of the scope of Chinese medical work.

Overall, however, this reevaluation of Chinese medicine was still guided by the larger goal of creating a new society and a new medicine. Noting that the experience of the preceding years demonstrated that the assumptions underlying current policies had been mistaken, Mao Zedong merely changed track and reversed the roles of student and teacher. From now on, Western medicine physicians would study Chinese medicine. These physicians, who through their studies and commitment would "abolish the boundaries between Chinese and Western medicine" (*jiu keyi ba zhongxiyi jiexian quxiao* 就可以把中西医界限取消), would form the spearhead of the new medicine.[19] As Taylor shows, Mao Zedong's goal at this stage clearly was not to ensure the independent survival of Chinese medicine as a stand-alone tradition. Rather he was trying to subordinate Western to Chinese medicine in an attempt to break existing patterns of behavior within certain institutions. The purpose was "to force doctors from the two traditions to work together in order to create, eventually, a medicine of China capable of serving as a world medicine."[20]

At Mao's specific behest young doctors of Western medicine from all over the country were summoned to Beijing in 1955 to be reeducated in the first experimental class of Western medicine doctors studying Chinese medicine (*diyijie xiyi xuexi zhongyi yanjiuban* 第一届西医学习中医研究班). Many of these young physicians, who shared with other intellectuals a perception of Chinese medicine as old and backward, were none too pleased about this invitation.[21] Later, however, the considerable status associated with this class allowed many of its graduates to advance into influential positions within the Chinese medical sector. A number of well-known Chinese medical practitioners, including Qin Bowei 秦伯未 and Zhang Cigong 章次公 from Shanghai, Pu Fuzhou 蒲辅周 and Du Zeming 杜自明 from Sichuan, Huang Zhuzhai 黄竹斋 from Shanxi, and Yue Meizhong 岳美中 from Hebei, were likewise called to Beijing as teachers and advisers to the MOH. The resulting concentration of senior practitioners in Beijing facilitated not only the establishment there of the Academy of Chinese Medicine in 1955, but also located these physicians, many of whom played a significant role in the subsequent transformations of Chinese medicine, much closer to China's political center of power.[22]

Soon, classes for Western medicine doctors studying Chinese medicine of various duration and quality had been established throughout China. Chinese medicine courses were integrated into the curriculum of Western medicine universities, colleges, and schools. By 1960 thirty-seven full-time courses had trained more than twenty-three hundred physicians, while an additional thirty-six thousand practicing Western medical doctors had received training in Chinese medicine.[23] Physicians of Chinese medicine were also admitted to existing Western medicine hospitals and clinics, and hospitals of Chinese medicine were founded. This strengthening of Chinese medicine's role within the health care sector was reflected in a new alignment between Western medicine and Chinese medicine. As a slogan used at the time proclaimed, "Chinese medicine must become scientific, Western medicine must become Chinese" (zhongyi yao kexuehua, xiyi yao zhongguohua 中医要科学化, 西医要中国化).[24]

"Integration of Chinese and Western medicine" (zhongxiyi jiehe 中西医结合), a concept initially developed by Mao Zedong in 1956 to describe the second attempt at creating a new medicine in China, was the new slogan that guided this policy from the mid-1950s onward. Unification of the two medicines remained the ultimate goal, but it was accepted that this would take longer than previously estimated. This new policy allowed Chinese medicine physicians to gradually reassert a certain degree of autonomy for their tradition. Taylor argues that this development was enabled by a coincidence of several interrelated events during 1955 and 1956. First, Mao Zedong's authority was threatened by a prolonged period of ill health. He therefore used Chinese medicine as a convenient tool to test the loyalty of leading party members. Mao's bad health also meant that overall responsibility for the development of Chinese medicine came under the direction of other CCP Central Committee members, in particular Zhou Enlai and Liu Shaoqi. Unlike Mao Zedong, both Zhou and Liu appear to have been much more favorably inclined toward the survival of Chinese medicine as an independent medical tradition.[25]

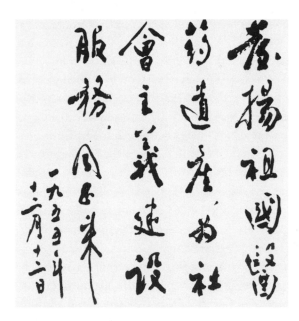

FIGURE 9. Calligraphy by Zhou Enlai celebrating the foundation of the Academy of Chinese Medicine: "Developing the roadbed of our fatherland's medicine serves the construction of socialism" (1955)

This newly asserted autonomy received a major boost in 1956 with the foundation of Chinese medicine colleges (*zhongyi xueyuan* 中医学院) in Chengdu, Beijing, Guangzhou, and Shanghai. By 1966 seventeen additional colleges had been set up in major municipalities and provinces.[26] Rather than reeducating practicing physicians as the old improvement schools had done, these colleges began training young people to become physicians of Chinese medicine. Initially, the teaching followed models established during the Nationalist period by physicians such as Ding Ganren 丁甘仁 (1865–1926) in Shanghai and Shi Jinmo 施今墨 (1881–1969) in Beijing, whose students and disciples became teachers and administrators in the new colleges.[27]

Students of the first courses taught at the Chinese medicine colleges still studied through reading and memorizing classical texts and following their teachers in the clinic. Such teaching methods, however, suited neither the needs of modern students nor the imperatives of their political masters. Unlike the scholar-physicians of previous times, the young recruits for the Chinese medicine colleges, and even more so the Western doctors who were studying Chinese medicine, did not possess the intellectual skill and patience necessary to work with medical books written in classical Chinese. Nor were these texts, with their many apparent contradictions, suited to facilitate the emergence of a single new medical paradigm. The development of teaching materials that aided the modernization (*xiandaihua* 现代化) and scientization (*kexuehua* 科学化) of Chinese medicine and sorted out the factionalism between contending traditions thus became an urgent political and practical need.

Various teaching materials had been compiled at the Chinese medicine improvement schools, often in cooperation between teachers and students, but the writing of the first national textbook, titled *Zhongyixue gailun* 中医学概论 (*Outline of Chinese Medicine*), was begun only in 1956 under the direct supervision of the MOH. Intended as a manual for Western medicine doctors studying Chinese medicine, the *Outline* was finally published in the autumn of 1958. This text presented classical sources only in excerpts and succeeded in pressing Chinese medicine into a more-or-less coherent system. Though quickly superseded by new and more specialized textbooks, the *Outline* has nevertheless been the model for later textbooks—and therefore in an important sense for Chinese medicine itself—ever since.[28]

From 1956 to 1960 advanced classes on special topics were established by teaching staff at various Chinese medicine colleges: on the *Neijing* in Beijing, on the *Shanghan lun* in Chengdu, on warm [pathogen] disorders and acumoxa in Nanjing. These classes began to define the content of the most important subjects (*men* 门) in the Chinese medicine curriculum in a systematic manner and to train a core of college teachers in them.[29] As I shall show in chapter 7, the resulting transformation of Chinese medicine reflected the pressure applied both from above (i.e., Maoist ideology and state-enforced modernization) and from below (the clinical and intellectual concerns of physicians of Chinese medicine).

Many of my informants participated in this transformation of Chinese medicine during the late 1950s and early 1960s. Their reminiscences speak of a period filled with the excitement of a new beginning accompanied by unprecedented cooperation within Chinese medicine circles, but also by chaos and uncertainty, personal struggle, and continued allegiances to older forms of personal relationships and local networks. In the summer of 1956, for instance, the Beijing College of Chinese Medicine, which was to begin teaching undergraduates on 1 September, had a provisional building only, no proper administration, and only two teachers. When the college opened, students complained vociferously about the conditions. In fact, it was only thanks to the personal intervention of Prime Minister Zhou Enlai that the entire project was not abandoned and the school moved to Nanjing. Instead, however, teachers were recruited from Nanjing through the help of Lü Bingkui 吕炳奎, who had helped to set up the Jiangsu Province Chinese Medicine Teachers Improvement School (Jiangsusheng zhongyi shizi jinxiu xuexiao 江苏省中医师

资进修学校) during the early 1950s. The young physicians who came to Beijing as a result made up the bulk of Beijing's most famous Chinese medicine academics and clinicians during the last quarter of the twentieth century.[30]

Despite the increasing political support Chinese medicine received during the period from 1954 to 1966, it continued to face opposition from the Western medical establishment and its allies. The number of Western medicine doctors studying Chinese medicine gradually declined, with the last full-time students enrolling at Shanghai in 1960. Following the disastrous Great Leap Forward and the resulting decline of Mao Zedong's influence, government policy shifted toward research and development in all spheres of production. Pressure was exerted on Chinese medicine to accelerate the process of its scientization and modernization. Politicians and bureaucrats inclined toward Western medicine once again asserted their dominance within the MOH, and Western medicine physicians who had studied Chinese medicine were placed in leading positions within the Chinese medical sector. By 1965 Minister of Health Qian Xinzhong could declare that the political misperceptions of the 1950s had been corrected. Chinese medicine was, he admitted, an essential aspect of the health care system. But he left no doubt about the need for its ultimate integration with Western medicine.

Thus, even though the position of Chinese medicine improved markedly during the 1950s, parts of the Chinese medical elite were quite aware of the dangers implicit in surrendering control over education, research, and medical practice to the state. Using the graduation of the first class of students from the new colleges of Chinese medicine as an opportunity to influence the future development of the profession, five of the most prominent scholar-physicians in Beijing—Qin Bowei 秦伯未, Ren Yingqiu 任应秋, Li Chongren 李重人, Chen Shenwu 陈慎吾, and Yu Daoji 于道济—sent a letter of protest to the MOH on 16 July 1962. In it they noted that modernization of teaching at the colleges threatened the continuity of Chinese medicine as a living tradition. They suggested raising educational standards by placing greater emphasis on the study of classical texts and reintroducing classical methods of learning.[31] This led to a revision of Chinese medical education following an MOH-sponsored conference in Beijing in September 1962. The Chinese medicine content of the curriculum was increased, though the overall policy did not change. Newly produced textbooks rather than classical texts increasingly became the foundation of all classroom teaching.[32]

Struggles between varying factions within the field of Chinese medicine were brought to a dramatic halt in 1965 when Mao Zedong criticized the MOH

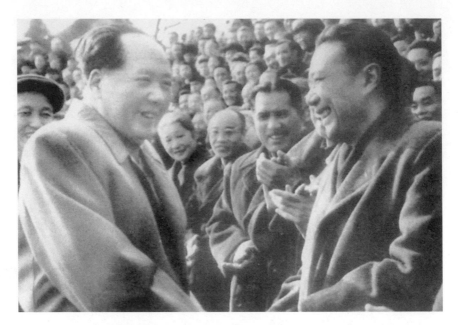

FIGURE 10. Mao Zedong shaking hands with Lu Zhihou, the first director of the Academy of Chinese Medicine, Beijing, 1956

for favoring health care in urban areas. He demanded radical change based on programs of mass action. The Cultural Revolution in the health sector had begun.

1966–1976: Ten Lost Years

The years of the Cultural Revolution are today referred to within Chinese medicine circles as "the ten years of going backward" (*daotui de shi nian* 倒退的十年).[33] Recollections about these years expressed in both official and private discourse emphasize a general sense of loss. In fact, Chinese medicine suffered institutionally and personally throughout this period on a scale far exceeding that of the Western medicine sector. As we shall see, however, some people and Chinese medicine in general also benefited from the upheavals of the time.

During the Cultural Revolution the full-scale integration of Chinese medicine and Western medicine into a "new medicine" became—for the second time in just over a decade—the politically correct way to develop medicine. Great efforts were made to integrate native pharmaceuticals and treatment methods such as acupuncture with basic Western medical science and to as-

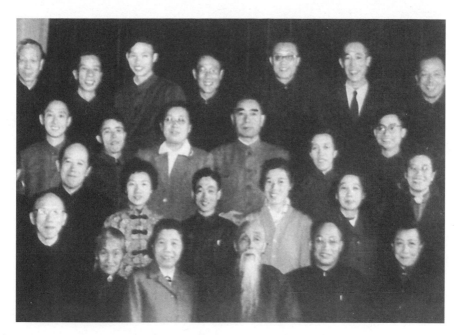

FIGURE 11. Zhou Enlai with famous *laozhongyi* Pu Fuzhou and others
at the Academy of Chinese Medicine, Beijing, 1961

similate these into the therapeutic repertoire of the new "barefoot doctors"
(*chijiao yisheng* 赤脚医生) and "half peasants–half physicians" (*ban nong ban
yi* 半农半医). Other aspects of Chinese medicine, however, were openly criticized. These included, on the one hand, its adoption of Western ideas of professional modernization during the previous decade, and, on the other, its attachment to "feudal" (*fengjian* 封建) and "superstitious" (*mixin* 迷信) theories.
Slogans such as "learning through experience" within an ethos of "mutual
study" (*xuexi huzhu* 学习互助), "mutual help" (*huzhu hezuo* 互助合作), and
"serving the people" (*wei renmin fuwu* 为人民服务) guided the establishment
of a medicine that in Mao Zedong's eyes attempted to meet the true needs
of the people. Research was still to be carried out, but it was to be based on
repeated practice rather than scientific protocol.[34]

As a consequence, formal education in the Chinese medicine colleges
ceased. The Academy of Chinese Medicine was closed. Publication of medical
journals was suspended, equipment disused. Medical infrastructure in general deteriorated, the Chinese medicine sector losing more than 30 percent
of its manpower. These losses must be considered especially serious in the
light of the large increases in the Western medical sector throughout the same
period. A survey commissioned by the MOH in 1978 established that between

TABLE 1. Number of Health Personnel in Health Institutions (in 10,000 persons), 1949–1996

	1949	1957	1965	1975	1980	1989	1990	1996
Total personnel	54.12	125.44	187.23	259.35	353.47	478.70	490.62	541.90
Doctors of Chinese medicine	27.60	33.70	32.14	22.86	26.22	36.95	36.85	34.78
Doctors of Western medicine	8.74	20.93	44.14	64.91	89.11	134.32	138.97	158.27
Senior doctors	3.80	7.36	18.87	29.30	44.73	102.25	105.85	120.73
Assistant doctors	4.94	13.57	25.27	35.61	44.38	32.07	33.12	37.54

Source: Chen Minzhang (1997: 294–95)

1959 and 1977 the number of people employed in the Chinese medical sector declined by one-third, from 361,000 to 240,000, while in the Western medical sector it almost quadrupled from 234,000 in 1959 to 738,000 in 1977 (see table 1).[35]

As Chinese medicine was no longer accorded any value in its own right, the Chinese Medicine Bureau at the MOH was absorbed into the new Office for Integrated Chinese and Western Medicine. Rural China in particular became the site where the new integrated medicine was implemented in practice within the wider context of cooperative health care (*hezuo yiliao* 合作医疗). Young and middle-aged doctors were sent to the countryside from town and city hospitals. Many venerated older physicians (*laozhongyi*) were dismissed from their jobs. Others were integrated into revolutionary health care as sources of empirical knowledge, even if the classical roots of this knowledge were now despised. A new brand of barefoot doctors was recruited from predominantly male youths of "good" political background and educated in intensive practice-oriented training courses lasting six to eight weeks.

The search for new treatment methods facilitated by revolutionary zeal and a genuine ethos of mutual assistance and help led to a general opening up, in the long term, of the borders that had hitherto defined Chinese medicine. Folk remedies were incorporated into the materia medica, and new acupuncture points and treatment techniques were discovered. Some of these achievements, such as the publication of the *Encyclopedic Dictionary of Chinese Pharmacology* (*Zhongyao dacidian* 中药大辞典) in 1977, have had a lasting impact on the practice of Chinese medicine.[36] Just as many widely proclaimed medical breakthroughs, however, were quickly discarded; revolutionary zeal all too often "passed off fish eyes for pearls" (*yumu hun zhu* 鱼目昏珠). Thus, on the one hand, the widespread repopularization of Chinese medicine, albeit in simplified form, may have ultimately contributed to saving it from becoming a treasured but practically redundant academic museum piece. On the other hand, the dissociation of medical practice from classical learning further accelerated the disintegration of older styles of therapeutic practice that had already been set in motion through the reforms of the previous decade.

As part of the general struggle against the "four olds" (old ideas, old culture, old customs, old habits), renowned physicians and leading cadres were branded "forces of evil" (niugui sheshen 牛鬼蛇神, lit. "bovine demons and snake goblins"), subjected to public abuse, and even physically attacked—sometimes by their students and even by their own children. Several famous physicians died as a result, other were banished to out-of-the-way provinces. Private practices and pharmacies were destroyed. The possession of classical texts found during house searches by Red Brigades constituted a reactionary offense, and classical medical texts were burned in public bonfires. In Beijing, victims of Red Guard fanaticism included Lü Bingkui and the "five elders who had made an official protest" (wu lao shang shu 五老上书) that is, the physicians who in their letter to the MOH had emphasized the importance of tradition in Chinese medical education. In many cases of prosecution the precise causes are difficult to establish. Ideological fervor, the settling of old scores, professional jealousies, and attempts to forestall more serious attacks on a person cherished or admired by means of preventive violence all played a part.

Data from Wujin County in Jiangsu provide a small snapshot of the destructive influence of this period on the lives of well-known members of the Chinese medical community. Of 156 physicians sent down to the countryside or victimized whose records were examined in 1978, more than 20 died of illness during this time and 5 died from the results of actual physical attacks. Of the remainder, 41 had to be retired due to incapacity to carry out their previous work duties, and 90 physicians were assigned to new positions on returning to their hospitals. Altogether the county employed 266 Chinese medicine physicians at the end of 1978 compared with 453 at the beginning of 1966, a decrease of more than 40 percent.[37]

The personal evaluation of this period by my informants, who were unanimous in their general condemnation, differed according to their individual experiences and outlook. Medical service in the countryside was despised by many for involving both physical labor and intimate contact with "dirty" and "backward" peasants. Up to the present day there remains much resentment about destroyed careers and opportunities. As we shall see in more detail later, one of the casualties of those years may have been a sense of trust and community within the emerging Chinese medical profession. Should one expect teachers with bitter memories of persecution by a previous generation of students to pass on the personal knowledge they worked so hard to acquire? And why should colleagues ever again trust and share information with one another, even if rules of scientific conduct require it?[38]

Some adapted better than others. For Dr. Yu, a consultant at a large Beijing hospital, the Cultural Revolution had at least one good aspect. As a young graduate with the wrong class background he had volunteered for service in the countryside. There he had found himself in great demand by villagers who quickly seized the opportunity of having access to an "educated" Chinese medicine physician. Dr. Yu recounted months of seeing patients from 5:00 A.M. to 11:00 P.M., treating many serious diseases which otherwise he might never have seen. Under pressure to produce results (and here he made a gesture of a throat being slit), he felt that this period had proved invaluable in raising his clinical skills. According to Dr. Yu (and many other older physicians with whom I spoke) young doctors nowadays see too few patients and have secure jobs where it does not matter whether patients get better or not. No wonder, he said, most turn out to be mediocre practitioners.

Professor Long, also with the wrong family background, was sent to an isolated province where he had much time to read and to acquaint himself with the medical traditions of local people. Of all the physicians I met in Beijing twenty-five years after the Cultural Revolution, he was not only one of the most erudite but also the one most open to other medical traditions. Yet, he was also deeply wounded and offended by the hardship his previously venerated teachers had been forced to endure and by the realization that, in some cases, his own classmates had had a hand in this.

Professor Xia, a graduate of the first class of the Beijing College of Chinese Medicine (*Beijing zhongyi xueyuan* 北京中医学院), did not have a single good thing to say of the time. She hated every day she had to work in the country because of the primitive living conditions. She regretted the loss of time, which according to her could have been spent much more usefully in postgraduate studies. She detested the violence and what physicians did to each other. And she bemoaned the resultant loss of trust within the profession.

Dr. Dong, who had been a teacher before 1966, used the upheavals of the Cultural Revolution to effect a change in career not otherwise possible in a planned economy. Interested in classical culture and Chinese medicine since his youth, he trained as a barefoot doctor and was soon running a successful rural practice. When the colleges reopened he managed to enroll for a postgraduate degree and is now working as a physician of Chinese medicine in the West. Outside of the Beijing elite there are today many physicians like Dr. Dong for whom the "ten lost years" opened up the possibility of an entirely new and different life. Within the state system, however, such physicians often remain disadvantaged. Although often they are excellent physicians, they fail to achieve positions of power due to their lack of official educational qualifications.

One such physician is Dr. Li, the heir of a long-established medical line who was educated as an apprentice of his father. The family medicine shop and practice, however, were destroyed during the Cultural Revolution. Dr. Li later managed to obtain a position within the state health care system and is now working within the Chinese medicine department of one of the smaller Beijing hospitals. Although he is well known and respected as a practitioner, he has never advanced beyond the position of assistant consultant (*fuzhuren* 副主任) and has to work under a physician younger in years and inferior in expertise.

1977 to the Present: The Establishment of Plural Health Care

With the fall of the "Gang of Four" in 1976 and the return to power of Deng Xiaoping, health care policies underwent yet another transformation. The "four modernizations" in agriculture, industry, science and technology, and national defense first proposed by Prime Minister Zhou Enlai now became the pillars of official discourse. Creating "socialism with Chinese characteristics" implied that Chinese classical culture could once more be valorized— though this time in order to effect a transition modeled on Western market economics.[39] The contours of post-1979 reforms in the health sector reflected these ideological reevaluations and tensions. They can be summarized by four new policies: (1) emphasis was to be placed on hospital-based services rather than primary or community care, thus reversing the priorities of previous policies; (2) moves toward the reprofessionalization of medicine were initiated, implying that specialist knowledge was to be valued above that of political cadres; (3) development was to be based on technology, including technology transfer from developed countries, in terms of both tools and personnel; and (4) a plural health care system was to be established.[40]

The acceptance of a fundamental plurality in health care emerged incrementally in a series of MOH meetings and conferences during the late 1970s and early 1980s. Once more, Lü Bingkui, who had been rehabilitated in 1977, played a pivotal role in the formulation of these policies. In a series of articles and speeches, Lü, on whom friends have bestowed honorary titles such as "the man who laid the foundation for Chinese medicine profession in the new China," argued for the restoration of Chinese medicine's infrastructure, which had been decimated during the Cultural Revolution. In doing so he set Chinese medicine apart from both Western medicine and the integrated Chinese and Western medicine that had been given priority during the Cultural Revolution.

In 1980 the MOH published a paper in which it confirmed Chinese medicine's independence while encouraging its modernization through the application of science and technology. In April 1982, after Lü's intervention, an MOH-sponsored conference convened in Hengyang, Hunan Province, established that Chinese medicine institutions should preserve and promote the independent character of Chinese medicine. Western medicine classes required at Chinese medicine colleges should not exceed five hundred hours. At a later conference at Shijazhuang, Hebei Province, in December 1982, it was decided that Chinese medicine, Western medicine, and integrated Chinese and Western medicine should have equal status and that work toward integrating Chinese and Western medicine should start from within Chinese medicine. Finally, a third conference in Xi'an in November 1983 determined that in all of its various aspects—clinical practice, teaching, and research—Chinese medicine was to be developed according to its own internal foundations and principles.

The "three paths" (san daolu 三道路) policy that guided these conferences is aptly summarized in a slogan formulated by Lü Bingkui following the Eleventh National Health Conference in 1979 but used by the MOH for the first time in 1980.[41] "Chinese medicine, Western medicine, and integrated Chinese and Western medicine constitute three great powers which all need to be developed and which will coexist for a long time" (Zhongyi, xiyi, zhong-xiyi jiehe sanzhi liliang dou yao fazhan changqi bingcun 中医, 西医, 中西医结合三支力量都要发展, 长期并存).[42] In the 1991 review of economic and social development for the next decade, "paying equal attention to Chinese and Western medicine" (zhongxiyi bingzhong 中西医并重) was once more affirmed to be one of the "great guiding principles" (da fangzhen 大方针) of health care policy.[43] Thus, after almost a century of struggle, physicians of Chinese medicine finally appear to have succeeded in carving out a secure and independent position in China's official health care sector. Western medicine and its supporters could not manage to ban Chinese medicine outright, and death by stealth—through the generation of a "unified" or "integrated" Chinese and Western medicine—was also averted.

What precisely is denoted by "Chinese medicine" and "integrated Chinese and Western medicine" and what distinguishes the two remains unclear, however. In Mao Zedong's initial formulation the latter referred to the goal of unifying Chinese and Western medicine. The same ideology also motivated the many attempts at integration carried out during the Cultural Revolution. Whether Chinese medicine was ever considered an equal partner to Western medicine in this process remains a disputed issue. Lü Bingkui and his supporters certainly did not think so, hence their demand for an independent Chinese medicine sector. American anthropologist Sidney White, on the other hand, interprets the practice of integrated medicine that emerged after the Cultural Revolution as a complex hybrid in which Chinese medical discourses occupied a by no means subordinate position. Western medicine, for instance, was incorporated by local practitioners in the Lijiang basin of Yunnan Province into various Chinese therapeutic discourses: both those derived from officially sanctioned transformations of Chinese medicine and those derived from the legacy of unofficial demonic medicine.[44]

Today, the term "integrated Chinese and Western medicine" appears to have at least four different meanings. In the widest possible sense it refers to the uptake of Western medical concepts and technologies by practitioners of Chinese medicine. In that sense almost all Chinese medicine is "integrated Chinese and Western medicine" these days. In a second sense, it refers to the conscious goal of developing Chinese medicine by importing Western medicine with the implication of creating a "new" medicine as a result. The third sense refers to the use of Western medical drugs and treatments by physicians of Chinese medicine, and Western medicine physicians' use of Chinese medicine. This, too, is extremely common. In a fourth sense, "integrated Chinese and Western medicine" denotes an institutionally separate sector of the health care system with its own degree courses, hospitals, journals, associations, and so on. In practice, however, degree courses in "integrated Chinese and Western medicine" are taught at Chinese medicine universities, "hospitals of integrated Chinese and Western medicine" are staffed by practitioners of Chinese medicine, journals of integrated medicine are published by Chinese medicine institutions, and members of associations of integrated medicine are usually also members of associations of Chinese medicine. In my opinion, it is therefore more useful to think of integrated Chinese and Western medicine as a subsector of the Chinese medicine sector. This view is shared by almost all physicians and students I have spoken to about this subject.

State policy at the beginning of the 1980s appears to have been influenced by the second sense of the term but afterward shifted to the fourth. At the time of this writing, moves were under way to classify all physicians as either "Western medicine," "Chinese medicine," or "integrated Chinese and Western medicine" by way of centralized state examinations. These classifications would in the future determine what drugs and treatments a physician is allowed to prescribe. However, neither the state nor the Chinese medicine establishment has arrived at a final definition of *zhongxiyi jiehe*. Due to the difficulties involved in clearly separating Chinese medicine from integrated Chinese and Western medicine, I therefore subsume the latter to the former both in the following discussion and in the remainder of this book.[45]

An analysis of the institutional organization of contemporary Chinese medicine seems to confirm these interpretations. Chinese medicine in contemporary China (including integrated Chinese and Western medicine) is supervised by its own department within the Ministry of Health, the State Administration of Chinese Medicine and Pharmacology (Guojia zhongyiyao guanliju 国家中医药管理局).[46] The department was established in 1986 as the State Administration of Chinese Medicine (Guojia zhongyi guanliju 国家中医管理局) under the leadership of Hu Ximing 胡熙明, then the vice minister of health, and charged with overseeing and controlling the practice and development of Chinese medicine.[47] To this function was added in 1988 the administration of drugs used in Chinese medicine. The Chinese medicine community attaches great importance to the state administration as a symbol and guarantor of its autonomy, as indicated in a letter sent to Jiang Zemin on 15 December 1992 by eminent Chinese medicine physicians concerned by the possibility of its possible reassimilation to the general office of the MOH.[48]

The organization of public health departments of provinces, municipalities, and autonomous regions mirrors that of the MOH. Chinese medicine is thus controlled by its own departments on lower administrative levels as well. In Beijing this entity is the Chinese Medicine Office of the Beijing Municipality Public Health Bureau (Beijingshi weishengju zhongyichu 北京市卫生局中医处). Physicians of Chinese medicine belong to the All-China Association for Chinese Medicine (Zhonghua quanguo zhongyi xuehui 中华全国中医学会) established in May 1979. The association fulfills the equivalent function accorded to the Chinese Medical Association in the Western medical domain. Both organizations are ultimately answerable to the MOH.[49]

Chinese medicine education today is independent of Western medicine education, though both are also interconnected within the overall health care and educational systems. Physicians of Chinese medicine are generally educated at universities (*daxue* 大学) or colleges (*xueyuan* 学院) of Chinese medicine. Secondary Chinese medicine schools (*xuexiao* 学校) train medical health personnel at the intermediate level. After the hiatus of the Cultural Revolution a second phase of expansion in the late 1970s and early 1980s saw the total number of Chinese medicine educational establishments rise to thirty-two universities and colleges and fifty-one secondary schools by 1989. In 1994 Beijing had one university, two colleges, and two secondary schools of Chinese medicine. Night schools and correspondence courses are also available to provide an entry into the medical profession for mature students. These were founded partially to increase the number of Chinese medical personnel, which in spite of state support had continued to decline in real terms.[50]

Chinese medical colleges have some influence on the development of their curriculum, and this allows them to establish particular local reputations. The Beijing University of Chinese Medicine (Beijing zhongyiyao daxue 北京中医药大学), for instance, is regarded by most students and physicians as rather traditional and conservative and as having a particularly strong *shanghan* department. The university in Shanghai, on the other hand, is seen as emphasizing modernization and the integration of Chinese medicine and Western medicine. Admission to tertiary education in Chinese medicine is via the yearly university entrance exams following completion of high school. In general, access to Western medicine schools is more difficult than access to comparable Chinese medicine schools. Most people I spoke to, including most teachers and students of Chinese medicine, considered studying Western medicine more prestigious, and most of the undergraduate students I asked said they would rather study Western medicine.

Many students at Beijing University of Chinese Medicine not ordinarily resident in Beijing had come there in the hope of obtaining a job in the capital after graduation. In 1994 the Beijing University of Chinese Medicine, in line with other major universities, began charging a fee to students (approximately RMB 1000 per annum in 1994, it had risen more than twofold by 1999). This makes it more difficult for economically disadvantaged students to apply for a place and is potentially threatening recruitment into the profession.[51]

Upon graduation physicians of Chinese medicine enjoy the same legal status as their Western medicine colleagues. Given appropriate postgraduate training they are entitled to practice medicine in whatever way they deem necessary for the health of their patients. This includes the practice of surgery and the prescribing of Western medicine drugs. Graduates in Chinese medi-

TABLE 2. Number of Chinese Medicine Institutions, Beds, and Personnel, 1952–1996

	1952	1963	1975	1980	1990	1993	1996
CM personnel	306,000	339,291	228,635	262,185	368,462	365,090	347,846
CM hospitals	19	124	160	678	2,115	2,418	2,526
At county level and above	19	124	160	647	2,037	2,305	2,398
Research institutes	0	33	29	47	55	67	66
Beds of CM hospitals	224	9,254	13,675	49,977	175,655	213,465	237,488
At county level and above	224	9,254	13,675	49,151	160,899	193,848	216,794

Source: Chen Minzhang (1997: 294–95)

cine can study for postgraduate degrees in Western medicine, and vice versa. Physicians of Chinese medicine may be employed in Chinese medicine hospitals, in Chinese medicine departments of Western medicine hospitals, and in Western medicine departments, or they may open their own private clinics. As a consequence, some undergraduates use a degree in Chinese medicine as a first step toward postgraduate education and a possible career in Western medicine.[52]

Data from a 1996 census conducted by the MOH indicate that there are 2,526 specialist hospitals for Chinese medicine in China (24 of them in Beijing), compared with only 19 such hospitals in 1952 and 160 in 1975 at the end of the Cultural Revolution (see table 2). These hospitals make up 3.8 percent of the total number of hospitals in China, provide 237,488 beds, and employ 347,846 medical workers.[53] Chinese medicine hospitals are run by different entities at various levels of state and regional administrative hierarchies. Of the four largest Chinese medicine hospitals in Beijing, the Dongzhimen Hospital (*Dongzhimen zhongyi yiyuan* 东直门中医医院) is affiliated with the Beijing University of Chinese Medicine, the Beijing City Chinese Medicine Hospital (*Beijingshi zhongyi yiyuan* 北京市中医医院) is jointly administered by the Public Health Department of the Dongcheng District of the Beijing Municipality and the Chinese Medicine College of Beijing Union University, and the Guang'anmen (*Guang'anmen zhongyi yiyuan* 广安门中医医院) and Xiyuan Hospitals of Chinese Medicine (*Xiyuan zhongyi yiyuan* 西苑中医医院) are run by the Academy of Chinese Medicine.[54]

Chinese medicine hospitals provide inpatient and outpatient services as well as neighborhood clinics. They are organized administratively and clinically according to medical specialities, about which more will be said later.

A small number of hospitals are designated combined Chinese and Western medicine hospitals. The largest of these hospitals in Beijing is the China-Japan Friendship Hospital (*Zhongri youhao yiyuan* 中日友好医院), which has a Western medicine–to–Chinese medicine ratio in terms of physicians and staff of approximately 2:1. The Chinese medicine and Western medicine sections of the hospital are organized as quasi-independent units, each providing specialist inpatient and outpatient services. In addition to specialist Chinese medicine hospitals, 95 percent of ordinary (i.e., Western medicine) hospitals have Chinese medicine departments providing outpatient services. In 1994 Chinese medicine hospitals treated more than 200 million outpatients and 2.5 million inpatients. In rural areas the Chinese medicine sector treats one-third of all outpatients and a quarter of all inpatients.[55]

With respect to research infrastructure Chinese medicine also enjoys relative independence. The Academy of Chinese Medicine, reopened in 1978, fulfills functions similar to those presumed by the China Academy of Medical Sciences in the Western medicine domain. Both academies are directly supervised by the MOII. By 1989 the Academy of Chinese Medicine controlled six specialist research institutes (*yanjiusuo* 研究所). A further 108 subsidiary research institutes are affiliated with various Chinese medicine colleges, hospitals, and regional or provincial public health departments throughout the country (see table 2).[56]

The economic reforms of the 1980s and 1990s have led to the emergence, in many areas of the PRC, of medical clinics run as private businesses and to an expansion of Chinese medical pharmaceutical production. According to MOII data the total output of Chinese medicine businesses in 1994 was worth 17.9 billion yuan ($2.1 billion).[57] Nevertheless, the state-supported Chinese medicine sector in Beijing remains well developed. As the state capital, Beijing concentrates significant political, economic, and educational resources. Access to state funding is facilitated not merely by Beijing's role as a national showpiece but also by its physical proximity to centers of power.

The number of private enterprises in the Chinese medicine sector in Beijing and other large cities thus remains relatively small. Shanghai, the most important center of Chinese medicine during the Nationalist period, for instance, had a total of 3,308 physicians of Chinese medicine at the end of 1948, of whom 98 percent worked in private establishments. From 1951 onward these physicians were assimilated into state-run clinics and hospitals while the new licensing regulations described above concomitantly reduced their overall number. Thus, by 1965 the number of Chinese medicine practitioners in the city totaled about 1,000, a reduction of more than 60 percent.

By 1990 this number had increased once more to 6,708, of whom only 266 (3.98 percent) worked in private practice. The majority of these were older retired physicians. My informants stated that the large number of hospitals and outpatient clinics in cities such as Beijing and Shanghai tied to insurance schemes and employing well-known physicians made it virtually impossible for young physicians to establish themselves in private practice there. In many areas physicians are also forbidden by their terms of employment to set up in private practice after retirement so as not to take away patients and revenue from their previous employers.[58]

Orchestrated Pluralism

In spite of its undoubted commitment to Chinese medicine, government policy is still clearly skewed toward the development of biomedical care. While the number of Chinese medicine doctors employed in official health institutions had risen from 276,000 in 1949 to 340,780 in 1996, the number of Western medicine doctors increased from 87,400 to 1,582,700 over the same period (table 3). The same disparity is found when comparing hospitals. In 1996 there were 2,398 Chinese medicine hospitals at county level and above compared with 10,681 Western medicine hospitals. Taking the number of beds as a measure, the total percentage of beds in Chinese medicine hospitals and departments actually fell from 4.2 percent of all hospital beds in 1978 to 3.4 percent in 1996 (see table 2).[59]

Such purely statistical data hide the true nature of Chinese medicine's role in the health care system because they paint a picture of separate and unequal systems. Nothing could be further from the truth. Chinese medicine today is deeply embedded within the global constitution of the Chinese health care system. From the perspective of the state, the "three great powers"— Chinese medicine, Western medicine, and integrated Chinese medicine and Western medicine—not unlike other natural resources, must be appropriately controlled if their productivity is to be fully marshalled. For Chinese medicine this translates into a state-directed obligation to "carefully sum up, study, and carry forward the medical heritage of our motherland in an effort to enrich the contents of medical science and to provide better health care for the people."[60] To this may be added a state-directed obligation to maximize revenue through structural reforms in the organization of health care delivery and the active economic expansion of the Chinese medical sector.[61]

The various catchwords that have guided the development of the Chinese medicine sector during the 1990s mark its penetration by and opening up to

TABLE 3. Number and Percentage of Personnel in Health Institutions in 1996

	Number	Total Personnel (%)	Health Professionals (%)
Doctors of Chinese medicine	257,285	4.7	6
Doctors of Western medicine	1,207,349	22.3	28
Doctors of integrated Chinese and Western medicine	10,598	0.2	0.2

Source: Chen Minzhang (1997: 294–95)

the forces of wider social and economic reforms. "One principal thread, three strengthenings" (*yitiao zhuxian, sange jiaqiang* 一条主线, 三个加强), a slogan coined in 1994, was intended to indicate that all policies concerned with Chinese medicine should be governed by the general thread of opening up thinking, being realistic and pragmatic in order to deepen reforms, while focusing on three specific areas of development: the strengthening of rural health care, the strengthening of the Chinese medical infrastructure, and the strengthening of a morally upright socialist culture. The "development and enhancement project" (*hongyang gongcheng* 弘扬工程), which summarizes plans for the development of Chinese medicine up to 2010, widens the scope of this development from China itself to a policy of active globalization, or "striding out into the world" (*kua shijie* 跨世界).[62]

In my opinion, therefore, Chinese medicine at the turn of the century cannot be understood as a semiautonomous part of the health sector. As analysts of other medical systems have noted, pluralism usually implies the existence of hierarchical relations between medical subsystems that tend to mirror the political, economic, and social relations of the larger society. It is an explicit assumption of such arguments that in modern or modernizing societies biomedicine enjoys a dominant status over heterodox and ethnomedical practices. The dominance of biomedicine is seen to be reflected not only in the support it receives from the state and its interweaving into the exploitative relation between industrialized and underdeveloped countries, but also in its ideological and practical infiltration of other health care practices.[63]

Clearly, such generalizations need to be revised with respect to the Chinese case. While my overview certainly demonstrates that biomedical ideas and institutions have exerted a significant influence on the development of Chinese medicine, it also shows that Western medicine, too, was repeatedly forced to accommodate to revolutionary medical reform. I shall therefore adopt Lock's notion of "orchestrated medical pluralism," a concept that emphasizes the structuring of local medical practice through globally constituted health care systems without insisting on the dominant role of biomedicine, as a more appropriate tool for the analysis of Chinese medicine's position in contemporary China.

According to Lock, "orchestrated medical pluralism" denotes that local medical practices are invariably transformed once they become "officially recognized and incorporated into the dominant institutionalized organization for the provision of health care."[64] The historical overview above established that accepting fundamental premises of what Chinese politicians considered to be the cornerstones of modernity (such as scientization and systematization) was the price Chinese physicians had to pay in order to secure the survival of their tradition. The policies of reform and opening up to the West instituted since 1978 have accelerated such modernization, albeit by diverting it from cooperative health care in the countryside back to the city hospitals; from an emphasis on mutual help to the generation of revenue; from the barefoot doctor medicine designed for the benefit of the masses toward a high-tech medicine aimed at those who can pay; from an emphasis on self-reliance and experimentation guided by self-reflective practice toward the integration of Chinese medicine into global economic, technological, and intellectual networks by means of scientific research.[65]

In spite of much outward change, two features of the relationship between Chinese medicine and the state remain unchanged. The first is the subservience, at least officially, of the Chinese medical establishment to the directives of CCP policy. Thus, in their letter to Jiang Zemin in which some of the most prominent physicians of Chinese medicine in contemporary China argue for the independence of their tradition, they also explicitly emphasize their loyalty to the state.[66] The second feature is the consistent effort on behalf of the state to bring under control the plurality of Chinese medicine—be it through the infusion of Western medicine, the simplifications of the barefoot doctors, or the bureaucratic regulation and commodification of the 1990s. Regulation of such plurality—diagnosed early on as sectarianism (*zongpaizhuyi* 宗派主义) by Mao Zedong—is necessary not only for ideological reasons. Much more important, it is only by way of such state simplifications that the global uniformities necessary for controlling a medical system from above and for marshalling its resources within larger schemes of planned progress can be realized. These forces, it should be noted, are imposed on the CCP itself by the demands of the system it is striving to create and do not simply flow from its political authority.[67]

There exist multiple instruments of social control by which all aspects of Chinese medicine, from its institutional structure to the content of its knowledge base, are manipulated from above, even if continued political mobilization has given way to control by means of bureaucratic mechanisms and market forces. As we have seen, state supervision extending from the licensing of physicians and clinics to the regulation of practice on both microlevels (e.g., what kind of drugs a physician of Chinese medicine was allowed to prescribe) and macrolevels (e.g., the formulation of policies concerning the modernization of Chinese medicine) began immediately after the founding of the People's Republic in 1949.[68] An exhaustive history of such regulation and its day-to-day practical implementation is neither possible nor necessary within the framework of the current investigation. Accordingly, I shall outline only a few mechanisms of state control in contemporary Chinese medicine that support my general argument.

Chinese medical education is administered by the Bureau of Medical Education, which is jointly managed by the Ministry of Education (MOE, Jiaoyubu 教育部) and the MOH. The MOE oversees general educational policies and financing, while the MOH is responsible for specific matters concerning teaching and school affairs.[69] Whereas the relevant departments of the MOH are staffed by cadres with a background in Chinese medicine, the MOE bureaucracy in general lacks such competence. The consequence is that Chinese medical education is influenced by civil servants not necessarily sympathetic to or understanding of its concerns. Course contents are formulated by specially appointed commissions whose members are drawn from Chinese medicine colleges and who carry out their task "under the guidance and with the support of the MOH."[70] The teaching plan for courses in Chinese medicine issued by the MOH in 1982 states that its aim is "to train socialist-minded doctors of Chinese medicine." Students are required "to support the leadership of the CCP, love the socialist motherland, . . . study Marxism-Leninism and Mao Zedong thought, possess the quality and ethics of a communist, observe discipline and the law, . . . and wholeheartedly serve the people and the cause of socialism . . . [and to possess and maintain] a sound physique."[71]

Almost the entire Chinese medicine infrastructure, from professional organizations to the publication of academic journals, is directly or indirectly controlled by the MOH or its regional branches. Of the 2531 work-units that constituted the official Chinese medical health care sector in 1989, 51 fell under the direct administrative control of the MOH or the State Administration of Chinese Medicine.[72] These 51 work-units comprise two of the four oldest and most influential universities and colleges of Chinese medicine (in Beijing and Guangzhou); eleven Chinese medicine journals; the country's most prestigious publishing house of Chinese medical books, the People's Health Press (Renmin weisheng chubanshe 人民卫生出版社); some of the country's largest and most important Chinese medicine hospitals and research institutes; as well as the Academy of Chinese Medicine and its affiliated work-units. The influence of the MOH is particularly pronounced in Beijing, where in 1989, 35 of the 60 Chinese medicine work-units came under the administrative control of the MOH and only 25 were under that of the Beijing Municipality.[73]

According to the founding decree of the Academy of Chinese Medicine by Premier Zhou Enlai (still quoted today), its purpose is "to develop the heritage of the medicine of the motherland and serve the establishment of socialism."[74] Given the nationalist connotations of this project, Chinese medicine was recruited already in the 1950s as a tool by which China's genius could be asserted at home and promoted abroad. The "Chinese medicine fever" (zhongyire 中医热) that has been spreading throughout the world since the 1970s has merely provided the state with more opportunities in this endeavor. In the foreword to a three-volume collection of medical cases by China's foremost Chinese medicine physicians published in 1986 and edited by Dong Jianhua 董建华, one of Beijing's most authoritative contemporary clinicians, the minister of health, at that time, Cui Yueli 崔月梨, wrote:

> From as early as the Tang dynasty, China was already established as the center of Asian medicine, which exerted an influence on the development of medicine in Asia and the world both profound and far reaching. . . . Recently, the influence of Chinese medicine and pharmacology on the international stage is becoming increasingly stronger, and "Chinese medicine fever" has erupted in quite a few countries. A number of internationally renowned scientists are of the opinion that Chinese medicine and pharmacology may bring about new breakthroughs in the life sciences. Many European, American, and Southeast Asian countries have strengthened their research efforts in this direction and several problems have already yielded definite results. For China, the birthplace of Chinese medicine and pharmacology, the vigorous promotion of the Chinese medical and Chinese pharmacological professions for the enrichment of humankind is an unshirkable [national] duty.[75]

International exchange and cooperation in the field of Chinese medicine are thus actively encouraged. Politically, the goal is to increase the influence of Chinese medicine around the world and to consolidate China's undisputed leadership in the field. Economically, every effort is made to expand the international market for Chinese medicine products with a goal set by the Ninth Five-Year Plan of generating an export volume of $800 million by the year 2000.[76]

MOH's power impinges on the daily life and work of all students and doctors of Chinese medicine in many ways. All physicians are obliged to attend an endless succession of meetings in which policies of all kinds are communicated and decided on and through which the health care sector can be mobilized to implement state-directed goals.[77] Two important examples of such MOH policies with direct effects on the practice of Chinese medicine at the microlevel are regulations regarding the keeping of medical records and efforts to standardize all aspects of Chinese medical practice. Regulations regarding the writing of case records (*bingli* 病历) stipulate precisely what information is to be recorded and how. In fact, most of the internship in the fifth year of undergraduate training seems to be spent in learning how to write accurate case histories. Chinese medical case records must carry a biomedical diagnosis. Several doctors informed me that while hospital authorities are lax about the Chinese medical diagnosis, a Western medical diagnosis is obligatory for all records (that is, not only for case records but also for outpatient treatment records, laboratory examination requests, etc.).[78]

The standardization (*guifanhua*) of Chinese medicine, a political imperative since the early 1950s, was accelerated in the 1990s. In order to eliminate the idiosyncratic use by physicians of classical labels for diseases, patterns, and symptoms and to facilitate bureaucratic control, the MOH actively promoted the development of a standardized system of disease classification. In 1996 National Standards for Clinical Diagnosis and Treatment Terminologies were published and formally implemented by the Department of National Standards of the State Bureau of Technical Supervision in the autumn of the same year.[79] The standardization of complex formulas in clinical practice is the next goal, and a pilot program examining methods to achieve this is listed as one of forty-six key scientific projects in the Ninth Five-Year Plan (1995–2000).[80]

Research goals in Chinese medicine and their financing are specified and controlled within the overall structure of five-year plans. The Eighth Five-Year plan (1991–95), for instance, specifically stressed the importance of the social and economic usefulness of any research undertaken. It specified pathologies and technologies on which research should be concentrated (malignant tumors, cardiovascular disease, hepatitis, and acupuncture anaesthesia) and emphasized the development of new technologies to facilitate the production and application of Chinese medicine drugs.[81] While lip service is paid to the special characteristics of Chinese medicine, research goals and research methodologies are by and large taken from biomedicine, often uncritically so. A draft report on acupuncture research to the WHO Regional Committee for the Western Pacific, which I helped to translate during my fieldwork, for instance, accepts randomized double-blind trials as the gold standard for improving acupuncture practice.[82]

As the government emphasizes scientific research and seeks to expand Chinese medicine internationally, such research is increasingly important for the career development of physicians and graduate students working in the state sector. This is particularly so in Beijing, where, as we have seen, opportunities for private practice remain limited. Attending physicians (*zhuzhi yisheng* 主治医生), the lowest rung on the career ladder, are expected to write one or more research papers a year. While I studied in the China-Japan Friendship Hospital young physicians complained to me about the constant pressure this generated. All of the senior physicians with whom I studied were engaged in research projects, and hospital departments as well as individual professors compete with one another for research funds.

Post-1979 reforms of the health sector indicate a gradual movement toward "dispersed competition" through macroeconomic control mechanisms and away from social control by means of bureaucratic hierarchies, solidarity mechanisms, or both.[83] Increasing pressure is placed on hospitals, for instance, to compete with one another and to generate a large proportion of their own revenue through increases in fees, drug sales, and chargeable diagnostic exams.[84] Hospitals transmit this pressure through a system of bonuses whereby individual physicians and entire departments receive cash payments according to the revenue they generate. As a consequence, physicians in Chinese medicine hospitals regularly use biomedical diagnostic devices from blood tests to MRI scans, while doctors outside these institutions seem to get by most of the time without them. Physicians also receive kickbacks ranging from dinner invitations to cash payments from pharmaceutical companies and apparently—though I was not able to confirm this and hospital authorities are making every effort to stamp out the practice—directly from patients hoping to buy preferential treatment or simply expressing their thanks in the form of "red envelopes" (*hongbao* 红包). The influence of the pharmaceutical industry is limited as long as physicians rely mainly on the use of crude drugs administered as decoctions (*tangyao* 汤药) individually composed for each patient. However, increasing promotional activity by drug companies for the use of ready-made drugs in conjunction with attempts by the state to standardize compound prescriptions and patients' preference for easily consumable (and good-tasting) medicines may profoundly change the practice of Chinese medicine in years to come.

Which doctor a patient sees is also influenced by state and hospital policies (see chapter 4). While I was studying at the China-Japan Friendship Hospital its administration shifted many cancer patients from Western medicine to Chinese medicine wards because the latter were rarely fully occupied. This annoyed Chinese medicine physicians, who felt they were given only the hopeless cases, but satisfied the hospital's accountants. Treatment on many of the Chinese medicine wards I visited was officially of the integrated Chinese medicine and Western medicine variety but in reality was often entirely biomedical. Students who spent their internship on these wards complained that they were studying Chinese medicine but learning Western medicine.

Many doctors, too, expressed their frustration at being used as second-rate Western medicine physicians or questioned the value for Chinese medicine of relying heavily on biomedical treatments. They were fully aware, of course, that placing surgery patients in Chinese medicine wards generated more revenue than would treating them with herbal decoctions. They acknowledged, too, that the boundaries of ethical Chinese medical practice were constantly evolving. While in the early 1980s Chinese medical doctors were still openly debating the benefits and risks of treating acute life-threatening diseases with Chinese medicine, few of the doctors I met in the 1990s considered it an option.[85] It might work, they said, perhaps even better than Western medicine. If someone died in your care, however, and you had relied on Chinese medicine alone, no authority would defend you against almost certain accusations of neglect by the family of the deceased. If you used only Western medicine, no one would dare to blame you.[86]

Pressure to use Western medicine seemed particularly acute for relatively less experienced junior doctors. One young physician working at the Beijing City Chinese Medicine Hospital told me, "It is very difficult for us young doctors. Most patients coming for Chinese medical treatment prefer to see an old, experienced doctor. When they come to us they don't trust us. Often they prefer me to treat them with Western medicine. You don't have much chance to improve your skills at a hospital such as this, where there are so many famous older doctors."

This is very frustrating for young doctors who have spent five years studying Chinese medicine and overcome ever-increasing obstacles in finding a job.[87] Those who work in the hospital wards rely on Western medicine because they do not trust their skill in Chinese medicine, while those working in outpatient departments find themselves pressured by patients to prescribe West-

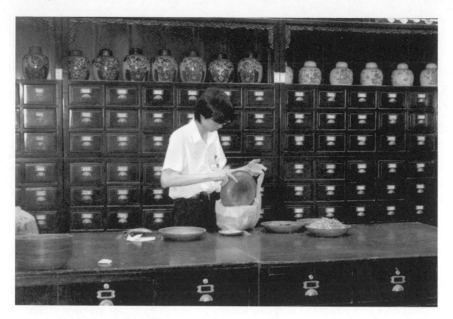

FIGURE 12. Pharmacy, Shanghai

ern medical drugs. On the other hand, as I was told in many conversations, the experience of the sometimes astounding efficacy of Chinese medicine in clinical practice—observed during twice-weekly ward rounds or achieved in one's own budding practice—convinces these younger physicians of the ultimate value of their career.

Transforming Chinese Medicine: The State as Disciplining and Disciplined Agent

The historical overview presented in this chapter established the state's leading role in shaping Chinese medicine since 1949—from defining its status as a science to defining its standing as a national treasure-house, from the creation of barefoot doctors as a vehicle for the mass campaigns in the 1960s to the recruitment of Chinese medicine into a high-tech hospital-based medical system in the 1990s. Contemporary Chinese medicine is thus not an autonomous medical tradition but rather one fully integrated into a larger state-orchestrated health care system. The various and ever-changing political, economic, bureaucratic, and cultural imperatives that govern the transformations of this system penetrate deeply into the constitution of Chinese medicine. They demand that it be at once traditional, so as to function as

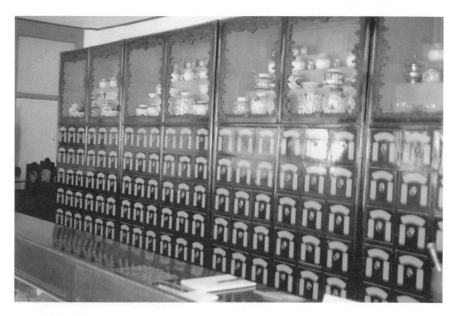

FIGURE 13. Old pharmacy, Shangdong

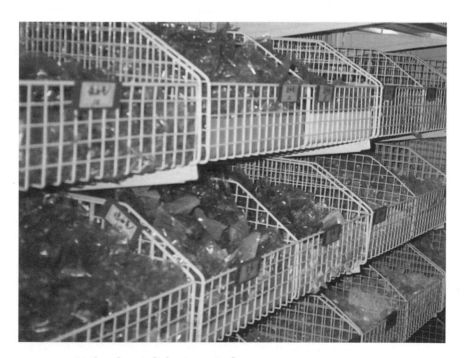

FIGURE 14. Modern hospital pharmacy, Suzhou

a visible embodiment of Chinese cultural ingenuity, and modern, flexible enough to reshape itself according to the current requirements of socialist modernization.

Chinese medicine has thus had to accommodate its theories, practices, and social networks to continually evolving interpretations of what precisely modernization and tradition stand for. Its flexibility in this regard has allowed Chinese medicine to succeed in forcing accommodation in return from the state. For instance, by defining Chinese medicine as a priori scientific—which is necessary to legitimize its inclusion within a modern health care system— and declaring that (at least where Chinese medicine is concerned) "practice [is] the only criterion to test the truth," the state has had to embrace official definitions of science and truth quite different from those dominant in the West.[88] Not only is this an outstanding achievement for Chinese medicine considering the fate of other medical practices around the world, but its secure position within China has also provided Chinese medicine with a platform from which it is busily realizing a global expansion befitting the 1990s.

The goal of the final section of this chapter is to link these observations to the general model of synthetic emergence developed in chapter 2. For this purpose I focus on one small area of practice, the recording of clinical information. For reasons of bureaucratic control (including the collation of epidemiological data; the evaluation and grading of hospitals, hospital departments, and individual physicians; economic indicators; protection of patients; etc.), the state has an active interest in accessing and controlling such information. Clear rules regarding the recording of clinical information have therefore been formulated and are continually being refined. These include the systematization of Chinese medicine diagnostic categories, treatment methods, and measurements of therapeutic outcomes as well as regulations regarding the recording of such information in clinical practice.[89] My argument is that the formulation of these rules, their implementation, and the writing of case records can all be understood as processes of synthesis in which the state is a powerful, but by no means an all-powerful, agent.

The state's influence on the recording of clinical information is strongest in institutions readily transparent to state bureaucratic control such as hospital inpatient departments, where the keeping of detailed medical records is legally prescribed. It is less developed in hospital outpatient departments, where medical records are often kept by patients themselves rather than the hospital, and almost nonexistent in private practice.

One acupuncturist I observed working from home, for instance, kept no records at all and relied solely on his memory. Another physician with whom

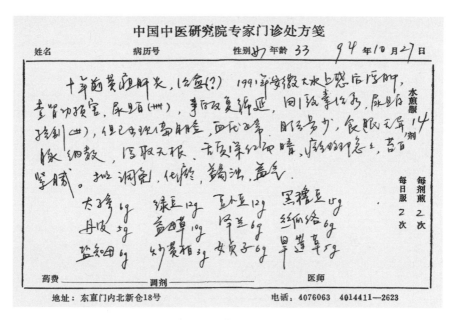

FIGURE 15. Modern outpatient case record and prescription

I studied in a pharmacy wrote out prescriptions (*chufang* 处方 or *fangzi* 方子) on preprinted forms (*tiaozi* 条子) and relied on his patients to keep these forms as medical records. This is a common practice, and many prescription forms contain a designated area where physicians can enter comments regarding symptoms and signs, diagnosis, or treatment principles. Some physicians keep copies of these annotated prescriptions for private use and possible publication at a later date. Annotated prescriptions are also the main means by which students and junior physicians acting as scribes for senior doctors during consultations record information for themselves (see chapter 6).

Most outpatients, however, own small medical history booklets (officially known as *bingliben* 病历本 but often referred to simply as *benr* 本儿), about fifteen by ten centimeters in size, which can be purchased when registering at hospital outpatient departments. These carry the name and work-unit of the owner on the front cover and are intended to document a person's medical history. Medical history booklets often get lost, however, and patients may decide to buy a new booklet when switching doctors or hospitals. Some outpatient case records are also kept on special hospital forms and stored in the hospital. This is the case for outpatients whose insurance contracts them to a particular hospital. The first page of such histories resembles those of inpatient case histories and requires the filling in of preprinted spaces. Later

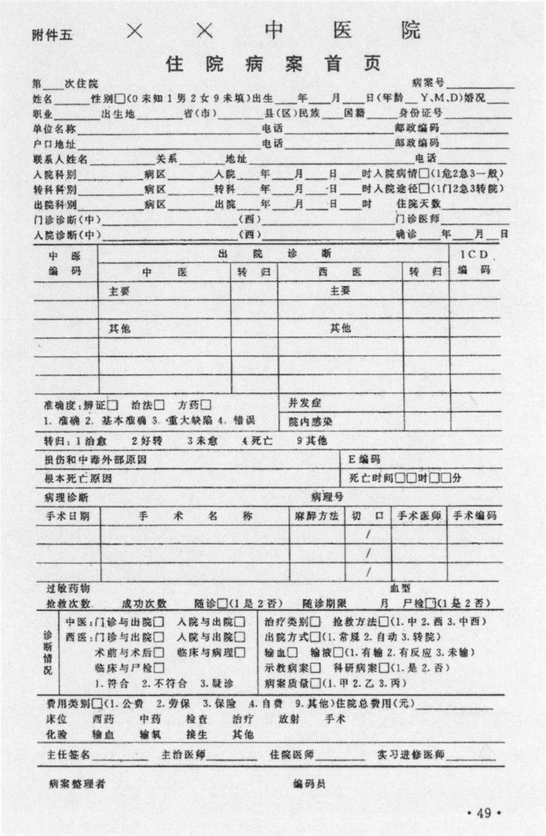
附件五　××中医院

住院病案首页

第___次住院　病案号___
姓名___性别□(0 未知 1 男 2 女 9 未填)出生___年___月___日(年龄__Y、M、D)婚况___
职业___出生地___省(市)___县(区)民族___国籍___身份证号___
单位名称___电话___邮政编码___
户口地址___电话___邮政编码___
联系人姓名___关系___地址___电话___
入院科别___病区___入院___年___月___日___时入院病情□(1危2急3一般)
转科科别___病区___转科___年___月___日___时入院途径□(1门2急3转院)
出院科别___病区___出院___年___月___日___时　住院天数___
门诊诊断(中)___(西)___门诊医师___
入院诊断(中)___(西)___确诊___年___月___日

中医编码	出院诊断				ICD编码
	中医	转归	西医	转归	
	主要		主要		
	其他		其他		

准确度：辨证□　治法□　方药□
1. 准确 2. 基本准确 3. 重大缺陷 4. 错误
并发症
院内感染
转归：1 治愈　2 好转　3 未愈　4 死亡　9 其他
损伤和中毒外部原因　E编码
根本死亡原因　死亡时间□□时□□分
病理诊断　病理号

手术日期	手术名称	麻醉方法	切口	手术医师	手术编码
			/		
			/		
			/		

过敏药物　血型
抢救次数　成功次数　随诊□(1 是 2 否)　随诊期限　月　尸检□(1 是 2 否)
诊断情况
中医：门诊与出院□　入院与出院□
西医：门诊与出院□　入院与出院□
术前与术后□　临床与病理□
临床与尸检□
1. 符合　2. 不符合　3. 疑诊
治疗类别□　抢救方法□(1. 中 2. 西 3. 中西)
出院方式□(1. 常规 2. 自动 3. 转院)
输血□　输液□(1. 有输 2. 有反应 3. 未输)
示教病案□　科研病案□(1. 是 2. 否)
病案质量□(1. 甲 2. 乙 3. 丙)
费用类别□(1. 公费　2. 劳保　3. 保险　4. 自费　9. 其他)住院总费用(元)___
床位　西药　中药　检查　治疗　放射　手术
化验　输血　输氧　接生　其他
主任签名___　主治医师___　住院医师___　实习进修医师___
病案整理者　编码员
· 49 ·

FIGURE 16. Modern case record form (cover page)

pages are simply glued to the existing history together with any examination results. Even though the pages used for this purpose often also have preprinted spaces with headings for symptoms and signs, diagnosis, treatment, and so on, most doctors I observed simply wrote over them.

The same regulations that govern the keeping of inpatient records mandate how records are kept on prescription forms and in booklets. Besides name, age, sex, and date of consultation, the data recorded should include information on symptoms and signs, medical history, examinations, the analysis of data, diagnosis (both Chinese and biomedical), treatment method, and prescription.[90] In practice, however, each physician interprets the amount of this information deemed necessary and the manner in which it is recorded differently. The records I saw varied considerably, ranging from a single sentence to an entire page complete with urine and blood examination record slips (*danzi* 单子) glued onto the opposing page.

Inpatient case records (officially called *bingan* 病案 but commonly referred to by physicians and students as *bingli* 病历) are written on special forms that comply with government and hospital regulations. These carry a unique identification number for each patient, are kept in the hospital, and require the documentation of information ranging from age, address, and occupation to the detailed recording of symptoms, signs, and examinations; biomedical and Chinese medical diagnoses; treatments; and treatment outcomes. Such case records consist of several portions. The first section, placed on the top and referred to as the *da bingli* 大病历 (big case history), is a double case history consisting of two parts: a Western medicine portion and a Chinese medical portion. This part is not actually written by the attending physician during the intake interview but rather is composed by students and interns within three days of a patient being admitted to the hospital. Its primary function, apart from serving as a legal document, thus appears educational. In addition to the *da bingli*, inpatient records contain illness progress notes (which are an amalgam of Chinese and Western medicine and contain the actual Chinese medicine prescription being used), lab reports, and medical orders (which contain information regarding prescribed Western medicine and Chinese patent medicines).[91]

The various forms of record keeping in contemporary practice all derive from classical clinical accounts. One can distinguish between two broad

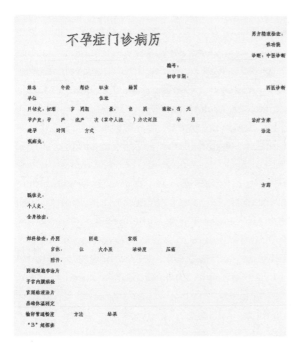

FIGURE 17. Modern case record form for treatment of infertility

genres: clinical stories (*yihua* 医话) and pulse records (*mai'an* 脉案). Clinical stories originated in the Song and Yuan periods as published records of clinical encounters. They are characterized by a prosaic mode of narrative, often documenting a particular treatment principle or a course of treatment rather than a single treatment episode. Pulse records represent a later style of writing originating in the Qing. In general, these are much shorter, consisting of the prescription and brief appended clinical information. Rather than giving longer elaborations of symptoms as the clinical stories do, pulse records provide only the information necessary to elucidate disease mechanisms and therapeutic principles. Clinical notes (*yi'an* 医案) are printed collections of pulse records by individual physicians sometimes annotated by their disciples or later editors. Although these genres differ in style and in the audiences for which they were intended, all three center on prescriptions as the pivotal embodiment of clinical skill and expertise in Chinese medicine. Even today, experienced physicians are still expected to be able to read from such prescriptions not only the condition as interpreted by the attending physician but also his or her particular style of treatment and its affinities to the various strands of the medical tradition.[92]

Contemporary clinical record keeping on prescription forms (*tiaozi*) and in medical history booklets (*bingliben*) resembles pulse records both in form and in the centrality of the prescription as the only invariable element. Where modern records differ from classical ones is in their frequent inclusion of biomedical diagnoses and examination results. Each note is still, however, a recording of the clinical encounter as understood by the physician and is thus a reflection of his or her subjectivity. We can distinguish two levels of such subjectivity. In its emphasis on prescriptions rather than the documentation of illness manifestations or diagnoses, each note reflects an understanding of Chinese medicine as the kind of "knowing practice" analyzed by Farquhar — a medicine rooted not in theory or system but in a self-conscious dialectic between personal insight and collectively owned methods of diagnosis and treatment. On a second level, each clinical record also constitutes a maneuver through which a physician seeks to project a particular image of himself to patients, students, and other physicians. These audiences are quite skilled at reading traces of a physician's skill, ability, and charisma in various aspects of a note besides the prescription at its core, from the recording of symptoms and signs to handwriting and linguistic style. Physicians are aware of this and act accordingly. Some choose to express themselves in an esoteric language that borrows heavily from medical classics while others document in great detail the results of blood tests and urine samples.

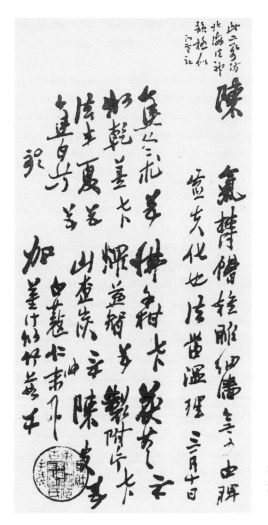

FIGURE 18. Qing dynasty
pulse record

Contemporary inpatient records are also consciously aligned with older genres of clinical accounts, though in a manner that is bureaucratically prescribed and embodies political and institutional rather than practical and subjective projections of agency. Medical anthropologist Shao Jing has provided a penetrating analysis of the historical emergence of these inpatient records as an aspect of Chinese medicine's entrance into hospitals since the late 1950s. Initially, inpatient records in Chinese medical departments of hospitals were kept only in Western medical terms. Their function was purely administrative, facilitating the integration of Chinese medicine into the overall organization of hospitals as at root biomedical institutions. For practical purposes physicians continued to rely on older ways of record keeping. Only since the

1980s—the historical moment at which China's plural health care system was officially established—has the state taken on an increasingly active role in the regulation of record keeping.[93]

Shao Jing argues that these regulations are not determined by administrative needs alone. They also reflect a political imperative to clearly define Chinese medicine's institutional boundaries in a context in which its spatial and practical disjunction from Western medicine are ever more difficult to ascertain. This is why inpatient notes consist of separate Western medicine and Chinese medicine parts even though in actual practice the two medicines are conjoined in multiple ways.[94] Shao Jing notes that while the Western medical part of the *da bingli* serves functional as well as practical needs (it enables the processing of patients through the hospital's administrative system and documents all biomedical examinations, diagnoses, and treatments), the composition of the Chinese medicine part is largely governed by aesthetic principles of narrative composition. For educational purposes, great emphasis is therefore placed in the writing of its main part, the "pattern differentiation analysis," on re-creating the archaic narrative of classical clinical accounts and minimizing contamination from Western medicine. This analysis is supported by the fact that the writing of case histories is carried out not by the senior physicians ultimately responsible for treatment but by clinical interns and young doctors, who spend most of their working time learning and rehearsing the skills necessary for composing such records. While on the outside each case history thus marks off the institutional distinctiveness of Chinese medicine, it functions on the inside as a disciplining mechanism in the education of Chinese medicine physicians.

Viewing these various types of clinical records and their integration into different practices and histories through the model of synthetic emergence helps us to put into perspective the agency of the state in the transformation of contemporary Chinese medicine. The multiple forms of record keeping that we have observed establish that state influence—powerful enough to create an entirely new genre of record keeping—is nevertheless not all-pervasive. For each actual clinical record constitutes a synthesis produced by the interaction of multiple locally efficient, heterogeneous infrastructures. These infrastructures include, besides the state, the physicians composing the records; their audience of physicians, students, patients, and hospital administrators; the vocabularies of Chinese and Western medicine and the practices they represent; and historical and contemporary narratives styles.

Other modalities of recording thus exist in those spaces into which government regulations do not readily penetrate. While the state has a clear interest in the way Chinese medicine is practiced, its interest manifests only in those contexts in which it actively engages with other agencies. Hospital inpatient departments—especially those of teaching hospitals where students and young doctors are trained and where the state has both administrative and educational influence—are the site at which that agency is most effectively deployed. Such deployment always encounters resistance, however. Shao describes how the residents and interns who must compose these accounts jokingly call them "fake archaic writings" (*jia guwen* 假古文) and how easily they slip back into modern language, which holds the promise of greater authenticity in the way it escapes the constraints of formulaic writing.[95]

The composition of case records in hospital inpatient departments requires a continual disciplining of their composers by the state. The agency of the state is translated into locally efficacious action in the supervision of interns and residents by physicians higher up in the hospital hierarchy. Exerting a similar controlling influence over outpatient or private practice would require economies of effort that the state would find difficult to sustain and justify. In these contexts the agency of individual physicians comes to the fore and projects onto each record a highly personal vision of medicine and self. But such self-projection is not autonomous either. Physicians enter the clinical encounter trained in a distinctive manner reflecting their own life journey and personal relations to teachers, colleagues, and students. They work within institutions that exert pressure on them to use biomedical technologies or, on the other hand, that cannot make available such technologies even if the physician desires to use them. Forms of linguistic expression are not fashioned by a physician ex nihilo but are pregiven in the language of the medical classics or contemporary discourse. Even a physician's handwriting—her bodily memories and habits—may resist her desire to create a particular image of herself.

Government regulations, in the same way, must react to what is already present in a situation. By deciding to maintain a distinctive institutional identity for Chinese medicine while at the same time demanding its scientization and modernization, the shaping of contemporary inpatient case records was, to some extent at least, predetermined. Many leading physicians consider understanding disease mechanisms (*bingji* 病机) to be the main purpose of a Chinese medical diagnosis. Maintaining the identity of Chinese medicine through the medium of the case record functions to assert the centrality of this principle. It furthermore demands that the state clear a space for the reinscription of classical clinical records into the modern hospital system. Time and space must be made available in the hospital's routine for the writing of these records, which takes place up to several days after a patient has been admitted and examined. Here, too, the state emerges as much as an agency that is disciplined as one that disciplines.

Future ethnographies will have to analyze the precise mimetic mechanisms whereby contemporary Chinese medicine has been fashioned out of its own past and future. The present chapter has documented in sufficient detail the agency of the state in this process as one that is simultaneously determining and determined, pervasive and limited, active and reactive. As the logical corollary, my own ethnography should examine in a similar manner those other infrastructures with which the state engages in the shaping of contemporary Chinese medicine. This is the topic of the following chapters, starting in chapter 4 with the agency of patients.[96]

4. DILEMMAS AND TACTICAL AGENCY
Patients and the Transformation of
Chinese Medicine   .

Patients are shaped by their encounter with Chinese medicine and, in turn, contribute to its ongoing transformation. In this chapter I illuminate how these processes constitute plurality in contemporary Chinese medicine. With the help of four case studies I elucidate the tactical agency deployed by patients in their quest for health and healing. I show that patients and their families do not encounter Chinese medicine as an abstract medical system but as health care practices embodied locally in individual physicians, hospitals, and therapeutic regimes. Choosing between alternative possibilities of treatment can therefore not be reconstructed as a choice between different medical systems or treatment modalities. Rather, it involves complex negotiations and struggles that become intelligible only as an unfolding of temporal synthesis. I next extend this analysis through a more general survey of changing presentations of being unwell based on participant observations, interviews, and other material collected during my fieldwork in Beijing. My examinations suggest that while patients must accommodate to medical practices in order to use them, they simultaneously change what they use in the act of its utilization.

I interpret these activities as characterized by processes of accommodation and resistance. Patients, their families, and the medical theories, practices, and institutions with which they come into contact mutually shape and transform each other within the context of a two-way dialectic. On the one hand, the objectively given institutional arrangements and demands implicit in Chinese medical practice structure patients' actions locally. Simultaneously, however, the requirements and needs that patients bring to bear on physicians and institutions in the context of local interactions can effect far-reaching transformations of medical practice if local accommodations are subsequently integrated into global syntheses.

Seeking Chinese Medicine: Four Case Studies

Only a few ethnographies that examine patient behavior in Chinese societies exist. They usually proceed from the assumptions that embarking on a course of therapy involves choices between competing medical systems and that such choices are guided by specific health beliefs. A survey carried out by the Beijing City Chinese Medicine Hospital, for instance, found that while lay-people still have a working knowledge of Chinese medicine, the majority of modern Chinese patients prefer Western medicine for treatment, particularly in the case of serious and acute illness. Western medicine is viewed as diagnostically more reliable and therapeutically quicker acting. Patients treated in Chinese medicine clinics thus tend to suffer from chronic diseases or from problems that have not responded to biomedical care.[1]

Popular perceptions regarding the properties of the different subsystems of the contemporary Chinese health care sector appear to confirm such data. Asked about their perceptions of Chinese medicine, the people of Beijing with whom I came into contact would usually recite one of a limited number of stereotypical efficacy attributions. These attributions invariably sorted effects and their causes into binary oppositions with Chinese and Western medicine constituting paradigmatic referents. The following is a list of the most common of these attributions.

> —Western medicine acts fast, Chinese medicine slow (*Xiyi kuai, zhongyi man* 西医快, 中医慢).
> —Chinese medicine treats the root, Western medicine treats ramifications (*Zhongyi zhi ben, xiyi zhi biao* 中医治本, 西医治标).
> —Western medicine often has side effects, Chinese medicine is free of side effects (*Xiyi chang you fuzuoyong, zhongyi meiyou fuzuoyong* 西医常有副作用, 中医没有副作用).
> —Western medicine is better for acute diseases, Chinese medicine for chronic diseases (*Xiyi jixingbing hao, zhongyi manxingbing hao* 西医急性病好, 中医慢性病好).

Roughly identical responses were reported by Ots from Beijing in 1984 and by Hsu from Yunnan in 1989–90.[2] They thus seem to reflect stable perceptions about the relative efficacy (real or imagined) of the two main therapeutic modalities within the Chinese health care system. It would be extremely unwise, however, to assume that these efficacy attributions reflect actual behavior, despite the intuitive appeal of this approach and the sound observational base of these surveys. As we shall see shortly, the actual processes whereby patients and their families arrive at decisions regarding health care choices are far more complex—simultaneously more confused and more enlightened—than such simple models would predict. Jia, for instance, describes how patients in Xiangfen, a county in rural Shanxi, shop for health care by taking into account not only perceived efficacy but also other criteria such as cost, quality of care, and service attitude. White, on the other hand, shows that in the Lijiang District of rural Yunnan elements of Western medicine have been assimilated into a Chinese medicine that is itself fundamentally shaped by the legacy of local spirit-based therapeutics and its own recent political history. The locality and historicity of all medical practice thrown into relief by these two studies asks us, if not to abandon comparisons between medical systems, then at the very least to specify the precise contexts in which they are made.[3]

A theoretical objection to research that takes patient statements regarding health care choices at face value concerns the belief/action model that constitutes its epistemological basis. This model holds that behavior is caused by (and can therefore be explained through) values, ideas, and meanings that reside in people's minds. The mentalism implicit in these formulations is derived from models about relations between knowledge and understanding, theory and practice, body and mind, as well as about what constitutes a person that are increasingly being challenged by recent scholarship.[4] As my first case study demonstrates, in making therapeutic decisions people not only draw on knowledge that they know to be illogical or contradictory, they also sometimes act contrary to their own explicit beliefs.

> CASE 4.1. *Zhennan's Mysterious Fever.* For more than a year, Mrs. Yan's five-year-old son, Zhennan, has suffered from repeated episodes of unabating fever. These episodes start suddenly with Zhennan's body temperature reaching up to 40.2° C. Zhennan also has lost his appetite and a considerable amount of body weight. His mother worries about him day and night. Mrs. Yan has taken Zhennan to many famous Beijing hospitals such as Tongren Hospital, Beijing University Hospital, the No. 3 Hospital, and Beijing Children's Hospital for treatment. Doctors have carried out repeated examinations and treated him with various injections. However, so far they have succeeded neither in discovering the cause of the fevers nor in bringing them under control.
>
> Nevertheless, every time Zhennan gets a fever he is taken to the outpatient department of a Western medical hospital. If treatment there does not help (and according to Mrs. Yan it never does), Mrs. Yan eventually takes her son to a doctor of Chinese medicine. On each occasion this doc-

tor has managed to cure the fever. He has offered Mrs. Yan an explanation for the repeated attacks and the loss of appetite (a spleen-stomach disharmony) that Mrs. Yan says makes sense to her. Even so, she has never embarked on a longer course of Chinese medical treatment with her son, always discontinuing the herbs once the acute fever has abated.

Mrs. Yan states that she believes in Chinese medicine and that she has been successfully treated with it for constipation and menstrual problems. She thinks the Chinese doctor would probably cure her son, too, provided the boy took his prescriptions regularly. Mrs. Yan's husband, however, is vehemently opposed to Chinese medicine. He thinks it is unscientific and based on superstitious theories. He also had a very bad personal experience with Chinese medical treatment when several years ago, under pressure from family and friends, he consulted a physician of Chinese medicine for gallstones and almost died as a result of his treatment.

Both Mrs. Yan and her husband think that Chinese medicine is troublesome to take. They say that it takes too much time to boil the medicines and that the decoctions taste unpleasant. They both think that Western medicine is far superior in treating acute diseases and symptomatic problems, and that Chinese medicine is more suitable for the treatment of chronic ailments and deep causes. They furthermore hold that Chinese medicine can be trusted, if at all, only if practiced by an experienced physician.

We already know that many Chinese share the evaluations of Chinese and Western medicine voiced by Zhennan's parents. In their opposition of the West, technology, and speed with tradition, craftsmanship, and slowness they capture an experience of modernization that can be imagined as having condensed into—take your pick—cultural stereotypes, folk theories, or semantic networks. These stereotypes (folk theories, semantic networks) appear stable in the face of contradictory experience (Chinese medicine consistently treats Zhennan's acute fever more successfully than Western medicine), thereby confirming their usefulness—to us as social scientists—as explanatory devices. Yet, they do not account for the actual behavior of Zhennan's parents. Mrs. Yan, eventually, and with the consent of her husband, who does not believe in Chinese medicine, will take Zhennan to a doctor of Chinese medicine. Zhennan's life, after all, is worth more than a belief. Mrs. Yan's husband's antipathy to Chinese medicine and the parents' shared perception regarding its inconvenience, however, prevents Mrs. Yan from trying to cure

Zhennan's illness more permanently with the help of Chinese medicine. This in spite of many factors that would suggest such a course of action: Mrs. Yan has accepted the Chinese doctor's explanation for the illness of her son and has herself benefited from such treatment in the past; treatment of the root (*ben* 本) of an illness is a commonly agreed upon strong point of Chinese medicine; and even Zhennan's father trusts the Chinese doctor, whom he regards highly.

Mrs. Yan informed us that she is finally considering a more prolonged course of Chinese medical treatment for her son, in spite of all the reasons that have made her avoid it so far. What seems to me to account for this conversion is not a change of a specific explanatory model or a sudden restructuring of Mrs. Yan's belief system, but a reevaluation of what is more and what is less important and a shift of balance in the various struggles she is engaged in: with her husband, who does not believe in Chinese medicine; with her son, who dislikes taking herbs; and with herself, for she must make time available to prepare the medicine. It is an understanding of these struggles (whose processual nature is all too obvious in Zhennan's case), not a mere mapping of semantic structures, that takes us closer to understanding why patients act the way they do.

My next case also speaks of struggles—struggles that characterize the interaction between patients and physicians during the clinical encounter. By using the word "struggle" I do not intend to portray this encounter as in any way confrontational. In fact, physicians of Chinese medicine and their patients appeared to me as mostly cooperative and as accepting one another's unique contributions to the health-seeking process. Nevertheless, as Zhennan's case has already taught us, there is more at stake in such encounters than the search for a prescription.

CASE 4.2. *Mr. Zhou Has To Take His Medicine.* Mr. Zhou is a tall and burly farmer in his sixties. Following a myocardial infarction he was treated as an inpatient on one of the Chinese medicine wards of the China-Japan Friendship Hospital. Mr. Zhou lived on the ward for more than three months. Such an extended period of treatment is not unusual, especially for those who come some distance to seek the capital's superior medical facilities. Allocation to this ward had not been Mr. Zhou's choice or that of his family but that of the hospital administration. At the time of admission there was simply no bed available in a Western medicine ward, the preference of Mr. Zhou's family. On the Chinese medicine ward he was treated with a combination of Western and Chinese medical drugs. I met Mr. Zhou during his first visit to the hospital as an outpatient following his release two weeks earlier. He consulted Dr. Guo, a doctor in his late fifties and assistant consultant (*fuzhuren* 副主任) in the hospital department to which the ward on which Mr. Zhou had been treated belongs. Mr. Zhou still suffered from high blood pressure, headaches, tinnitus, and leg edema. Dr. Guo made a Chinese medical diagnosis of kidney and liver *yin* depletion (*shen gan yinxu* 肾肝阴虚), ascendant liver *yang* (*ganyang shang kang* 肝阳上亢), and phlegm and [blood] stasis obstructing the network vessels (*tanyu zu luo* 痰瘀阻络). He explained the diagnosis to his students and wrote out a herbal prescription to be decocted, a variation of *Qi ju dihuang wan* 杞菊地黄丸 (Lycium Fruit, Chrysanthemum, and Rhemannia Pill).[5] Mr. Zhou politely declined. He indicated that he prefers Western drugs because they are more convenient to take. A short discussion ensued about the benefits and disadvantages of Chinese medicine. At its conclusion Dr. Guo, a very gentle and nonaggressive person, surrendered to Mr. Zhou's demands and prescribed a beta blocker and a diuretic. After Mr. Zhou had left, Dr. Guo explained to us that there is no use arguing with a person who is unlikely to comply with treatment he does not like.

Several weeks later I was studying with another physician, Professor Sun. Professor Sun, fifty-eight, is the senior consultant (*zhuren* 主任) of another ward within the hospital's Chinese medicine section. She is a considerably more forceful person than Dr. Guo, who, in spite of his age, occupies a relatively junior position in the hospital's hierarchy. Professor Sun also seemed to be a much more popular and successful physician. During an average morning session she always treated more than twenty patients and had to turn away many others, while Dr. Guo never had more than five or six patients. Mr. Zhou had transferred to Professor Sun because his symptoms had not substantially improved since his consultation with Dr. Guo. He therefore had decided to pay slightly more for a consultation with a more senior physician. Again he asked for Western medicine drugs. Professor Sun, however, was quite adamant that Mr. Zhou should take Chinese medicine in addition to his other drugs. She told him that otherwise he would not get better. At first Mr. Zhou resisted, but in the end Professor Sun won the argument. Professor Sun's Chinese medical diagnosis was similar to that of Dr. Guo although in her therapeutic approach she placed greater emphasis on treating phlegm and blood stasis. This was reflected in the fact that she used a variation of *Danggui shaoyao san* 当归芍药散 (*Tangkuei* and Peony Powder), a blood-

and fluid-regulating formula, as the basis of her treatment.[6] Mr. Zhou went home with Chinese medicine sufficient for two weeks' treatment. He returned a fortnight later. Because he felt significantly better, he asked for more of the decoction.

Mr. Zhou's case reminds us that therapy is an open-ended process involving performative choices at various levels. The authority that Professor Sun displayed in her encounter with Mr. Zhou exceeded that of Dr. Guo because, unlike the latter, she could and did marshal resources (her personal charisma, her patient's fears, her status in the hospital hierarchy, her greater confidence in her clinical skills) that encouraged Mr. Zhou's compliance with her treatment. Both physicians practice Chinese medicine, but their craft is clearly not the same. Professor Sun's task was considerably facilitated, of course, by the fact that Mr. Zhou's symptoms had not improved after treatment with Western medicine alone.

Clinical encounters thus become intelligible only as particular constellations in space-time, conjunctions of the temporal development of a patient's quest for health and the trajectory of a physician's career as well as the institutional spaces in which therapeutic encounters take place. Mr. Zhou came to see Dr. Guo not because of his status as a practitioner of Chinese medicine but because Mr. Zhou had previously been treated successfully in the department of which Dr. Guo is a member. He now had a personal relationship with this department and, by implication, its physicians. It is for this reason that he did not go to the Western medicine department even though he wanted Western medicine.[7] Due to the hospital's administrative setup, the physicians who had treated him on the ward were not available for consultations in the outpatient department. This meant that Mr. Zhou had to seek out a new physician. Had Mr. Zhou's symptoms improved after his first visit, he most likely would have returned to the care of Dr. Guo. Had Dr. Guo been a more effective or more charismatic physician, he might have been able to do for Mr. Zhou what Professor Sun did for him later on.[8]

Mr. Zhou's preference for Western medicine treatment, finally, was based not primarily on considerations of efficacy but on matters of convenience. Economies of effort linked to evaluations of pleasure or discomfort play an important role in choosing where and when to consult a physician and what course of treatment to pursue. When I visited an acupuncture department at a Chinese medicine hospital in Chengdu in 1992 I was surprised at the small number of patients. "It's raining," I was told. "It's simply too troublesome for patients to come." Whether or not, where and when one should go to see a doctor depends on whether the effort justifies the expected outcome. Mr. Gao, a fifty-eight-year-old researcher I interviewed, had been successfully treated by acupuncture for his shoulder pain. Nevertheless he decided to discontinue his treatment. "I was supposed to go back for another ten times, but the weather got colder," he told us. "I was too lazy to go to the hospital. I practiced *taiji-quan* 太气拳 every morning. It, too, helped my shoulder."

Anybody who has ever been to China knows the effort involved in organizing even the most ordinary lives. Getting up early, traveling to the hospital, and having to wait in a long line to register with a physician and later to collect one's prescription adds considerably to this burden. Patients who attended Dr. Zheng's Tuesday morning surgery in a pharmacy in a busy Beijing shopping precinct did not necessarily come to see him personally as "their" doctor or as a "physician of Chinese medicine." They came because it was more convenient to go to the pharmacy—and perhaps combine it with some shopping—than to queue up at the hospital. Hence, although Dr. Zheng was officially running a Chinese medicine surgery (opened by the pharmacy to increase its sale of Chinese medical drugs), many patients asked for Western drugs. Dr. Zheng, who had studied Western medicine before being ordered to study Chinese medicine in 1956, had no ideological problems with this. Nevertheless, he prescribed Chinese drugs whenever possible. After all, this was what he had been hired to do.[9]

Patients like Mr. Zhou have their own ideas of what treatment should be like based on what has been effective in the past, what has helped a neighbor, or what causes the least disruption to their daily routines. They may ask for a particular prescription, or for pills rather than decoctions because they do not want to be bothered with boiling herbs. Their physicians have to respond, sometimes giving in, sometimes not, adapting individually but, as we shall see in due course, changing the practice of Chinese medicine cumulatively in the process.

Physicians and patients do not meet one another in a vacuum. They meet within physical and institutional spaces created for them rather than by them. Struggle, then, is not an engagement merely with self (case 4.1) or other (case 4.2), but also with the spaces in which the two meet. This is exemplified particularly clearly by case 4.3.

CASE 4.3. *Mr. Ke's Search for the "Eleventh-Floor Ward."* Mr. Ke, forty-nine, suffers from chronic nephritis. I met him in the outpatient clinic of Professor Zhu, a specialist who treats the disease with integrated Chinese and Western medicine. Previously, Mr. Ke had been treated as an inpatient in the ward of which Professor Zhu is director (located on the eleventh floor of the hospital). In the course of our conversation Mr. Ke told me repeatedly that "the eleventh-floor ward" had saved his life. It transpired that prior to his admission to Professor Zhu's ward he had been treated for several months on a Western medicine ward on the sixth floor of the same hospital. Before that, he had been an inpatient for several months of another Beijing hospital of Chinese medicine. Treatment at these institutions had produced no notable results. Only after admission to Professor Zhu's ward had his condition (the most notable symptoms of which at the time of his admission had been severe edema of the entire body and loss of mental functioning) begun to improve.

Mr. Ke's first choice of hospital had been determined by the fact that his work-unit has a contract with this institution. He had then moved to the Western medicine ward of Professor Zhu's hospital because it is widely known to be one of the most modern and technologically well-equipped hospitals in Beijing. His transfer within that hospital from the sixth-floor Western medicine ward to the eleventh-floor Chinese medicine ward had been his wife's decision, based on word-of-mouth recommendation from other patients within the hospital. At each point of his journey Mr. Ke had been treated with Western medical drugs. In the Chinese medicine wards he had also taken Chinese medical decoctions. What medicines or combination of medicines he had been treated with seemed of secondary importance to Mr. Ke and his wife. What they had searched for and ultimately found was "the eleventh-floor ward," an institution capable of producing the desired outcome. Now that they had found it, they expressed their appreciation and loyalty by heaping praise on Dr. Zhu in front of his other patients.

Mr. Ke's initial choice of institution was determined by structural factors operating through the health insurance system. Of the three major types of health insurance found in modern China, worker insurance for enterprise workers (laodong baoxian 劳动保险) was the most common in Beijing during the period of my fieldwork.[10] It is funded by the organization, department, or enterprise (referred to in Chinese as gongzuo danwei 工作单位, work-unit), which provides it to employees in the form of individually variable benefits attached to a basic salary. According to the financial resources of each individual work-unit as well as a person's job status, insurance companies refund a fixed share of employee's health care expenses, which can range from 10 to 100 percent under the terms of such policies. In order to reduce a growing burden placed on insurers by epidemiological changes, demands for "high-technology medicine," and the rising costs of drugs, work-units have instituted a series of restrictive measures over recent years: cutting the share of the insurer's contributions, monitoring treatment by work-unit physicians, and entering into contracts with specific hospitals and clinics to buy health care at discounted rates. As a result, patient choice has been severely curtailed. It is becoming increasingly common, for instance, for work-units to vet therapeutic procedures, a measure that had caused a significant drop in patient numbers at all the Chinese medicine clinics I visited. Furthermore, many patients are now limited to care at contracted institutions.[11]

This had been the case with Mr. Ke, who had been admitted to a Chinese medicine hospital not because of his preference for Chinese medical care but because it provided the facilities he needed under the terms of his insurance. Only as his condition deteriorated did Mr. and Mrs. Ke begin to mobilize alternative resources. This included the private financing of inpatient care at another hospital and the selection of an appropriate institution. This time the choice was guided by the second hospital's reputation for having available high-tech diagnostic resources. Mr. and Mrs. Ke believed that these facilities might detect what had gone unnoticed at first hospital. The sixth-floor ward was chosen because it dealt with the "disease" from which Mr. Ke was suffering. It was only after Mr. Ke had been an inpatient at the second hospital for some time that, motivated by continued treatment failure, he and his wife began to discern differences within that institution of which they previously had not been aware. This, finally, initiated the move to the eleventh-floor ward.

Mr. and Mrs. Ke's choices at each stage of their journey depended on events that evolved as treatment unfolded: continued therapeutic failure, sourcing of funds, making contact with other patients, getting to know the institution. Efficacy attributions concerning the supposed properties of specific medical practices directed the decision-making process at some of its stages. At no point of their peregrination, however, did such beliefs exhaust the input into this process. The final case study, in which I was myself involved as an actor, makes this particularly clear. It shows that patient behavior, at any moment in time, emerges as the tactical utilization of a variety of available resources by the ill and their social networks.

CASE 4.4. *Mr. Li Attempts to Cure a Cold.* Mr. Li, thirty-one and originally from the countryside near Chongqing, Sichuan Province, suffers from a chronic knee ache. At the time I met him he worked as a handyman at the university. His income was very low (about Y200 per month in 1994) and did not include any health insurance. His sister worked as a porter in the guest house in which I lived during my fieldwork and Mr. Li and his wife occupied a bedroom in the same building. Thus, we got to know each other quite well. One day Mr. Li asked me if I might be able to help his knee pain. Previously, he had tried Western medicine and had also received acupuncture from another student at the guest house, neither of which had relieved his pain. I agreed and, fortunately, my acupuncture proved more successful. After that (and also because my services were provided free of charge), I was adopted as occasional physician by a small circle of family members and friends.

About two months after I had treated him for his knees Li got a summer cold. One evening he came to my room and asked if I could write out a prescription for him. The cold had started two days previously and bothered him because of the relative severity of the symptoms. These included renewed aching in the knees, headache, fever, daytime sweating, extreme lethargy, thirst, and a bitter taste in the mouth. After the onset of the first symptoms Li had self-prescribed a combination of Western (aspirin) and Chinese medicines (*Yin qiao wan* 银翘丸 (Honeysuckle and Forsythia Pills).[12] Both are common household remedies for colds and flu. The symptoms got worse, however, and he consulted a Chinese medicine physician (a friend of a friend) at the outpatient clinic attached to the university located about two hundred meters away from our building.

This doctor's prescription also had no effect. At this point Li turned to me for help. I treated him with acupuncture and also wrote out a Chinese medicine prescription. In order for him to buy these drugs at the dispensary of the university clinic rather than at the nearest pharmacy (more than a kilometer away), Li needed to procure for me an official prescription form from the clinic. This took about half a day and required Li to utilize various personal connections. Following my treatment his severe symptoms got better. He came back the next day, and I gave him another prescription, but this time it took him a day and a half to buy the herbs. Over the weekend the pharmacy at the university clinic was closed, Li was in bed, his wife was at work, and he did not find anyone else to buy the herbs for him. Li thus self-prescribed some more drugs he had at home (aspirin, Contac, *Yin qiao wan*, and *Huoxiang zhengqi pian* 藿香正气片, or Agastache Tablet to Rectify the *Qi*).[13] After three days his fever and aches had gone but he now had a cough and was still sweating. At this point he returned to the doctor at the university clinic and asked for antibiotics as well as Chinese medicine. After four more days of taking a combination of prescribed and self-prescribed drugs his symptoms had cleared sufficiently for him to declare himself well again and discontinue treatment.

Throughout the course of his short illness, Li's choice of practitioner and treatment failed to conform to academic and popular explanations of illness behavior in Chinese cultures. These hold that Western medicine is generally preferred over Chinese medicine treatment, particularly in the treatment of acute diseases and where quick results are desired. Mr. Li, however, never even looked for a Western medicine physician. This was not because he had any particular ideological or experiential attachment to Chinese medicine. He told me that although his native village had a good Chinese medicine doctor, he personally had never consulted him. He had taken antibiotics on several occasions. He was conversant with basic concepts of Chinese medicine theory but had little systematic knowledge of it. Whatever he knew of *yin/yang*, hot/cold, and seasonal influences was of a practical nature and applied to basic rules regarding diet and lifestyle.

Li's therapeutic quest, I believe, acquires meaning only if it is viewed like any other task he might be engaged in. It was directed toward achieving an effect and implied the negotiation of simultaneously or successively occurring dilemmas of various kinds. Choices had to be made regarding expenditure of money and effort, and real and potential efficacy had to be evaluated. Face had to be negotiated. Social networks had to be brought into play, calling in previously accumulated debts and making new ones.

Li first treated himself. He seemed to be suffering from a minor illness, and self-medication required the utilization of the least number of resources. Only when the symptoms persisted did he seek professional help. The easiest option for Li was to go to the university clinic where he had connections to a physician. I am not sure why he did not come to see me first, as he had done so for several minor complaints up to then. The difficulty in obtaining the herbs I prescribed is one possible explanation and certainly was a main reason why he reverted back to his first doctor. Efficacy attributions of which I am not aware are another. Each switch of practitioners was also influenced by his evaluation of how they were managing his case and what drugs they could prescribe.[14]

Li's case also highlights patients' scant regard for the sanctity of medical traditions. Li was eclectic in combining the tools at hand until he achieved what he desired. Being less severely but more acutely ill than Mr. Ke allowed but also demanded of him to be more flexible in changing practitioners quickly. Unlike Mr. Zhou, the relations he mobilized predated his illness rather than emerged from it. Whether or not clinical results were due to aspirin, *yin qiao wan*, a needle, time, the skills of particular physicians, or a combination of some or all of the above mattered less to Mr. Li, Mr. and Mrs. Ke, and Mr. Zhou than that something worked at all.[15] Drug manufacturers understand this and supply combinations of popular Chinese medicine and Western medicine drugs (e.g., aspirin, vitamin C, and *yin qiao san*) in one product. Physicians understand this, too, of course. Both Chinese medicine and Western medicine physicians routinely combine Chinese medicine and Western medicine drugs. It is a practice firmly established in the Chinese medicine canon since the turn of the century and something about which I shall have much to say later.

Patients in China, furthermore, do not perceive medical traditions as homogeneous. As the common proverb, "If you are thinking of having Western medicine take care to examine the institution; if you are thinking of having Chinese medicine take care to examine the physician" (*Xiyi kan men, zhongyi kan ren* 西医看门, 中医看人) indicates, Chinese people take great care in choosing practitioners and hospitals. Knowledge about the skills and background of individual physicians and the advantages and disadvantages of attending specific hospitals or clinics circulates widely in the public domain and is actively utilized as a resource for making therapeutic decisions. The Guang'anmen Hospital 广安门医院 in the south of Beijing thus is known for its treatment of hemorrhoids, while the Beijing City Chinese Medicine Hospital has famous liver disease specialists. Some doctors I observed treated more than seventy patients during a morning session and turned away many more, while others in the same department rarely saw more than half a dozen.

Another proverb dating back to the Spring and Autumn period but still in common usage admonishes: "Do not take the drugs of a physician who is not practicing in the third generation" (*Yi bu san shi, bu fu qi yao* 医不三世, 不服其药).[16] Physicians, now as ever, emphasize their pedigree through real or invented genealogies and connections to famous teachers. If no descent can be claimed, special therapeutic techniques and the possession of secret prescriptions will do. A doctor in the Chinese medicine department of a small hospital close to Xidan, in the west of the city, claimed to have invented thirty prescriptions that were so successful that he could not use them in his hospital because it would make his colleagues jealous. Individual physicians and entire hospital departments are engaged in research projects searching for formulas that will establish their fame and reputation. In waiting rooms all over Beijing patients trade information about the doctors they see and make mental notes of what is said about whom.

As the vision of a socialist new medicine in which everyone is treated equally and has access to the same resources gives way to medical care based on the forces of a (socialist) market economy, difference is not only emphasized by physicians but sought after and created by the consumers of health care themselves. Newly rich patients display their wealth by purchasing expensive tonics, often presented as gifts, and by consulting famous physicians at extravagant expense.[17] The wife of a rich businessman in Shenzhen regularly flies to Beijing to be treated by one of my teachers even for minor colds. She is joined there by patients from Singapore, Hongkong, Taiwan, Vancouver, and the highest Beijing cadres. I noted above that some practitioners have opened lucrative private practices. Hospitals compete for the services of *ming laozhongyi* by allowing them to keep their consultation fees, while the institutions profit from the sale of medicines and an increase in corporate status.[18] Certain sections of the contemporary Chinese medicine world, it appears, have joined Rémy Martin, Mercedes Benz, and the latest medical technologies from the West in functioning as expensive consumer items through which the new Chinese elite defines itself.

Changing Presentations of Being Unwell

My analysis so far has focused on individual behavior in order to argue against simplistic oppositions between distinct alternatives in a pluralistic Chinese health care system. Furthermore, I have presented patients not as passive recipients of therapy or, at best, as rational choosers or creative resisters, but as agents who actively participate in their quest for therapy.[19] I now affirm and extend this shift of perception by examining briefly how individually and locally realized patient pressures can effect transformations that may appear —from a different perspective—as transformations of cultural forms. Changing presentations of being unwell and the adaptations this has demanded and is demanding from Chinese medicine practitioners provides a convenient focus for such an inquiry.

Although health preservation constitutes an important aspect of Chinese popular culture, its practice—with the exception of state-controlled disease prevention programs such as mass immunization and pest control—is a private matter. Contrary to certain Western stereotypes, Chinese patients visit their doctors only when absolutely necessary.[20] Expenditure of money and effort, unwillingness to admit weakness in a culture where the endurance of physical discomfort has often been viewed as a virtue, and "white coat syndrome" (feeling uncomfortable in the presence of physicians) all are relevant factors.[21]

Patients thus come to Chinese medicine clinics for the relief of symptoms and the curing of disease. In observing more than four thousand individual consultations I never once witnessed a person attending merely for illness prevention. It was always a bodily function experienced as disordered, a problem interfering with daily activities, or a sudden medical emergency that necessitated the visit to a hospital or clinic. The language through which these patients expressed their discomforts conjoined discourses on illness with distinctly different roots. Many symptoms were reported in terms synonymous with the specialist lexicon of Chinese medical symptoms and signs: *fanzao* 烦燥 (vexation), *paleng* 怕冷 or *pafeng* 怕风 (aversion to cold or wind), *xiongmen* 胸闷 (a stifling sensation in the chest), *suantong* 酸痛 (muscle aching as distinct from pain), *erming* 耳鸣 (tinnitus), and so on. At other times, the standard opening question of the Chinese medicine physician, "What's wrong with you today, then?" (*Jintian shenme bu hao* 今天什么不好) or "What's bothering you?" (*You shenme bu shufu* 有什么不舒服) elicited answers in which a physical sign reported by the patient named the disease in the lexicon of Chinese medicine. Such answers can thus be translated without loss of meaning as both; for example, "My periods are irregular" and "irregular periods" (*yuejing bu tiao* 月经不调), "I've got a stomachache" and "stomach ache" (*weiteng* 胃疼), "cough" (*kesou* 咳嗽), and so on.[22]

Description and analysis in Chinese medicine thus continue to remain close to the body experienced by its patients.[23] Hence, as Farquhar has already shown, patients of Chinese medicine in contemporary China retain a considerable degree of authority in delimiting the parameters of their illness, and the close match between lay and professional vocabularies can be interpreted as a condensation of this cooperative effort.[24] These close articulations between lay and professional discourse are changing rapidly, however. The patients I observed in Beijing had begun to integrate into their understanding and presentation of being unwell categories of experience that were neither specifically "Chinese" nor resonant with modes of explanation in classical medicine. While languages of body were still replete with classical idioms, biomedical signs and disease categories—more distant from the acute experience of the lived body—made up an increasing percentage of the complaints of patients arriving for their first consultation. A patient might present with dizziness (*touyun* 头晕)—according to Ots a category that can be properly understood only in relation to Chinese concerns with balance and equilib-

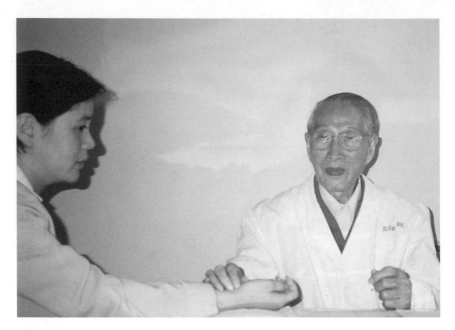

FIGURE 19. Pulse diagnosis by famous *laozhongyi* Shen Zhongli, Yueyang Hospital, Shanghai

rium—but mention equally quickly that he had high blood pressure and proteinuria.[25]

The same syncretism can be observed in the kinds of investigative procedures demanded by patients. Those who consult a Chinese medicine doctor want to have their pulse taken. "Have a good feel of my pulse" (*Haohao mo mai* 好好摸脉), they urge their physicians encouragingly. They still expect their doctor to arrive at a profound diagnosis by this most emblematic of Chinese medicine diagnostic technologies.[26] But increasingly they also bring to the clinical encounter evidence from previous biomedical exams with which they expect their Chinese medicine physicians to be conversant: X-rays, CT scans, ECGs, ultrasound, blood and urine tests. If such tests have not already been carried out, they demand them, particularly in the larger teaching hospitals that have the necessary technological resources.[27]

Chinese patients enjoy relatively free access to their medical records and are surprisingly familiar with the quantitative parameters of their problems (surprisingly, of course, only if compared with the average patient in Britain). Patients in contemporary China take a keen interest in their bodies. They are able to provide their physicians with information about the functioning of various physiological processes that demand detailed attention and mental record keeping. Chinese patients spontaneously differentiate whether they sweat excessively during the day (*zihan* 自汗) or at night (*daohan* 盗汗), whether their chest feels stuffy (*men* 闷), distended (*zhang* 胀), or full (*man* 满). Women know precisely on what day their last menstrual bleeding started, when it finished, and how long their menstrual cycle is—details that in my own clinical experience require American, British, or German women to check their calendars.

Whether or not this kind of bodily awareness indicates a tendency of Chinese patients to somatize their disorders, whether it is a habit reflecting centuries of Chinese medicine diagnostic practice that begins its own inquiries from the experienced body of its patients, or whether it reflects more general cognitive skills is not a question I wish to pursue at this juncture.[28] It is sufficient to note that an interest in and mental record keeping of biomedical disease parameters is not, in principle, different from tracking and communicating subjectively defined signs. As a result, Chinese medicine physicians increasingly must convince their patients not only by reducing dizziness and stopping diarrhea but also by lowering blood pressure, keeping blood sugar levels within expected limits, and reducing immunoglobulin plasma concentrations. With respect to causal explanation such syncretism has moved even further in the direction of biomedical models. Biomedical disease labels can

FIGURE 20. Pulse diagnosis, Longhua Hospital, Shanghai

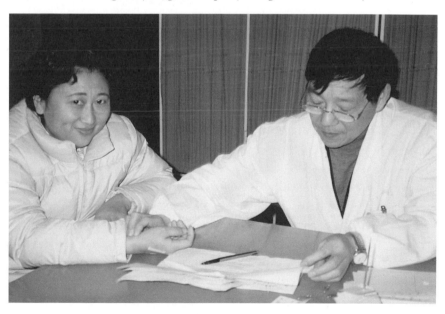

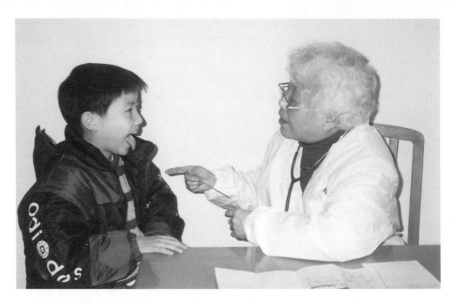

FIGURE 21. Tongue diagnosis, Longhua Hospital, Shanghai

become overarching organizational categories in people's illness narratives to which other concepts are subsumed.

"Two years ago I got a shoulder inflammation [*jianyan* 肩炎]. It hurt severely." This is a description of a medical problem offered during a consultation I observed. The patient here labels his problem first using a bio-medically derived explanatory concept and only then goes on to describe its experiential dimensions. "Coronary heart disease" (*xinzangbing* 心脏病), "diabetes" (*tangniaobing* 糖尿病), and "hepatitis" (*ganyan* 肝炎) were common complaints with which patients introduced their health problems. Many patients, of course, began their narratives not with a disease label but with experiential accounts. Chinese medical diagnostic patterns (*zhenghou* 证侯) such as "spleen depletion" (*pixu* 脾虚) or "static blood" (*yuxue* 瘀血), however, were never put forward as reasons for attending a doctor during any of the consultations I observed.

Many doctors, especially those less experienced and still struggling to find their feet, lamented that patients no longer understand the meaning of Chinese medical patterns. They felt that they could not explain to their patients what was wrong in Chinese medical terms and that—at least for the purpose of explanation—they needed to fit Chinese medicine pattern differentiation into Western disease models. Older doctors rarely made such complaints. This may be because they commanded more respect from their

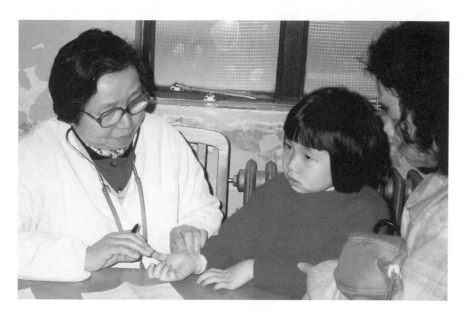

FIGURE 22. Hand diagnosis, Longhua Hospital, Shanghai

patients, or perhaps they were simply more experienced in providing satisfactory explanations. They, too, confirmed to me, however, that as time goes by, the man and woman in the street know less and less about Chinese medicine.

Historical comparisons show how profound the changes are. Case histories from the end of the Republican era, for instance, still contain numerous examples of debates between physicians and family households over a particular diagnosis or choice of drugs. At that time it was not unusual for a family to invite several physicians to "submit a record" (tou an 投案) of the patient's case outlining diagnosis and treatment recommendations, on which the family would then deliberate before choosing which course of treatment to follow. The doctors themselves frequently used these records in their writings as evidence for the superiority of their own knowledge. The following case by Zhang Xichun 张锡纯, one of the most influential physicians of the time, provides a telling example: "On examination the [patient's] pulse was thin like a thread, even more so on the right hand. I [immediately] knew that this was [a case of] sinking of the great qi and intended to treat it with the [appropriate] formula. The patient's household asked in disbelief: '[Among] previous physicians, no one ever spoke of so called sinking of the great qi. And even if the cause of the disease were sinking of the great qi, how could it account for the various symptoms?'"[29]

Needless to say, Zhang managed to convince the household of his new

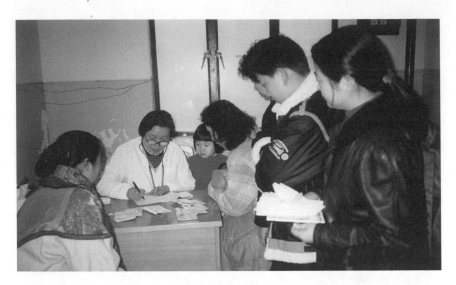

FIGURE 23. Writing a prescription, Longhua Hospital, Shanghai

theory and cured the patient. During almost eighteen months of fieldwork I encountered only four patients who displayed the necessary erudition to engage their physicians in similar discussions.[30] The knowledge of Chinese medicine possessed by most patients seemed to be limited to a basic familiarity with concepts like *qi,* "kidneys" (*shen* 肾), and "depletion" (*xu* 虚). These still carry important connotations in popular discourses about health, disease, and aging that are derived from Chinese medicine but are not synonymous with it. If a commercially produced tonic, therefore, carries on its label the claim that it "supplements *qi* and blood, strengthens kidney *qi,* eliminates wind damp, removes cold obstructions, moves *qi* stagnation, transforms blood stasis, firms and strengthens the back and knees, fortifies the bones and rejuvenates the disposition," this does not necessarily imply an intimate familiarity with Chinese medicine theory on behalf of its consumers. In fact, the list of indications (rather than actions) is more likely to read as follows: "Back and knee pain and a general decrease of vitality. (Corresponding to Western medicine diagnoses such as hyperplastic inflammation of the spine, rheumatoid arthritis, sciatica . . .)."[31]

That presentations of being unwell in China have changed over time and continue to do so today is beyond doubt. Linking individual acts of symptom reporting to global changes of practice may seem more difficult to substantiate. Unequivocal evidence attesting to just such an influence, however, can be found in the writings of some of modern China's most influential physicians and teachers of Chinese medicine. From the 1950s onward, leading faculty at the Beijing College of Chinese Medicine, including Qin Bowei 秦伯未 and Zhu Chenyu 祝谌予 (of whom we shall learn more in chapter 7), began to argue for the assimilation of biomedical diagnostics into Chinese medical practice, specifically noting that in order to retain the trust of a clientele increasingly consulting them for biomedically defined problems, it was insufficient merely to be familiar with Western medicine theory. Rather, such theory had to be actively integrated into the delivery of Chinese medicine in clinical contexts.[32]

Qin and Zhu quickly turned these pronouncements into practice, although their individual syntheses did not, therefore, totally agree.[33] By the time I carried out my fieldwork almost forty years later, the assimilation of Western into Chinese medicine had become routine. It was visible not only in clinical practice (described in detail in chapter 5) but also in the ways physicians advertised themselves to their patients. This can be easily observed, for instance, in the entrance lobbies of hospitals and clinics, where the names of all consultants are listed together with their specialities and surgery hours. Descriptions of such specialities can be sorted into three large groups:

1. Terms indicating expertise in the treatment of specific classical nosological entities such as "obstruction patterns" (bizheng 痹证) or "atrophy patterns" (weizheng 痿证) or in a distinctly Chinese medical speciality such as "miscellaneous diseases" (zabing 杂病).
2. Terms indicating expertise in the treatment of biomedically defined

FIGURE 24. Acupuncture treatment, Mingyitang Clinic, Shanghai

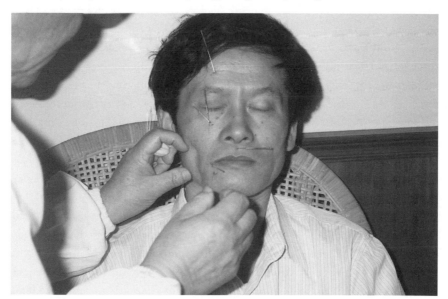

disorders such as "diabetes" (*tangniaobing* 糖尿病) and "thyroid disorders" (*jiazhuangxian jibing* 甲壮腺疾病), or systems such as "diseases of the respiratory system" (*huxi xitong bing* 呼吸系统病).

3. Polysemic terms that may be taken to refer to either Chinese or Western medicine, such as "kidney disease" (*shen bing* 肾病) or "gynecology" (*fuke* 妇科), or terms that are, strictly speaking, Chinese medical terms but evoke biomedical disease names. An example is "wind damp" (*fengshi* 风湿), which evokes "rheumatoid arthritis" (*leifengshi* 类风湿).[34]

Almost all physicians use terms taken from groups 2 and 3. At the Dongzhimen Hospital I found only one practitioner who advertised himself entirely with terms from group 1, while at the China-Japan Friendship Hospital I found none. The only addressees of such advertisements arc, of course, patients. Taken together with the statements discussed above, this allows me to argue with some conviction that political process—on which previous commentators have concentrated—is an important but by no means exclusive factor shaping contemporary Chinese medicine. Grassroots pressure for a more modern Chinese medicine expressed locally by patients through such mechanisms as practitioner selection, demand for certain kinds of diagnosis or treatment, or simply through bringing to the clinical encounter certain kinds of problems cannot be ignored.

Tactics, Performances, and Dilemmas

That patients actively shape the medical systems they employ is not yet widely accepted in anthropological theory. Initial accounts of illness behavior in plural medical systems were based on rational choice models that saw patients as choosing between objectively existing alternatives on the basis of their health beliefs. The complicated plurality of actual health care systems and the complexity of patient behavior in contemporary China seriously undermines the validity of such models and confirms similar criticisms that have been advanced on the basis of ethnographic observations of therapeutic practice in many other contexts.[35]

The structure/agency dilemma at the heart of classical social theory has been identified as generating the contradictions intrinsic to all health belief and culture theory models of health-seeking behavior. In response, critical medical anthropologists have tried to produce accounts of medical systems that collapse local and global levels of explanation through ethnographies that create a continuum stretching from the phenomenology of individual life-worlds to the local and global political forces that order, destabilize, and

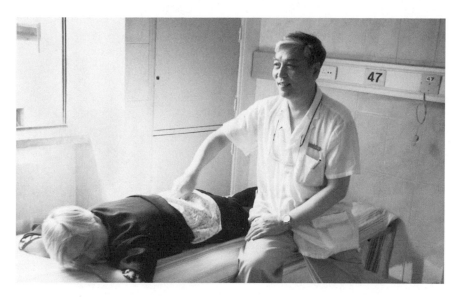

FIGURE 25. Tuina treatment, Anhui University of Chinese Medicine, Hefei

often violate these worlds. These anthropologists have thereby succeeded in showing how macrosocial forces insert themselves, often obliquely, into personal worlds of suffering and local therapeutic actions. Local experiences of body/self are commonly identified as potential foci of critique and resistance to such domination, and patients' agency is sometimes depicted as one of heroic struggle against such domination. Generally, though, a more pessimistic undertone questions the real power of this resistance. In the end, marginalized and dominated people can undermine but not ultimately overcome the global powers that shape their lives.[36]

The work of critical medical anthropologists, like that of other postcolonial and poststructural writers, thus takes up a politically problematic stance. Wishing to appear progressive by identifying hegemonic regimes of power, many authors working within these traditions nevertheless appear to accept the ultimate fallibility of grassroots power. Hence, critique rarely leads to actual models for how change might realistically be accomplished. Furthermore, by construing the outsider/anthropologist as capable of transcending the limited perspectives of local actors, critical medical anthropologists all too often perpetuate the problematic emic/etic discourse of previous social theory. Finally, the particular view of resistance implicit in these models—romanticizing it without according to it real and autonomous power—is a sign that in the end they do not succeed in overcoming the monist discourse of all world systems narrative.[37]

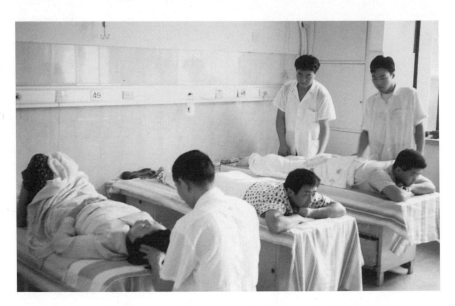

FIGURE 26. Tuina department, Anhui University of Chinese Medicine, Hefei

I do not for a moment deny the political and economic powers of globally operating forces such as the biomedical-industrial complex. Yet, as recent grassroots activism in the Western world demonstrates, I believe one does not have to be quite as pessimistic about the effects of local agencies on global regimes of power.[38] Here, my model of emergent synthesis offers a viable alternative. The evidence I have presented allows me to argue that what is available to individual patients in the official health care sector and the options they choose between are the resources of specific institutions and the skills of individual physicians. Such institutions and physicians represent globally constituted powers inasmuch as they are integrated into health care systems at national or even international levels of synthesis formation. When they come into contact with individual patients, however, each physician and each hospital constitutes a local infrastructure.

At the global level of synthetic emergence, the input of individual patients into the transformation of medical systems or traditions is usually negligible.[39] Hence, patients did not feature in chapter 3, where I discussed the transformations of Chinese medicine from a political and economic perspective. At the local level of the concrete clinical encounter, patients' influence on health care delivery becomes increasingly stronger, however. This influence is amplified in health care systems in which patients can draw on real alternatives, where they can easily move from one physician and one style of therapy to another. By demanding of physicians and institutions certain kinds of treatment and diagnosis and refusing others, patients can and do shape the delivery of local health care practice. These local changes can feed back into syntheses operating at higher levels of organization (most easily into local institutions but also into the more global syntheses) because local physicians and health care providers are infrastructures that participate in their formation. It is thus that patients, too, shape the transformation of medical systems over time.

I have used the assimilation of Western medical disease categories and diagnostic technologies into Chinese medicine as examples to demonstrate this process. The physicians I cited as responding to patient pressure, Qin Bowei and Zhu Chenyu, were opinion formers whose influence extended from personal teaching and the writing of textbooks to the formulation of health care policy. As such they were exposed to patient pressure not merely in their own practices but also in the demands transmitted through students, colleagues, and politicians. All of the physicians with whom I spoke in China agreed that patients' demands for the use of modern technology in diagnosis and treatment (such as electro-acupuncture) or for more modern types of drug application (pills rather than awful-tasting and difficult-to-prepare decoctions) have had a definite impact on the shaping of Chinese medicine. Nor is such pressure a new phenomenon in the history of Chinese medicine, as an example taken from the case histories of Fei Shengfu 费绳甫 (1851–1914) demonstrates.

Fei Shengfu, a famous physician of the influential Menghe 孟河 medical stream, practiced in Jiangsu and Shanghai toward the end of the imperial era. At the time, patients throughout the Jiangnan 江南 region (the lower valley of the Yangzi river roughly corresponding to southern Jiangsu and Anhui and northern Zhejiang) appear to have been adverse to taking harsh-acting drugs such as *mahuang* (Ephedrae Herba) or *guizhi* (Cinnamomi Ramulus), the use of which was typical of the *shanghan* 伤寒 (Cold Damage) scholarly stream in Chinese medicine. Southerners believed they had more delicate constitutions and were affected by different climatic pathogens than people from the north, where *shanghan* therapeutics were widely believed to have originated in response to penetration into the body of cold and wind. The reasons for the emergence of these beliefs and their conjunction with issues of local identity formation in late imperial China are too complex to discuss here in detail. Suffice it to say that in the domain of medicine they involved the input of previous generations of Jiangnan physicians such as Ye Tianshi 叶天士 (1667–1746), Xue Shengbai 薛生白 (1681–1770), and Wu Jutong 吴鞠通 (1758–

1836). The treatment style of these physicians, referred to as the *wenbing* 温病 (Warm [Pathogen] Disorder) scholarly stream in Chinese medicine, was characterized by a preference for light and gentle drugs and came to dominate local practice in the Jiangnan region.[40]

Fei Shengfu's own medical line, though very much part of the southern tradition, advocated the flexible use of both *shanghan* and *wenbing* approaches. Discussing the clinical application of *shanghan* formulas, Fei lamented how difficult it had become to use harsh-acting drugs with his southern clientele. Even physicians who knew that the use of such drugs might clinically be indicated often did not prescribe them for fear of losing their patients. His own strategy, therefore, was "first to employ light and mild substances to achieve a small yet visible effect and only then add strong drugs. In this way the mind of [his] patients" remained "tranquil" and he relied "for help on people's will to get better."[41]

Fei Shengfu was not alone in encountering resistance. The physician Ma Yuanyi 马元仪 apparently devised a strategy whereby he soaked soybeans in a decoction of Ephedrae Herba and then prescribed the soybeans to his unsuspecting patients.[42] Ding Ganren 丁甘仁 (1865–1926) explicitly referred to the use of mild drugs and formulas to allay patients' suspicions as part of the craft (*shu* 术) of medicine.[43]

The patients and physicians in this historical example—like those I describe in my own ethnography—are influenced by institutional arrangements, ideology, power, and economic factors as well as the desire to heal and be healed. It would be unwise, therefore, to accord excessive agency to patients or to neglect how they themselves are shaped by the infrastructures with which they engage in their quest for health. The preference for gentle drugs exhibited by Jiangnan patients in late imperial China did not come from nowhere. It stemmed to a considerable extent from the doctrines and aesthetic preferences of the Suzhou physicians mentioned above. Likewise, as I noted in chapter 3, patients who visit Chinese medicine departments of urban hospitals in contemporary China are increasingly diagnosed by biomedical techniques and expensive drugs not because they or their condition demand it but because it increases the income of physicians and institutions.

The impermanence of patients' agency nevertheless evades all attempts at monocausal explanation. Rather, it emerges tactically and performatively in concrete local contexts, reacting to but also changing the forces that shape it.[44] In their quest for health, patients employ and encounter infrastructures such as efficacy attributions, the physical arrangements and locations of treatment spaces, physicians with varying degrees of skill and charisma, different medical systems, and different treatment modalities within each system. Inasmuch as these infrastructures are objectively given, patients and their families experience them as resistances to which they must accommodate. They have to make the necessary financial arrangements, pull *guanxi*, be cooperative, defer to authority. Yet, they are not infinitely flexible and adaptable. They have their own desires, needs, and pride. These, in turn, are experienced by other agencies as resistances to which they themselves have to accommodate—by exerting pressure, by using guile or the powers of persuasion, by changing the way one practices, or by removing patients from the field of practice, declaring them to be incurable or outside one's area of expertise.[45]

As studies of culture demonstrate, texts, consumer goods, and cultural performances are given diverse significations by individual readers, customers, and audiences. In an important sense they are newly synthesized within each individual act of consumption, utilization, and reproduction, and thereby are also reshaped.[46] The same applies to medicine. The particular advantage that such modeling supplies to my own investigations is that it makes available a mechanism for understanding how Chinese medicine is changing in response not only to political process but also to patient use. For within each individual consultation patients can bring to bear on their physicians pressures that find their cumulative expression in global changes of practice. Such changes and reinterpretations of Chinese medicine on the level of clinical practice constitute the topic of the next chapter.

5. SHAPING CHINESE MEDICINE
Integration, Innovation, Synthesis

Medical anthropologist Judith Farquhar has examined the practice of Chinese medicine in contemporary China with great perception and clarity. Based on a detailed analysis of the clinical encounter Farquhar locates the specific agency of contemporary physicians in their strategies to produce desired effects in the complex, overdetermined, and often internally contradictory contexts of everyday practice. She sums up these efforts "as a definite struggle for personal excellence, historical contribution, and genuine moral efficacy."[1]

My intention in this and the following chapters is to extend Farquhar's account in two complementary directions. First I will examine in greater detail the actual diversity of the agency she describes; then I will explore physicians' agency in relation to that of other infrastructures. The infrastructures I describe are physically, socially, politically, and textually embodied—thereby extending Scheper-Hughes and Lock's influential tripartite division of medical bodies into a fourth, the body of the medical canon.[2] The necessity of such an examination for the wider analysis of plurality is clear. For unless agency itself can be shown to be plural, relational, and by implication emergent, we are immediately returned to an anthropology of culturally bounded practices (from which I am trying to escape), rather than moving toward one of lived practice that constantly defines its own boundaries (as is my stated goal).[3]

Methodologically, this chapter examines the agency of one physician, Professor Zhu, through a series of four case studies that focus on Professor Zhu's relation to physical and textual bodies. This is not to say that practitioners of Chinese medicine (contrary to what is sometimes claimed) do not also engage with their patients as social and emotional beings.[4] They do, and at least some of these interactions surface in my narrative. However, every ethnography needs self-imposed boundaries. In the present case these exclude the complexities of patient-practitioner interactions. This is not because the analysis of such interactions would not contribute to our understanding of the problems at hand but because it would take us far beyond the scope of what is possible in the context of this investigation.

I was assigned to Professor Zhu by the administration of the Beijing University of Chinese Medicine during the first week of my fieldwork in 1994 and studied with him throughout the remainder of my first year in Beijing. I attended his outpatient clinics once or twice a week, occasionally followed him on his ward rounds, and was a frequent guest at his home. I have had an ongoing relation with Professor Zhu ever since, including an invitation to visit my own practice in Great Britain, where I had the opportunity to work with him without interruption for an entire month. I have come to know his wife and family, his students, and the staff of his hospital department. Thus, not only have I had ample opportunity to observe Professor Zhu's clinical practice, I have also been able to supplement these observations through conversations with him on all aspects of medicine, autobiographical data, and third-person reports. If familiarity is a precondition for observing both the stable and the contextual aspects of individual agency, then of all the physicians of Chinese medicine with whom I am acquainted, Professor Zhu is the most familiar to me.

Professor Zhu's Background and Views on Medicine

Professor Zhu was born in 1942. This means that his life has been lived almost entirely in postliberation China and that he belongs to the first generation of physicians educated at the newly established colleges of Chinese medicine. Professor Zhu is the first physician of Chinese medicine in his immediate family, though one of his uncles did apparently practice medicine. Born into a family of intellectuals and scholars, he entered the Nanjing College of Chinese Medicine (*Nanjing zhongyi xueyuan* 南京中医学院) in 1959 and graduated in 1965 with the highest marks in his class. He met his wife at college, but they spent the first ten years of their marriage mostly separated. Neither possessed the inclination or the class background necessary for active participation in the Cultural Revolution. Professor Zhu's wife was thus posted to a hospital in the south, while he remained in and around Jiangsu Province — in his own words, "reading rather than making revolution." He studied with famous older doctors at the hospital in Nantong, where he was employed, got to know biomedical investigative techniques while collaborating with physicians at a Western medicine hospital in nearby Shanghai, volunteered for medical service in the countryside, and employed his artistic skills as a painter of Mao Zedong portraits in order to survive attacks on his political background.

After the universities were reopened in the late 1970s Professor Zhu studied for a master's degree in integrated Chinese and Western medicine at the Beijing College of Chinese Medicine. His supervisor was Professor Ming, *xi xue zhong* 西学中 (that is, a graduate of the Chinese medicine classes for biomedical physicians established in the 1950s who were by then advancing into senior positions within the Chinese medicine sector). For his master's thesis Professor Zhu carried out research on the treatment of cardiovascular disease, a subject that has since become his speciality. After two more years of postgraduate specialization in cardiology at a medical school in Japan, he took up a position in one of Beijing's most prestigious hospitals.

Professor Zhu's hospital was established in 1988 as a class III hospital, the highest class of hospitals in China, and as a key institution for the integration of Chinese and Western medicine. It is one of the technologically best equipped hospitals in Beijing, owned and administered directly by the Ministry of Health. Physicians at older and more established institutions such as the Dongzhimen Hospital and the Beijing City Hospital of Chinese Medicine sometimes speak of their colleagues at Professor Zhu's hospital as second-class Chinese medicine physicians, implying that the domination of the hospital by Western medicine accords Chinese medicine an inferior position. Professor Zhu, who on his return from Japan was also offered a position at the older Dongzhimen Hospital, explained that he opted for his current position because of its better biomedical facilities. Today, Professor Zhu is the chief consultant of an internal medicine ward that specializes in the treatment of heart and kidney disease (*xinshen neike bingfang* 心肾内科病房) and a professor of integrated Chinese and Western medicine at the Beijing University of Chinese Medicine.[5]

The direct care of patients on Professor Zhu's ward is in the hands of ordinary consultants and junior physicians. Professor Zhu's main task is to manage the ward and supervise student research. He has few inpatients of his own, but conducts a twice-weekly ward round to supervise the clinical work of his staff. Professor Zhu also holds a surgery at the hospital's outpatient clinic twice a week, treating between ten and fifteen patients during the four-hour morning session.[6] Most of the patients in Professor Zhu's care are seriously ill. Many have passed through a number of different clinics and hospitals before attending his surgery. A good number come from outlying districts or even from provinces as far away as Shaanxi and Shandong.

Professor Zhu, who describes himself as a practitioner of integrated Chinese and Western medicine, claims to utilize both the most advanced scientific knowledge and a broad range of resources from the Chinese medical tradition. He eschews linkage with any one school or doctrine of Chinese medicine, yet holds that integration is best advanced from a firm foundation within Chinese medicine: *zhongyi xuexi xiyi* 中医学习西医 (practitioners of Chinese medicine studying Western medicine) rather than Mao Zedong's *xiyi xuexi zhongyi* 西医学习中医 (practitioners of Western medicine studying Chinese medicine) formulation.[7] Accordingly, he pays close attention to patients' biomedical diagnoses and case histories. Besides examination by the four methods of Chinese diagnosis (*sizhen* 四诊), he routinely orders ECGs, blood and urine tests, X-rays, and CT scans. Biomedical physical examinations are carried out whenever they are considered necessary.

On the ward and in the outpatient clinic, patients are sometimes treated by either Western medicine or Chinese medicine alone, but in most cases a combined approach is used. In the outpatient clinic the emphasis is reversed, with Western medical treatment used more often as an adjunct to Chinese medicine. In what follows I present only observations from these outpatient clinics. My reasons for doing so include space (which is limited), topicality (I am concerned with Chinese rather than Western medical practice), and expertise (I lack the competence required to analyze Professor Zhu's cardiological skills and compare them with standard practice in the West).

The explanations Professor Zhu gives to his patients about their illness in these outpatient clinics draw on both Chinese and biomedical reasoning. Comparisons between Chinese medicine and Western medicine constitute a recurring theme. As an advocate of the integration of Chinese and Western medicine, Professor Zhu directs his rhetoric against two adversaries at the same time: conventional biomedicine, which, according to him, understands much about isolated areas but little about complex processes, and the conservative (*baoshoude* 保守的) Chinese medicine of many older doctors, which—in his opinion—fails to develop the valuable knowledge it possesses in the light of ever-advancing scientific progress.

Individual treatment strategies depend on Professor Zhu's assessment of how he can most effectively manage the patient's complaint. When Professor Zhu assumes that biomedicine has little or no more to offer than Chinese medicine (e.g., for insomnia, menstrual irregularity, some types of headache, certain heart conditions, common colds) he uses Chinese medicine by itself. A few problems are treated with biomedical drugs alone, either for reasons of convenience (e.g., minor skin rashes for which a steroid cream works quicker and is more convenient than bitter decoctions) or to manage a problem for which Chinese medicine is considered a less effective therapeutic modality (e.g., in the management of severe hypertension). If he decides that neither approach would be sufficient on its own, he prescribes both Chinese herbs and biomedical drugs. Professor Zhu always follows a clear plan when using this approach. Biomedical drugs are deployed to manage a particular symptom or sign that is usually biomedically defined (e.g., hypertension), while Chinese medical drugs are prescribed to deal with what Professor Zhu sees as the underlying cause specified in terms of Chinese medical doctrine (e.g., kidney *yin* depletion with ascendant hyperactivity of liver *yang: shenyin xu, ganyang shang kang* 肾阴虚, 肝阳上亢). Sometimes biomedical drugs are chosen to achieve a quick effect in the initial stages of treatment with herbal medicines following to consolidate the effect. These treatment strategies recall previously mentioned popular stereotypes of Western medicine as rapidly treating surface manifestations while Chinese medicine excels at treating the root of a problem, even though it may take some time (*zhongyi zhi ben, xiyi zhi biao* 中医治本, 西医治标).

When I asked Professor Zhu why he thought it important to assimilate Western medical knowledge into Chinese medicine he gave two reasons. The first concerned efficacy. As the essence of medicine is to help people get better, it matters little *how* patients are cured provided they *are* cured. However, there are particular advantages to Chinese medicine. It frequently helps when Western medicine fails, and if used correctly it has no side effects.[8] Thus, when both systems offer treatments for a given problem, Chinese medicine is always preferable. Chinese medicine must not merely be kept alive as a tradition, Professor Zhu believes, but should be developed to treat ever more problems successfully.

Professor Zhu's second reason for promoting assimilation concerned social and technological change. He argued that biomedicine presents Chinese medicine with a vast array of new data that cannot be ignored. Chinese medicine must integrate modern technologies and the data they produce within its modes of practice or run the danger of being left behind in the society China is constructing. Like all his colleagues, Professor Zhu is daily confronted with the fact that while classical medical doctrine does not speak of proteinuria, blood sugar levels, and occluded arteries, modern Chinese patients certainly do. As we saw in chapter 4, progressive doctors have long argued the need to bring such data within the scope of Chinese medical doctrine and practice. They claim that in some instances the reality of Western medicine transcends that of Chinese medicine. A patient may suffer from proteinuria without having any subjective symptoms. Relying solely on pulse diagnosis and tongue inspection betrays not only ignorance but, more important, fails the patient.

Professor Zhu is representative of these progressive physicians. For the last twenty years he has applied himself to projects ranging from biochemical research into the action of herbal drugs, such as measuring the effects of particular drug constituents on platelet agglutination and other aspects of blood rheology, to the redefinition of theoretical concepts in the classical literature such as a novel interpretation of the concept of *wuxue* 污血 (polluted blood). He has engaged in various clinical trials and clinically applied historical studies such as an exploration of the use of the formula *Shengmai san* 生脉散 (Generate the Pulse Powder). He has become a national expert in his speciality, the treatment of *yuxue* 瘀血 (static blood), and has been awarded several national prizes for his achievements.

Professor Zhu is in addition a man of many interests, in art and philosophy as well as medicine, who emphasizes the need for the wide-ranging perspective and combination of modern and classical thought and practice his profession and hobbies have taught him. He is an accomplished painter who never fails to impress on his students (including myself) the close relation between medicine and art. He frequently recounts how his ability to paint helped him (literally) to survive a time when merely being a doctor was not enough. And he claims that it provided him as well with dexterity and an ability to look at things simultaneously from different perspectives.[9] In his teaching he emphasizes the importance of both modern and classical thought. Elucidating a treatment strategy, Professor Zhu might thus discourse on the crucial importance of balance and the Doctrine of the Mean (*zhongyong* 中庸), on the principles of action without interference (*wu wei* 无为), and on the importance of learning by heart, while citing Hegel and Marx in order to emphasize the importance of dialectical contradiction (*maodun* 矛盾) for medical practice.

Four Case Studies

I concur with Farquhar's opinion that "much of the intellectual life of Chinese medicine revolves around the reading and writing of prescriptions." Prescriptions directly help people and thus constitute medicine as practiced benevolence. They reflect a practitioner's affiliation to teachers and medical traditions, aesthetics, and even political commitments.[10] Professor Zhu's prescribing thus provides a convenient focus for the examination of his clinical agency. The following case studies are derived from observations of patients treated by the professor at the internal medicine outpatient department of his hospital between May and December 1994 and supplemented with information from conversations with Professor Zhu. My intention is to present the widest possible overview of the clinical strategies utilized by Professor Zhu. Space limitations forced me to select the cases that condense the most information into a few surface events. This ruled out (in spite of the many advantages such presentations would have had) following lengthy treatment episodes or documenting how Professor Zhu dealt with treatment failure.

The orthodox practice of writing a prescription (*chufang* 处方) consists of choosing a basic formula from the extensive medical archive of Chinese medicine and "to add and subtract" (*jiajian* 加减) drugs to these as required by circumstance.[11] In practice, physicians also compose complex prescriptions by combining various pairs or triplets of drugs. Although they are not, strictly speaking, following the classical method of adding and subtracting (because they create new formulas rather than varying existing ones), physicians often claim that they are doing so.[12] The following is a list of the main resources on which Professor Zhu draws when prescribing in his outpatient clinic:

1. Courses on formulas (*fangjixue* 方剂学) taught at Chinese medical colleges.

2. The *Shanghan zabing lun* (*Discussion of Cold Damage and Various Disorders*). This text from the late Han is the foundation of applied Chinese pharmacotherapy. Many older and some younger doctors know the entire text by heart. Professor Zhu can quote, if not the entire text, many passages. He still uses his heavily annotated copy of the original text from which he studied during his college days.

3. Zhang Xichun's 张锡纯 *Yixue zhongzhong canxi lu* 医学衷中参西录 (*Records of the Assimilation of the Western to Chinese in Medicine*) compiled between 1900 and 1934. Zhang Xichun was one of the first physicians to consciously and practically assimilate Western medical knowledge to Chinese medicine, an attitude much admired by Professor Zhu. Professor Zhu thinks that Zhang's works are particularly useful for contemporary physicians because Zhang practiced at the beginning of the twentieth century when illnesses and the people who had them were more like those of today than those of the Han or the Yuan.

4. A number of formulas formulated in Shanghai in the 1950s and 1960s that have since become "classical" and are directly influenced by biomedical thinking. The Shanghai College of Chinese Medicine (in keeping with the political avant-gardism of the city) had a pioneering role in the integration of Chinese medicine and Western medicine and is still considered more "modern" than "conservative" Beijing (chapter 3). Professor

Zhu worked in Nantong during his early years as a physician. Nantong is located on the northern side of the Jiangzi River, about fifty kilometers north of Shanghai. During his Nantong period, Professor Zhu was thus physically as well as intellectually close to Shanghai.

5. Less often, but not infrequently, formulas from other classical sources such as Gong Tingxian's 龚廷贤 *Wanbing huichun* 万病回春 (*Restoration of Health from the Myriad Diseases*) dating from 1587 or Li Gao's 李杲 *Neiwaishang bianhuo lun* 内外伤辨惑论 (*Clarifying Doubt about Injury from Internal or External Causes*) from 1247.

6. Several of his own formulas.

7. A number of synergistic drug combinations known as *duiyao* 对药 (lit. "complementary drugs") commonly used by contemporary physicians.[13]

We shall now observe the composition of formulas in actual practice.

CASE 5.1. *Diarrhea* (*la duzi* 拉肚子). A sixty-six-year-old woman attends the clinic for diarrhea. It started a week ago in the wake of a feverish cold and has not responded to self-treatment with dietary changes and over-the-counter drugs. She reports four loose bowel movements per day, constant nausea, bloating, and an aversion to cold. She has no more fever but upon questioning says that she sweats easily. Professor Zhu interprets her pulse as wiry (*xian* 弦) and her tongue as having a thin, greasy coat (*bo ni tai* 薄腻苔).[14] After a brief abdominal examination he diagnoses "[simultaneous] great *yang* and *yang* brightness disease" (*taiyang yangming bing* 太阳阳明病) to be treated by "Pueraria, Scutellaria, and Coptidis Decoction" (*Gegen huangqin huanglian tang* 葛根黄芩黄连汤). He explains that evil *qi* (*xieqi* 邪气) has penetrated from the surface (the greater *yang*) to the interior (the *yang* brightness), as indicated by simultaneous sweating (a greater *yang* sign) and diarrhea (a *yang* brightness sign). He then writes out the following prescription:

> *gegen* 葛根 (*Puerariae Radix*) 15 g
> *huangqin* 黄芩 (*Scutellariae Radix*) 15 g
> *huanglian* 黄连 (*Coptidis Rhizoma*) 8 g
> *muxiang* 木香 (*Aucklandiae Radix*) 10 g

Pueraria, Scutellaria, and Coptidis Decoction treats a disease pattern known as "complex dysentery" (*xiere li* 协热痢) first described in the *Shanghan lun:* "In [a case of] greater *yang* disease with Cinnamon twig [decoction] pattern the physician purges [although it is] contraindicated. [There ensue] incessant dysentery [and] a skipping pulse (*cumai* 促脉) [indicating] that the exterior has not [yet] been resolved. Such cases [where there may also be] panting and sweating are mastered by Pueraria, Scutellaria, and Coptidis Decoction."[15]

Professor Zhu memorized this pattern during his studies of the *Shanghan lun* at college. He now identifies it via the key presenting symptoms of his patient (simultaneous sweating and diarrhea) occurring in the wake of an acute infectious disease, the paradigmatic case of a *shanghan* disorder. His skill as a physician thus consists of two interrelated activities: sorting out the important symptoms (those reflecting the underlying disease process) from the less important ones (such as tongue and pulse), and making a small modification of the original formula (which has *gancao* 甘草 [*Glycyrrhizae Radix*] instead of *Aucklandiae Radix*) so as to respond to the slightly changed actual symptomatology. *Glycyrrhizae Radix* is cloying and would increase the nausea and abdominal fullness of this patient, whereas *Aucklandiae Radix* moves *qi* (*xingqi* 行气), thus treating these symptoms. It also combines well (as a *duiyao*) with *Coptidis Rhizoma* in the treatment of diarrhea.

Professor Zhu indicates to his students and patients that this is a straightforward and easy case to treat. He prescribes three bags of the decoction and instructs the patient to return only if the illness has not cleared up within three days. He then uses this case to lecture to his audience of students and patients on the fact that Chinese medicine, contrary to popular stereotypes (chapter 4), is very adept at treating acute diseases.

In private conversation Professor Zhu repeatedly returned to this observation. He explained that until very recently Chinese medicine had mainly treated acute diseases. All four of Beijing's *si da mingyi* 四大名医 (four famous physicians of the Republican and immediate postrevolutionary era still known to present-day Beijingese), for instance, and many present-day *laozhongyi* made their names treating infectious diseases.[16] Only with the advent of antibiotics had this changed. Chinese medicine, he insisted, needs to adapt to these changing realities without forgetting what it is capable of.

This particular patient did not return for treatment. I cannot, therefore, report what the effects of Professor Zhu's treatment were. Given that he had asked the lady to return if her symptoms had not cleared up, Professor Zhu, at least, assumed his prescription had worked.

CASE 5.2. *Abdominal Distension* (*fuzhang* 腹胀). The patient is a forty-five-year-old male chauffeur who is thin and looks older than he is. He says that he has suffered from abdominal distension for many years. It is very uncomfortable and is aggravated by work and cold. He has tried many Western and Chinese medical doctors without success. Upon questioning he says that he has no abdominal pain, that his stools are small and dry, that he fears cold, that he has a dry and bitter mouth and likes to drink cold drinks, that he dreams a lot, and that he tires easily. His pulse, according to Professor Zhu, is deep (*chen* 沉), weak (*ruo* 弱), and hesitant (*bu liuli* 不流利), and his tongue coating white and greasy (*bai ni tai* 白腻苔). The patient's medical records indicate a biomedical diagnosis of functional gastritis and treatment by various Chinese physicians for stomach depletion cold pattern (*weixu han zheng* 胃虚寒证). Professor Zhu explains to his students and the patient that this is a complicated disease that has not responded to previous treatment because none of the physicians understood its complexities. He notes four interrelated pathomechanisms:

1. Phlegm-rheum (*tanyin* 痰饮) in the stomach due to stomach depletion cold. This is indicated by the greasy, white tongue coating. Professor Zhu quotes a famous passage from the *Jingui yaolue* regarding the treatment of phlegm-rheum that all his students, too, know by heart: "For those with phlegm-rheum disease one should employ warming drugs to [achieve] harmonization of the condition."[17] In spite (and because) of this accumulation of pathological fluids the proper fluids (*jinye* 津液) are not ascending and moving downward, causing dryness (i.e., thirst and constipation). Taken together these symptoms indicate spleen-stomach disharmony (*pi wei bu he* 脾胃不和) and spleen movement failure (*piyun bu jian* 脾运不健).

2. Disordered ascending and directing downward (*shengjiang shichang* 升降失常). Even though the stomach is distended the patient does not burp. This is explained by Professor Zhu in biomedical terms as a combination of weak peristalsis and ptosis and in Chinese medical terms as a combined depletion of spleen and stomach. Peristalsis in Western medicine equals downward moving (governed by the stomach) in Chinese medicine. Lack of peristaltic movement leads to a buildup of gas, which causes bloating. This peristaltic weakness is an expression of a general lack of muscle tone reflected also in ptosis of the stomach, the presence of which he demonstrates to his students by palpation. Ptosis in Western medicine is spleen *qi* sinking downward (*piqi xiaxian* 脾气下陷) in Chinese medicine. Because

the stomach is low and utterly weak it cannot vent its gas upward. Professor Zhu then outlines how this condition should be treated: "For there to be ascending there must also be downward movement. Many doctors say, if there is prolapse use *Buzhong yiqi tang* 补中益气汤 (Supplement the Middle and Benefit *Qi* Decoction).[18] But this is not true. The success is not always that good. You must sometimes first help downward movement to make things go up. Hence, it is important to treat the stomach [which according to Chinese medical doctrine governs downward movement] as well as the spleen [which governs ascending]."

3. *Qi* stagnation blood stasis (*qizhi xueyu* 气滞血瘀) and food stagnation (*shizhi* 食滞) secondary to the spleen-stomach disharmony.

4. Dryness from blood stasis corresponding to circulatory problems in Western medicine.

Thus, the entire problem is one of depletion complicated by repletion (*xuzhong jia shi* 虚中夹实), a heat-cold complex (*hanre jiaza* 寒热夹杂), and simultaneous dryness (*zao* 燥) and damp (*shi* 湿) indicated both by the chronicity of the illness and by the many contradictory symptoms and signs (aggravation of the symptoms by cold yet desire for cold drinks; distension yet no belching or pain; a greasy and white tongue coating indicating repletion; yet a deep, weak, and hesitant pulse indicating depletion). Professor Zhu argues that the treatment must address the case in all its complexity, requiring the formulation of an individually tailored prescription. Treating just one aspect would not work, as the patient's medical history demonstrates. Professor Zhu's own prescription reads as follows:

> *huangqi* 黄芪 (*Astragali Radix*) 10 g
> *chaihu* 柴胡 (*Bupleuri Radix*) 10 g
> *shengma* 升麻 (*Cimicifugae Rhizoma*) 10 g
> *quangualou* 全瓜蒌 (*Trichosanthis Fructus*) 30 g
> *banxia* 半夏 (*Pinelliae Rhizoma*) 15 g
> *zhishi* 枳实 (*Aurantii Fructus immaturus*) 10 g
> *jineijin* 鸡内金 (*Gigeriae galli Endothelium corneum*) 10 g
> *sanleng* 三棱 (*Sparganii Rhizoma*) 10 g
> *ezhu* 莪术 (*Curcumae Rhizoma*) 10 g
> *juemingzi* 决明子 (*Cassiae Semen*) 15 g
> *dingxiang* 丁箱 (*Caryophylli Flos*) 6 g
> *rougui* 肉桂 (*Cinnamomi Cortex*) 2 g

Based on Professor Zhu's own explanation the formula is composed of four parts. The first three drugs (*Astragali Radix, Bupleuri Radix,* and *Cimicifugae Rhizoma*) are a condensation of Li Gao's *Buzhong yiqi tang* (Supplement the Middle and Benefit *Qi* Decoction), which supplements the spleen and raises what has sunken (*bupi juxian* 补脾举陷).[19] The next three drugs (*Trichosanthis Fructus, Pinelliae Rhizoma,* and *Aurantii Fructus immaturus*) are a variation of *Xiao xianxiong tang* 小陷胸汤 (Minor Sinking into the Chest Decoction) from the *Shanghan lun,* in which *Coptidis Rhizoma* (*huang lian*) has been replaced by *Aurantii Fructus immaturus.* The original formula treats pain and fullness in the chest and upper abdomen due to accumulation of phlegm heat. According to later commentators it promotes flow (*tong* 通) and regulates spleen and stomach (*tiao pi wei* 调脾胃).[20] The next four drugs (*Gigeriae galli, Sparganii Rhizoma, Curcumae Rhizoma,* and *Cassiae Semen*) are used to resolve stasis of *qi,* blood, and food following the maxim that "freeing [medicinals] can eliminate stagnation" (*tong ke qu zhi* 通可去滞). The choice of these drugs (rather than others that might achieve a similar effect) originates, in the first place, in Professor Zhu's engagement with the works of Zhang Xichun.[21] Secondarily, it derives from his preference for herbs that quicken blood (*huoxue* 活血) in addition to their primary effect. In the present prescription, *Gigeriae galli* is used to resolve food stagnation, *Astragali Radix* to supplement and uplift *qi,* and *Trichosanthis Fructus* to transform phlegm and open the chest. According to Professor Zhu these three drugs also quicken blood. The combination of the final two drugs is known as *Ding gui san* 丁桂散 (Clove and Cinnamon Powder) and is a modern prescription for stomach cold developed in Shanghai.[22] It is used here to warm the stomach and thereby aid the transformation of phlegm-rheum (in Chinese medical terms) and to encourage peristalsis and the secretion of stomach acid (in biomedical terms).

As Professor Zhu finishes writing out his prescription one of his students indicates that she does not follow his thinking. Why, if the main pattern is one of stomach depletion cold, did he not use a prescription indicated to treat that pattern such as *Lizhong wan* 理中丸 (Regulate the Middle Pill)?[23] Professor Zhu points out to her the need to understand and regulate the entire pathomechanism, not merely to match a prescription to a pattern. He explains again his appreciation of this mechanism, emphasizing the importance of harmonizing opposites. The student clearly has some difficulty grasping his train of thought because she repeatedly goes back to asking about *lizhong wan*. Other students get excited about the flexibility of their teacher's practice. Professor Zhu explains that the ability to see a situation from different perspectives at once comes with experience but is also an advantage of Chinese medicine. Integrating Western medical knowledge (such as about ptosis of the stomach, peristaltic functioning, or hypoacidity) into such an understanding is not a hindrance but instead adds potentially useful vistas.

The patient himself follows the discussion attentively although clearly he does not understand all of it. Nevertheless, he takes the herbs and on his return one week later reports an improvement in his condition that continues over subsequent visits.

CASE 5.3. *Joint Pain* (*guanjie tong* 关节痛). Mrs. Huang is a forty-one-year-old woman suffering from joint pains in her fingers and feet that have been diagnosed as rheumatoid arthritis (RA). The pains started six years ago, and since then she has consulted both Western and Chinese medical practitioners. Despite several courses of steroids her condition did not significantly improve. Besides swollen, red, and painful joints aggravated by cold Mrs. Huang complains of low-grade fever, constipation, slight dizziness, and chest oppression (胸闷 *xiongmen*). Physical examination reveals low blood pressure (90/70 mm Hg); a deep, weak, and wiry pulse; and a pale tongue with a white, greasy coat. Professor Zhu sends her for a blood test and asks her to return to his surgery the following week. The blood test reveals the presence of rheumatoid factor, a raised ESR (25mm/h), and raised plasma viscosity supporting the diagnosis of RA,[24] while a hematology report was normal (RBC 5.2 × 10^{12}/l, WBC 4.5 × 10^9/l, PLT 208 × 10^9/l).

During the next visit Professor Zhu diagnoses the condition as painful obstruction pattern (*bizheng* 痹证) on the basis of both *qi* and blood depletion (*qi xue liang xu* 气血两虚). His prescription, as listed below, is a variation of *Duhuo jisheng tang* 独活寄生汤 (Duhuo and Mistletoe Decoction), a standard formula for the treatment of this pattern in contemporary Chinese medicine.[25]

duhuo 独活 (*Angelicae pubescentis Radix*) 10 g
qianghuo 羌活 (*Notopterygii Rhizoma seu Radix*) 10 g
sangjisheng 桑寄生 (*Taxilli Herba*) 10 g

sangzhi 桑枝 (*Mori Ramulus*) 30 g

fangji 防己 (*Aristolochiae fangchi Radix*) 10 g

haifengteng 海风藤 (*Piperis kadsurae Caulis*) 10 g

cansha 蚕沙 (*Bombycis Faeces*) 10 g

yiyiren 意苡仁 (*Coicis Semen*) 10 g

niuxi 牛膝 (*Achyranthis Radix*) 10 g

huangqi 黄芪 (*Astragali Radix*) 15 g

shengdihuang 生地黄 (*Rehmanniae glutinosae Radix*) 10 g

danggui 当归 (*Angelicae sinensis Radix*) 20 g

danshen 丹参 (*Salviae militiorrhizae Radix*) 30 g

There is nothing remarkable about this prescription other than that *Piperis Caulis* is chosen here because it exhibits, according to Professor Zhu, a steroidal action, and that the combination of *Angelicae sinensis Radix* and *Salviae Radix* is evidence, once more, of the influence of Zhang Xichun.[26] More interesting is the additional prescription of forty milligrams per day of a standardized extract of the drug *leigongteng* 雷公藤 (*Tripterygii Radix*), a highly toxic drug. Due to potentially lethal side effects (which include internal bleeding and kidney damage) it has been assimilated into the actively used pharmacopoeia of Chinese physicians only very recently. It is used today for the treatment of RA, where its clinical efficacy was demonstrated by several studies in the 1980s.[27] Interestingly, although Chinese medical practitioners include it as a drug in their materia medica (Professor Zhu certainly thinks of it as a *zhongyao* 中药, a "Chinese drug"), it was available at his hospital only as a standardized preparation from the Western medicine pharmacy.

Professor Zhu routinely uses *Tripterygii Radix* in the treatment of RA. He also employs other toxic drugs such as *dafengzi* 大风子 (*Hydnocarpi Semen*), *maqianzi* 马钱子 (*Strychni Semen*), and *liuhuang* 硫黄 (Sulphur) whenever he considers their use necessary and appropriate to a given case. Aware of potential side effects, he regularly monitors patients taking these drugs by means of biomedical investigative techniques as part of his treatment regime. In the present case, he asks for another hematological exam, a liver function test, and an ECG to be carried out prior to Mrs. Huang's next consultation a fortnight later. On that visit Mrs. Huang's joints are significantly less painful and her bowels regular. She still has a mildly raised temperature. The various tests reveal no abnormality and Mrs. Huang reports that she is feeling well. Professor Zhu is pleased about the

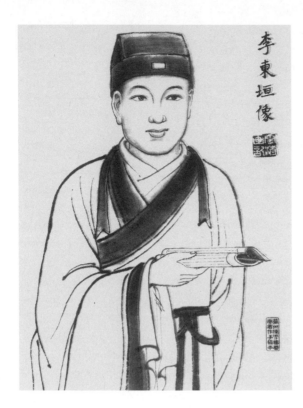

李東垣像

FIGURE 27. Li Gao
(1180–1251)

improvement but considers the low-grade fever to be a sign that the inflammation is still active. He therefore doubles the dosage of *Tripterygii Radix* to eighty milligrams per day and makes a small adjustment to the herbal formula. He increases the dosage of *Angelicae sinensis Radix* to thirty grams and of *Rehmanniae glutinosae Radix* to fifteen grams in order to enhance the blood cooling (*liangxue* 冷血), quickening and supplementing effects of the formula. He also adds ten grams of *lüdouyi* 绿豆衣 (*Glycinae Pericarpium*), a blood-nourishing and liver-pacifying (*yangxue pinggan* 养血平肝) drug, because in Professor Zhu's opinion it synergistically supports the therapeutic effects of *Tripterygii Radix* while counterbalancing its side effects.

On Mrs. Huang's third visit one month later the joint pain and inflammation have entirely subsided. ESR and plasma viscosity are normal, and Mrs. Huang reports feeling better than at any time since the onset of her illness. Professor Zhu, distinctly pleased, discontinues the previous prescription. He finds that the pulse is still thin, weak, and rough (*se* 涩), which indicates to him that the original *qi* (*yuanqi* 元气) is still depleted and needs support. He therefore prescribes a variation of *Si junzi tang* 四君子汤 (Four Gentlemen Decoction), a major *qi*-supplementing formula.[28] Shortly afterward I returned to the United Kingdom, but according to Professor Zhu's information the patient continued to do well.

In various contexts Professor Zhu gave the following explanations for his use of toxic drugs despite his claims that Chinese medicine should be side effect free. First, he followed the experience of physicians such as Zhang Xichun, who extolled the virtues of sulphur for severe cases of *yang* depletion.[29] Second, he felt it to be his duty as a physician to help his patients with all the means at his disposal. Third, the use of these drugs was part of his wider goal of integrating Chinese medicine and Western medicine. Fourth, competent physicians should not be afraid to use powerful toxic drugs where they are indicated. He ridiculed younger physicians who immediately look to Western medicine if they encounter a serious problem, though he admitted it is a fault of the system, which allows or even requires them to do this (chapter 3), as much as of individual doctors.

A little medical history will make it easier to appreciate the rhetorical

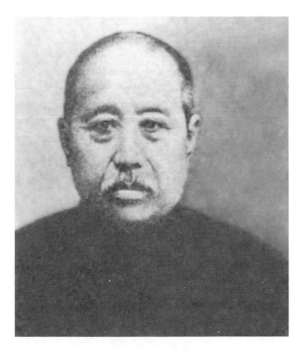

FIGURE 28. Zhang Xichun (1860–1933)

power of Professor Zhu's argument and the multiple forces that shape his actions. According to a statement attributed to the famous Tang physician Sun Simiao 孙思邈 (581–682), the first Chinese doctor to concern himself explicitly with medical ethics, a good physician is characterized by four attributes: he is morally honorable in his actions (*xing fang* 行方), has a comprehensive knowledge (*yuan zhi* 圆智), and is careful (*xin xiao* 心小) yet also courageous (*dan da* 胆大).[30] This statement is attributed to Sun Simiao by Song Qi 宋祁 (998–1061) in the *Xin tang shu* 新唐书 (*New Tang History*) and is regularly cited by later physicians lecturing on good practice in texts that contemporary students read as part of their training in classical Chinese and medical ethics.[31] In an extensive discussion elucidating the meaning of the passage in the *Yizong bidu* 医宗必读 (*Essential Readings from the Medical Ancestors*) of 1637, courageousness is explicitly exemplified by the use of poisonous herbs such as *fuzi* 附子 (*Aconiti Radix lateralis praeparata*) and of harsh draining formulas such as the various *Cheng qi tang* 承气汤 (Order the *Qi* Decoctions).[32] Within one statement Professor Zhu thus achieves at least, four effects: (1) he asserts his own status as an exemplary practitioner of Chinese medicine and, vice versa, (2) the contemporary relevance of long-established ethical values; (3) he distances himself from his students (which he has to do as their teacher) and other physicians (with whom he competes for prestige); and (4) he assimilates the use of a biomedical preparation into Chinese medical practice not merely on the grounds of efficacy but also those of morality.[33]

CASE 5.4. *Ménière's Disease* (*meinierbing* 美尼尔病). The fourth case study does not follow the treatment of an individual patient. It discusses, instead, Professor Zhu's treatment of Ménière's disease. I have selected this case because it reflects in exemplary fashion Professor Zhu's innovative theoretico-practical integration of Chinese and Western medicines.

Ménière's disease, which affects the inner ear, is characterized by bouts of vertigo, nausea, and vomiting. These symptoms are accompanied by tinnitus, partial loss of hearing, a sensation of fullness in the ear, and sometimes a continued rapid oscillation of the eyeballs (nystagmus). Biomedicine describes its pathology, a progressive distension of the endolymphatic fluid, but determining its precise cause has proved more elusive and treatments to date remain palliative.[34] Contemporary Chinese medical textbooks—even those organized according to biomedical diseases—place Ménière's disease under the classical disease category "dizziness" (*xuanyun* 眩晕).[35] The standard therapeutic approach is to use different treatments for different patients according to a pattern differentiation of dizziness.[36] Textbooks of integrated Chinese and Western medicine break up the disease into several types (xing 型) such as "ascendant hyperactivity of liver yang type" (ganyang shang kang xing 肝阳上亢型) or "phlegm turbidity obstructing the middle type" (tanzhuo zhongzu xing 痰浊中阻型) that are derived from (and sometimes identical with) the more classical patterns.[37]

Professor Zhu criticizes the variety of "types" of Ménière's disease put forward in the literature. His argument that it is possible to discover a much closer match between Western and Chinese descriptions of the disease leads to a novel method of treatment. The following analysis of his reasoning is derived from extensive discussions and the observation of six cases of Ménière's disease treated by Professor Zhu.

In Professor Zhu's opinion more than 80 percent of all patients diagnosed as suffering from Ménière's disease also exhibit a consistent pattern of disharmony according to Chinese medicine. Not only do these patients have a stable set of symptoms (nausea, vertigo, tinnitus, or deafness), they also show a wiry and slippery pulse (mai xian hua 脉弦滑) and a greasy tongue fur (ni tai 腻苔). The wiry pulse indicates phlegm (tan 痰) or wind (feng 风) as pathogenic qi (xieqi 邪气) and points to impaired functions of liver (gan 肝) or gall bladder (dan 胆). Professor Zhu argues that the biomedical localization of the problem in the inner ear as well as the symptoms of tinnitus and impaired hearing also indicate a liver or gall bladder problem. The ear relates to the foot lesser yang gall bladder vessel (zu shaoyang dan jing 足少阳胆经), which stands in an internal/external relation (biaoli guanxi 表里关系) to the foot-attenuated yin liver vessel (zu jueyin gan jing 足厥阴肝经). "The liver opens into the eyes" (gan kaiqiao yu mu 肝开窍于目) explains why there should be nystagmus. Dizziness and loss of coordination signify internal wind (neifeng 内风) caused by ascendant liver yang (ganyang shang kang 肝阳上亢), liver fire (ganhuo 肝火), or both; according to Chinese medical doctrine, the two are closely related.[38] This liver pathology is complicated by phlegm as indicated by the nausea, dizziness, and greasy tongue fur.

According to Professor Zhu, Ménière's disease is the consequence of disordered ascending and directing downward (shengjiang shichang 升降失常) involving jueyin (attenuated yin or the liver visceral system) and yangming (yang brightness or the stomach visceral system).[39] As ascending and directing downward involve many other visceral functions apart from liver and stomach, their specification as the core of the present problem is a crucial aspect of Professor Zhu's diagnosis.[40] The liver is often in abundance (*gan chang you yu* 肝常有余) while the stomach governs directing downward of the turbid (*wei zhu jiang zhuo* 胃主降浊). If the relationship between the two is disturbed, it can lead to an upward surge of *qi* (*qi shangchong* 气上冲) and harm due to turbid pathogen (*zhuoxie* 浊邪) in the head and particularly the inner ear. Phlegm is the actual manifestation of this turbidity. Its presence is explained here both by the disordered function of the middle (*zhong* 中), namely the stomach or the *yang* brightness, and by a disturbed *qi* dynamic due to an abnormal upsurge of liver *qi*. Professor Zhu cites Pang Anshi 庞安时 (1044–1099), who is usually known by his literary name Anchang 安常: "Someone who is good at treating does not treat phlegm but *qi*. [Once] *qi* flows in the right way the fluids of the entire body follow the *qi* and also flow in the right way."[41]

In his analysis Professor Zhu draws in particular on theories of disordered ascending and directing downward developed by Li Gao in the Jin dynasty and Zhang Xichun in the early twentieth century that we encountered in case 5.2 above. Thus far, the analysis includes only one element of biomedical knowledge: an awareness of the anatomical location of the disorder in the cochlear and vestibular sensory apparatus of the inner ear. In Ménière's disease the excessive pressure and dilation of the endolymphatic system causes damage to these organs. The definition of phlegm and its relation to other substances such as water (*shui* 水), rheum (*yin* 饮), and dampness (*shi* 湿) in the classical literature of Chinese medicine is far from precise, while modern textbooks define it as a pathological body fluid. Without a great leap of imagination Professor Zhu now relates the phlegm, which manifests itself in vertigo, nausea, a wiry pulse, and greasy tongue fur, to a dysfunction of the fluids of the endolymphatic system, thereby establishing a conceptual link between the anatomical body of biomedicine and the functional body of Chinese medicine.

This link is important to Professor Zhu because he perceives it as resolving the problematic tension in contemporary Chinese medicine between tangible, or formed (*you xing* 有形), and intangible, or formless (*wu xing* 无形), phlegm. The former can be seen on expectoration, while the presence of the latter is deduced from symptoms and signs such as numbness of the extremities, lumps in various locations of the body, a sense of disorientation, mania, depression, and, in many cases, greasy tongue fur.[42] The structural opposition between tangible and intangible phlegm seems to be quite recent in origin. In the classical literature, phlegm was defined pathophysiologically as a process of condensation and congealing. The new interpretation perhaps reflects modern theoreticians' desires to move Chinese medicine closer to a reality capable of objective representation rather than delineation as a process.[43] The Ming author Feng Zhaozhang 冯兆张, for instance, wrote:

> When phlegm is created by disease from the viscera's body fluids and follows the rise and fall of *qi*, this is standard pathology. But when it is between the skin and the membranes or in where the joints bend and stretch, how could this be the phlegm from the viscera flowing and reaching into these places? It is, in fact, the local body fluids of these places being affected by heat or cold which then congeal, knot, and create phlegm pathologically. It certainly is not phlegm created by disease in other parts leaving that original place and shifting to this one. Not to mention, *qi* by nature has no form [*wu xing* 无形] and thus there is no place, however tiny, which it cannot reach; body fluids follow the *qi* in its circulation. But if it comes to disease causing this fluid to become phlegm, then it transforms into [something] formed [*you xing* 有形], congealing, obstructing. How could this follow the *qi* flow through into the tiniest most secret parts of the body?[44]

Professor Zhu explained to me on several occasions that the phlegm that causes dizziness and is described as intangible phlegm in contemporary Chinese texts, in fact, possesses a form, which in the case of Ménière's disease presents as the thickened lymphatic fluid in the inner ear. This is made visible by modern scientific technology. In our discussions, Professor Zhu used this as one example to demonstrate that biomedical technology does not of necessity stand in opposition to Chinese medicine. Rather, it can affirm and strengthen it. Something previously related functionally by analogical reasoning can now be seen to be related in a visibly materialistic sense. In a social context where objective knowledge is frequently equated with the perceptually visible and where there is pressure on Chinese medicine to increase its objectivity, Professor Zhu thinks that this affirmation is no small achievement.

Based on his analysis, Professor Zhu developed a herbal formula for the treatment of Ménière's Disease that reads as follows:[45]

dai zhe shi 代赭石 (*Haematitum*)
xiakucao 夏枯草 (*Prunellae Spica*)

huangqin 黄芩 (*Scutellariae Radix*)
fuling 茯苓 (*Poriae*)
banxia 半夏 (*Pinelliae Rhizoma*)
tiannanxing 天南星 (*Arisaematis Rhizoma*)
quangualou 全瓜蒌 (*Trichosanthis Fructus*)
cheqian zi 车前子 (*Plantaginis Semen*)

The main action of this formula is to direct *qi* downward (*jiangqi* 降气) by regulating the *jueyin* and *yangming*. Its secondary action is to transform phlegm (*huatan* 化痰). It thereby reconstitutes harmony between ascending and directing downward and reestablishes the correct balance between the clear (*qing* 清) and the turbid. The formula draws inspiration in its selection of specific drugs from a variety of sources: (1) from Zhang Xichun, the deployment of *Haematitum* as a sovereign (*jun* 君) drug to direct *qi* downward;[46] (2) from established classical strategies, treating phlegm with *Poriae*, *Pinelliae Rhizoma*, and *Arisaematis Rhizoma* and treating liver disorders with *Prunellae Spica* and *Scutellariae Radix*;[47] (3) from Professor Zhu's interest in the integration of Chinese and Western medicine, the use of *Plantaginis Semen* and from his own clinical experience, the use of *Trichosanthis Fructus*.[48] A genealogy of the formula is graphically displayed in figure 29.

The exact composition of Professor Zhu's formula need be of no further concern beyond the deployment of *Plantaginis Semen* as another example of the integrative reasoning by means of which Professor Zhu and many of his colleagues are currently developing Chinese medicine. Classical and modern pharmacopoeias give as the main actions of *Plantaginis Semen* its capacity to disinhibit water (*lishui* 利水) and to dispel dampness and clear heat (*qushi qingre* 祛湿清热). Although some sources state that it transforms (*hua* 化) or dispels (*qu* 祛) phlegm, it is not usually considered a primary drug for this purpose. Where the literature indicates its use in phlegm disorders, it refers to cough with copious sputum, especially when this is due to lung heat.[49] As indicated above, phlegm constitutes a problematic entity in Chinese medical doctrine. Like dampness, phlegm is an excessive accumulation of the turbid and is discussed under the rubric of fluid physiology and pathology.[50] Both phlegm and dampness are sometimes seen as having their cause in rheum. Rheum is often described as a fluid accumulation less dense than phlegm with which it combines in the paired term phlegm-rheum (*tanyin* 痰饮).[51] Phlegm is also described as originating from damp. Thus, it is sometimes said that "with-

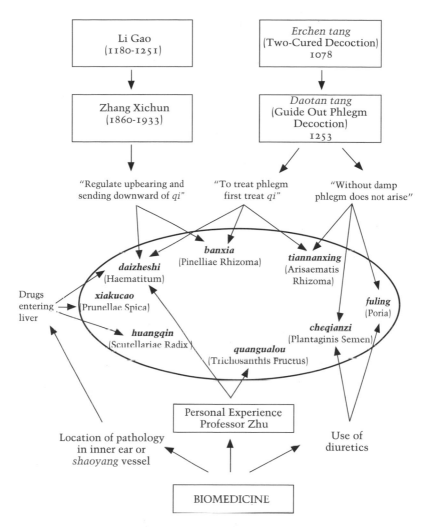

FIGURE 29. The genealogy of Professor Zhu's formula

out [the prior existence of] dampness phlegm does not arise" (*wu shi bu cheng tan* 无湿不成痰).[52]

If, as biomedicine holds, Ménière's disease is due to increased endolymphatic pressure, temporary relief, at least, may be attained by reducing the total amount of fluid in circulation. Some biomedical authorities administer intravenous diuretics to achieve this effect.[53] Professor Zhu explained that this was one reason why he used *Plantaginis Semen*. I had previously observed Professor Zhu to employ *Plantaginis Semen*, *yimucao* 益母草 (*Leonuri Herba*), *niuxi* 牛膝 (*Achyranthis Radix*), *zelan*

泽兰 (*Lycopi Herba*), and other drugs with a known diuretic effect as assistant (*zuo* 佐) drugs in the treatment of essential hypertension. I had also observed a similar choice of drugs when studying with a physician from Chengdu in the late 1980s who explained to me that his strategy was derived from the biomedical use of diuretics in the treatment of hypertension. Professor Zhu also admitted to the influence of biomedicine. Both physicians pointed out, however, that the drugs chosen were not selected because of their diuretic effects alone. Rather, they were integrated into a prescription because they combined a diuretic action along with others that were important from a Chinese medical point of view, such as quickening blood (*huoxue*), directing *qi* downward (*jiangqi*), or because they entered into a particular vessel (*guijing* 归经).

According to modern Chinese textbooks *Plantaginis Semen* belongs among the drugs that disinhibit water and percolate damp (*lishui shenshi yao* 利水渗湿药). The capacity of a drug to "disinhibit water" seems to encompass that of biomedical diuretics (*liniaoyao* 利尿药, lit. "drugs [to] disinhibit urine") while extending its effects to a wider fluid metabolism. Thus, these drugs have the biomedical function "of increasing the volume of urine, promoting and extending urinary flow," and also the Chinese medical function of "expelling water damp stagnating and accumulating in the interior of the body."[54] Inducing diuresis is thus not only biomedically indicated, but just one further aspect of the Chinese medical "disinhibition of water and percolation of damp."

Increasing urination has long been one of the most important methods for removing the turbid from the body in Chinese medicine. Thus, in a second step that takes the action of *Plantaginis Semen* in Professor Zhu's prescription even further away from its use as a simple diuretic, the drug is integrated into a treatment strategy informed by classical assumptions about the cooperation of drugs within a formula as sovereign (*jun* 君), minister (*chen* 臣), assistant (*zuo* 佐), and envoy (*shi* 使). Here, *Plantaginis Semen*, in its "disinhibition of water and percolation of damp," assists the more important phlegm-transforming action of *Pinelliae Rhizoma* and *Arisaematis Rhizoma*. It has been noted that dampness is widely assumed in Chinese medical thinking to be a source of phlegm. Classical formulas to treat phlegm therefore often include drugs that disinhibit damp (*lishi* 利湿) in order to assist their principal phlegm-transforming drugs. Both *erchen tang* 二陈汤 (Two-Cured Decoction) and *daotan tang* 导痰汤 (Guide [Out] Phlegm Decoction), which are important influences on the formulation of Professor Zhu's own prescription, employ *Poriae* for this purpose. In the words of a contemporary teaching manual: "Phlegm is engendered from dampness, [while] dampness itself comes from the spleen. Therefore, one uses *Poriae* as an assistant to strengthen the spleen and disinhibit damp, so [that when] dampness has gone the spleen becomes effulgent and there is no longer anything from which phlegm could be produced."[55] *Plantaginis Semen* is added to *Poriae* in Professor Zhu's formula primarily for this effect but *also* because it can be understood as a diuretic in the biomedical sense. In addition, it enters the liver (*gui gan* 归肝) and brightens the eyes (*ming mu* 明目) and thus supports the dynamic of the entire formula both physiologically and symptomatically.

To sum up, we can say that in his treatment of Ménière's disease Professor Zhu collates symptoms and signs into a pattern of disharmony that is accessible to manipulation via treatment strategies recorded in the archives of the Chinese medical tradition. He also adds to this archive by strategically employing biomedical knowledge when connections can be established between both frames of reference. Biomedicine is used as a tool that confirms Chinese medical knowledge, but also as one that makes possible new ways of reacting to a complex and ever-changing world. Furthermore, the strategies Professor Zhu applies to Ménière's disease do not represent an isolated effort by a single physician. Studying with different doctors at different institutions I came across many similar attempts to develop Chinese medicine. Some examples are the interpretation of proteinuria (abnormal protein in the urine) as loss of essence (*jing* 精), formulas for female infertility based on an understanding of estrogen and progesterone cycles, the treatment of male infertility based on investigations of sperm counts and sperm motility, and the use of ultrasound as an essential aspect of Chinese medical diagnosis. Physicians regularly include drugs in their prescriptions because they are antiviral, spasmolytic, or antihypertensive. Nor is this a historically new phenomenon. Professor Zhu's training relates him to physicians in Shanghai in the 1950s who developed now classical formulas such as *Tianma gouteng yin* 天麻钩藤饮 (Gastrodia and Uncaria Drink) for the treatment of biomedically defined problems such as hypertension;[56] and even further, to Zhang Xichun at the turn of the century, who not only integrated biomedical knowledge into his clinical strategies but also used biomedical drugs whose actions he had translated into Chinese medicine functions.[57]

Professor Zhu has subtle strategies for appropriating from biomedicine that which he perceives as desirable because efficacious without surrendering what he values in his own tradition. While previous studies have focused on the corrosive impact of Western knowledge on Chinese medicine, my own fieldwork demonstrates that its import can equally stimulate the development of local practice.[58] What anthropologists have documented for other Asian medicines thus also holds true for contemporary China. Syncretisms abound while relationships between different medical practices can be both complementary and competitive, invigorating as well as nocuous.[59]

Integration as Synthesis: An Analysis of Professor Zhu's Agency

As in previous chapters, I shall use the concluding section to tie the ethnography of Professor Zhu's plural agency as a physician to the theoretical discussion of synthesis presented in chapter 2. The most important observation in this context is the presence of multiplicity even within a single person. Nothing we have encountered in Professor Zhu's agency as a physician might justifiably be described as the expression of a single style of reasoning, a single form of medical practice, a single kind of aesthetics, a single medical gaze, a single symbolic system.

On his ward Professor Zhu sometimes practices only Western medicine. He also routinely prescribes Western medical drugs in the outpatient clinic.[60] In case 5.1 he was seen matching symptoms and signs to a prescription as dictated by a two-thousand-year-old text. In case 5.2 his agency was much more complex. It consisted not merely of unraveling a disease mechanism from an intricate and contradictory set of symptoms and signs, but also of responding to it by means of formulating an equally intricate and complex prescription. This form of prescribing is a continuation of the medicine of neo-Confucian scholar-physicians created during the Jin-Yuan period, which itself was a complex reaction to and further development of the Han-derived medicine of its time.[61] In case 5.3 Professor Zhu combined the prescribing practice of case 5.2 with the use of a standardized drug extracted from a Chinese herb for the treatment of a biomedically defined disease. In case 5.4 he constructed an entirely new nosological hybrid and corresponding treatment strategy.

Professor Zhu's multiple agency as a physician emerges in the course of his encounter with a complex ensemble of other infrastructures that populate the field of contemporary Chinese medicine. In each of the four case studies we saw Professor Zhu interacting with the physical bodies of his patients, whose being (both present and in the past) shaped what he did.[62] We perceived him as being motivated, guided, and disciplined by the experiences, theories, and treatment strategies of his medical ancestors and teachers; by cultural conceptions about what constitutes a good and powerful doctor and his desire to be just such a physician; by historically specific notions regarding the integration of Chinese medicine and Western medicine; by a desire to heal and to help shaped by subjective dispositions as much as by an ethos of "serving the people" prominent during his formative years; by a desire to innovate that might be part of his character but also resonates with the current telos of Chinese medicine and Chinese society; and by the availability of particular technologies of diagnosis and medical care such as hospital wards, sphygmomanometers, hematological tests, and the laboratories necessary for their evaluation.

Professor Zhu experiences all of the infrastructures listed above as factors that he manipulates in the course of expressing his medical art. From a more global perspective, however, the very same infrastructures can also be seen as shaping Professor Zhu. His use of classical formulas is a good example. Professor Zhu interacts with his patients through the use and modification of formulas available to him in the medical archive. In Chinese medicine such formulas are not merely therapeutic tools, they also shape diagnosis and the understanding of pathology. In committing himself to the use of these formulas he is thus shaped by how these formulas synthesize symptoms and signs, disease processes, treatment strategies, and medicinal drugs.

Like Professor Zhu these infrastructures have histories that document the syntheses through which they have been constructed. Contemporary applications of formulas from the *Shanghan lun*, for instance, are derived not from direct readings of the original text but from the interpretations of later scholar-physicians who are today remembered collectively as the Cold Damage scholarly stream (*shanghan xuepai* 伤寒学派). Song dynasty interest in the *Shanghan lun*, as well as its original inception in the Han, was mediated, among other factors, by general concerns about pathogenic *qi* (*xieqi* 邪气) that entered the body from outside. Such types of pathogenic *qi* included not merely cold and wind but also ghosts and demons.[63] The modern reception of these interpretations is influenced by the sorting out of the Chinese medical tradition in progress since the 1920s. One aspect of this current reworking of the *shanghan* tradition is its reconciliation with dialectical materialism in which ghosts and demons no longer exist. Another aspect is its integration with the *wenbing* tradition, or Warm Pathogen [Disorder] scholarly stream (*wenbing xuepai* 温病学派), that emerged during the Qing as an explicit challenge to *shanghan* therapeutics.[64]

Professor Zhu thus sometimes merges formulas from both the *shanghan* and *wenbing* traditions, while at others he is guided by one or the other or rejects both in favor of a novel Chinese-Western medical approach. Before a particular patient enters his surgery and the case unravels over successive treatment episodes, however, it is impossible to predict just how the treatment will evolve. Whether or not Professor Zhu becomes a representative of the *jingfang* 经方 stream (i.e., physicians frequently associated with the *shanghan* stream who match clinical realities to classical formulas: case 5.1), the *shifang* 时方 stream (i.e., physicians frequently associated with the *wenbing* stream who formulate prescriptions by the skillful combination of herbs to match clinical realities: case 5.2), or the *zhongxiyi jiehe* 中西医结合 stream (i.e., physicians who formulate prescriptions so as to derive from clinical realities a new medicine: cases 5.3 and 5.4) is not determined by the disease, the patient, Professor Zhu, the institution in which he works, or any other single factor alone. What determines it is the coming together of all these elements into a complex and complicated ensemble, an ensemble that is, by definition, a spatiotemporally singular event. This local coming together—which is governed neither by the ensemble as a whole nor by any one of its constitutive elements—is what I refer to as synthesis.

The case histories I have collected and analyzed in the present chapter allow us to examine the process of emergence and disappearance at the heart of such synthesis. Professor Zhu's integration of Chinese and Western medicine is a case in point. As it stands, this certainly represents a heterogeneous and unfinished project. At the simplest level a combination of the two medicines is practiced concurrently but without any noticeable degree of interpenetration. Inasmuch as such practice must be structured to be usable, it seems to be guided by Chinese medical concepts about the relationship between root (*ben* 本) and branch (*biao* 标). Whenever a more self-conscious interpenetration takes place, Professor Zhu marshals the resources of biomedicine within a process of practice exhibiting Pickering's mechanisms of accommodation and resistance.

Professor Zhu's reinterpretation of classical anatomy in the light of biomedical information is one example. The cochlear and vestibular sense organs he treats are neither entirely the brain or vessels of the *Huangdi neijing* 黄帝内经 (*The Inner Classic of the Yellow Lord*) and other canonical works, nor are they what a neurologist or ENT specialist would see—though they can be either. They are constituted by a mode of reasoning that has assimilated biomedical ideas of endolymphatic fluid to Chinese medical ideas of phlegm and of the inner ear to the lesser *yang* vessel. The body of Professor Zhu's patients is still recognizable as the body of viscera and vessels. It is still brought to life by the metabolic transformation of *qi,* blood, and body fluids. Yet, it has also accommodated to approximate more closely the body that is revealed by biomedical technology.

The selfsame process occurs on the level of treatment formulation. The new formula composed by Professor Zhu represents an accommodation of the Chinese medical pharmacopoeia to resistances encountered in the course of clinical practice that manifested as repeatedly unsatisfactory applications of older formulas. The concepts on which these older formulas were built remain operative, but their combination has accommodated to a reality of disease made visible by a medical technology that was not available to physicians in the Han or the Yuan.

Once new formulas and views of the body are constructed they compete with the older ones they seek to replace. There is no mechanism in place, however, by which Professor Zhu could impose his reasoning on his colleagues even though he is gradually moving into positions associated with considerable influence and prestige. The systematization of Chinese medicine that has taken place since the 1950s on the level of education and theory has been counterbalanced by an equally strong emphasis (especially during the late 1980s and the 1990s) on individual skill and experience. Pressure on physicians to treat patients according to one strategy rather than another is still mediated by personal relationships (of teacher to student, superior to inferior) rather than by explicit or implicit professional rules of conduct and their policing by professional bodies. Accordingly, what changes in the process of innovation is not Chinese medicine as a system but the practices and views of individual physicians.

This has two important consequences for our understanding of contemporary Chinese medicine. First, it draws our attention to the importance of personal relationships in the transmission and practice of Chinese medicine. Second, the location of Chinese medicine in locally specific syntheses rather than global modes of reasoning or habitus supports my claim that thinking of Chinese medicine as a continually evolving field of practice provides us with a more adequate understanding of its actual practice. Some infrastructures in this field connect with more infrastructures than do others. For this reason some persons, living and dead, are more influential, some concepts more true, and some formulas more efficacious than others. Thinking in this way about synthesis formation permits a view of medical practice that allows the input of biological, social, and cultural infrastructures without privileging one above the other.

Of thirty-one new formulas for the treatment of dizziness published in Chinese medical journals between 1980 and 1991, twenty-five treat phlegm-dampness and twenty-five treat liver disharmonies—the very same disease mechanisms treated by Professor Zhu's formula. Those that treat phlegm-dampness draw their inspiration from one or more of three classical formulas: fourteen from *Er chen tang* or one of its derivatives such as *Wendan tang* 温胆汤 (Warm the Gallbladder Decoction) and *Banxia baizhu tianma tang* 半夏白术天麻汤 (Pinellia, Atractylodes, and Gastrodia Decoction); fourteen from *Zexie tang* 泽泻汤 (Alismatis Decoction), and five from *ling gui zhu gan tang* 苓桂术甘汤 (Poria, Cinnamon, Atractylodes, and Liquorice Decoction).[65] Liver treatment strategies are only slightly more varied. Biomedical influence exhausts itself in the use of a small number of drugs such as *Puerariae Radix*, *Salviae militiorrhiziae Radix*, *Lycopi Herba*, and *Plantaginis Semen* for their vasodilator or diuretic effects.[66]

All patients suffering from Ménière's disease share certain biological malfunctions. Patients furthermore have symptoms and signs in common that will invariably lead physicians relying on the same tools of examination toward broadly similar diagnoses. Yet, the biological dysfunctions of Ménière's disease are also complemented by additional symptoms and signs, bestowing on each case at each moment in time a very specific character and presentation. Each physician, in turn, has been disciplined in the use of Chinese medical diagnosis and therapeutics within individually specific social relations and institutional contexts resulting in inclinations to use some tools and concepts more than others. Physicians have idiosyncratic preferences and tastes, and institutional facilities differ in some aspects. Finally, documentation of treatment effects in Chinese medicine does not insist on the homogenization of local contexts of practice but admits single case narratives and clinical studies without the use of control groups.

Here, too, then, the observation of chapter 4 is confirmed: Local interactions that are not directed by any single organizing principle can nevertheless lead to accommodations that from a global perspective appear as changes of cultural form. Innovations in the treatment of Ménière's disease differ from each other yet do not differ all that much because the resistance patients offer to the drugs and formulas that physicians employ in their treatment are similar but not alike. The adjustments physicians make to their formulas in accommodating to these resistances are also filtered through disciplined modes of perception and understanding that are similar but not alike. Finally, the social mechanisms of control that structure Chinese medicine as a field of practice tolerate the coexistence of certain degrees of diversity.

There remains one further issue that deserves attention. It might be argued that the accommodating strategies I have described are evidence of the increasing domination of Chinese medicine by Western medicine rather than of the independent survival of the former. I would concur with such a view insofar as science in general and biomedicine in particular constitute reference points of such power in contemporary China that Chinese medicine physicians simply cannot ignore them. However, the outcome of this confrontation is no foregone conclusion. As I have shown, the local is not simply dominated by the global, but rather has the power to make the global local by assimilating it. Professor Zhu, in particular, shows that the clinical gaze of biomedicine is not the natural outcome of viewing the body through the instruments of biomedical technology; as we know from Kuhn, Foucault, and others, it is the result of distinctive disciplinary practices. Practitioners of Chinese medicine in contemporary China have learned to subject themselves to these disciplines but also know how to escape from them. The inner ear is filled with endolymphatic fluid, but it can also be full of phlegm. *Plantaginis Semen* is a diuretic, but that does not mean that it does not also enter the liver, clear the eyes, and eliminate damp.

To argue that contemporary Chinese physicians are losing, or may already have lost, touch with "traditional" medicine misses a more significant point—namely, that it is possible to communicate effectively across apparently incommensurable paradigms, that horizons are essentially open, that plurality is practicable. Even though—or rather because—it emerges from a position of weakness, the integration of biomedical practices and concepts into the field of contemporary Chinese medicine teaches us much about how to engage with the other without abandoning the integrity of the self.

6. STUDENTS, DISCIPLES, AND THE ART OF SOCIAL NETWORKING
Becoming a Physician of Chinese Medicine

The present chapter continues my exploration of plurality in contemporary Chinese medicine by examining the connection between medical practice and social relationships. Given the vastness of cultural space and the complexity of the contemporary in modern China I have opted, once more, for a case study approach. The individual I have placed at the center of this study is Professor Rong, a leading physician, author, and educator. Professor Rong's multiple involvement in the practice, transmission, and transformation of Chinese medicine over the course of four decades bears witness to how doctrine and practice are continuously reconstituted through a plurality of social interactions. My case study depicts how, within the small space of a consulting room in the north of Beijing, a multiplicity of heterogeneous social relations converge on and radiate out from a single center. This center is Professor Rong. From a different perspective, however, Professor Rong will seem to be merely a convenient intersection of networks through which different kinds of things (information, emotions, favors, capital of various kinds) travel and are exchanged.

To reduce the complexity of the undertaking and thereby make it practicable I have chosen to concentrate on the social relations implicated in becoming a physician. I speak about "becoming a physician" rather than "knowledge transmission" to avoid the cognitivist bias and reliance on mystifying notions of internalization implicit in the latter. Paying attention to how one becomes a physician rather than on how knowledge is transmitted shifts attention to the investigation of development and learning as an intrinsically open-ended process in which identity, knowing practice (to use Farquhar's term), and membership of social groups forever entail one another.[1]

Such a perception of learning and understanding accepts that plural ways of knowing (like those we encountered in chapter 5) are not merely possible but highly practicable. Knowing and understanding are seen as emerging in local syntheses in which people engage with the agency of other people and things. One particular characteristic of human agency is its ability to insert itself simultaneously into many syntheses by relating itself to many different infrastructures at once. This understanding of human agency is reflected in an emerging research tradition in anthropology and related disciplines that argues that analyses of social behavior must allow for the possibility of a non-unitary individual composed of or existing as "a set of multiple and contradictory positionings."[2] Conceptually, this is expressed in an explicit desire to move away from explanations of behavior centered on the universalized Enlightenment subject as the "gold standard for successful personhood" toward analyses of "subjectivity" or "subject positionality."[3]

Exploring agency as mediated by "subjectivities" or "subject positionalities" naturally leads to the exploration of social space. At the end of chapter 2 I delineated this space in terms of fields of practice that are populated by human and nonhuman infrastructures integrated into or excluded from processes of synthesis. I argued that fields of practice determine agency and subjectivity, while agency and subjectivity reciprocally construct the fields of practice in which they are located. Such mutual construction may be usefully explored by means of a mode of analysis that explores not only the spacial relation of infrastructures in relation to each other but also the performativities that establish, maintain, and rupture them. I employ the notions of topography and topology to describe these modes of analysis. The *Oxford English Dictionary* defines topography as mapping the surface of a body with reference to the parts beneath it, making it a particularly fitting term for my examination of syntheses built from infrastructures. However, the mapping of a body or field of practice is as dependent on how the observer constructs a place through observation and analysis than it is a function of the organization of space itself. My awareness of this effect is indexed by reference to the notion of topology.[4]

I begin this chapter by describing the field of practice of contemporary Chinese medicine in its relation to professional development, highlighting three distinct forms of learning and the kinds of social relations they embody and support: discipleship, studentship, and social networking, or *guanxixue* 关系学. I adduce each type of relationship in Professor Rong's own professional development and that of his students and disciples. This methodological device enables me to undercut the separation of social relations into mutually exclusive types and the organization of fields of practice into clearly bounded terrains. In the final section of this chapter I draw on the notions of topography and topology as defined above in order to understand how the plurality of Chinese medicine in contemporary China is socially constructed.

Let me begin, then, by introducing my main actor. From September to December 1994 I was privileged to study with seventy-three-year-old Professor Rong, one of Beijing's *ming laozhongyi*. The following is an account of a typical day in the working life of Professor Rong, his students, and his disciples.

CASE 6.1. *A Day in the Life of Dr. Rong.* At about 7:30 A.M. Professor Rong and his son and disciple Dr. Rong Jr. are picked up at their home by the professor's three Ph.D. students. The students have come to escort their teacher to his surgery, where ten or more patients, Dr. Lu, and I await his arrival. Dr. Lu, a gray-haired woman in her early fifties and a professor at Beijing University of Chinese Medicine, is the second disciple of Professor Rong. As Professor Rong and his entourage approach the building that houses the clinic, his students, who usually file behind their teacher, quickly move to the front. As one opens the door for the professor and helps him take off his coat, the other two busy themselves with arranging the consulting room: placing chairs for Professor Rong and his patients, making sure he is supplied with boiling water for his tea, sorting patients' files, preparing prescription blocks. As soon as Professor Rong has seated himself he begins his consultations. By lunchtime he will have attended to between sixty and seventy patients.

Professor Rong's small consulting room is sparsely furnished with a large rectangular wooden table, several chairs, and a coat rack. The furniture, in the classical heavy Chinese style, is new. In its contrast to the cheap fittings of most ordinary clinics it obviously has been chosen to underline the status of Professor Rong and his colleagues who see patients in this room. The east side of the table is placed against a mirrored wall that makes the room appear larger. Professor Rong occupies its north side, facing south toward the only window. A chair for the patient is provided at the corner of the table next to Professor Rong. On the south side, opposite Professor Rong, sit one of his disciples and a student; the other two students and I are crammed next to the patient. The remainder of the room is filled with waiting patients and their relatives and friends.

Each consultation proceeds according to the same pattern. Professor Rong examines the patient's pulse and tongue, asks a few questions, and then writes out a one- or two-line diagnosis followed by a prescription into the case history booklet that serves as the treatment record. The booklet is then passed to the student seated opposite, who copies the prescription on a prescription pad. He keeps one copy for himself and passes another to the patient, who has already vacated the chair for the next person in line. The two other students also copy Professor Rong's prescriptions and notes. Occasionally they ask a supplementary question of patients who are waiting for their prescriptions. If the need arises, they deal with patients' queries and problems, ensuring that as few as possible intrusions are made into Professor Rong's precious consulting time.

The role of Professor Rong's two disciples is different from that of his students. On alternate days one of them sees a small number of Professor Rong's patients in an adjacent windowless cubicle toward the rear of the building. Professor Rong decides which patients these will be. Most often he chooses new patients whose intake interview would make excessive demands on his time. The consultation of these patients follows the same pattern established by Professor Rong, though his disciples take considerably longer to arrive at a prescription. The patient then takes this prescription to the main room, where, following a short inspection of pulse and tongue, Professor Rong makes a few alterations to his disciple's prescription. He crosses out some of the drugs and replaces them with others in a gesture that has educational as well as social significance. The student may have made a mistake, but patients coming to Professor Rong for treatment would not be happy if they received only the benefit of his disciples' knowledge.

The second disciple, meanwhile, also makes copies of Professor Rong's notes and prescriptions. Sometimes Dr. Lu or Dr. Rong Jr. retains a patient's case history booklet in order to translate its content into a detailed case history for Professor Rong's archive. If Professor Rong is out of town attending a conference or giving a lecture, as happens frequently, his disciples treat his patients in his absence. His students do not attend on these days. His son also assists his father during the surgeries he holds at his home in the evenings and on Sundays, where Professor Rong treats many high-standing cadre and business leaders.

During consultations, Professor Rong focuses his attention entirely on his patients, sporadically interrupting his treatment to light yet another cigarette. Only three or four times during the entire four months I studied with him did he teach his students or disciples verbally. Considerable time was devoted, instead, to instructing his patients individually or as a group on issues of diet and lifestyle or on the special characteristics of Chinese medicine. Without surrendering his gravity he did everything his patients expected from an exemplary physician: he entertained them from time to time with little stories from his life or accounts of the many famous people he treats, or briefly played with a baby and reassured its mother.

In order to gain an audience with Professor Rong patients must purchase a numbered ticket (*guahao* 挂号) on the previous evening. Professor Rong allows fifty such tickets to be sold for each morning session. Toward the end of the morning patients without tickets begin to appear, those who were too busy the night before or who live too far away to buy a ticket. They know that, being a benevolent physician, Professor Rong will do his best to treat them, too. Although it is Professor Rong who decides how many extra patients he treats on a given day, it is the task of his students to make sure that no one's feelings are hurt and that a proper balance is achieved between demonstrating Professor Rong's benevolence and his need to get home in time for lunch and some rest before his afternoon schedule. Shortly before or after 12:00 noon, when the last patient has left, Professor Rong sets out for home. Having cleaned up, his students and disciples follow him in a small procession back to his home.

In the afternoon, Professor Rong usually attends a meeting of one of the many committees of which he is a leading member. On some afternoons he holds surgeries at another clinic in Beijing to which he is accompanied by his disciples. His disciples also attend to the archive of their teacher's case records and assist him with the writing and preparing of manuscripts. The students are busy with their own doctoral dissertations; the topic of each is research into formulas designed by Professor Rong. Such research involves tracing the historical lineage of the formula as well as research extending from biochemical analyses and animal experiments to the documentation of case histories, clinical experiments, and clinical trials.

Discipleship: The Past Endures

My Chinese informants clearly distinguished between the students (*xuesheng* 学生) and disciples (*tudi* 徒弟) of a given teacher. The present section deals with Professor Rong's relation to his disciples, but also draws on observations from other discipleships to which I gained access during my fieldwork.

Perhaps the most common route to becoming a physician of Chinese medicine until the end of the nineteenth century was by way of apprenticeship.[5] The modernization of Chinese medicine attempted from within the Chinese medicine circles during the late Qing and Republican eras led to the opening of schools and colleges in many cities and provinces that modeled themselves on universities and technical colleges and sought to emulate Western medical training. Apprenticeship nevertheless continued as a mode of teaching and learning, with the boundaries of modern schooling and classical learning not always clearly defined and separated.[6] The particularistic nature of older-style master-disciple relationships and the private monopoly of knowledge thereby retained by teachers were not ideologically approved of after the establishment of the new China in 1949. Nevertheless, discipleship was integrated into the state-controlled education system and even expanded in the latter half of the 1950s in an effort to increase the total number of physicians practicing Chinese medicine.[7] Under a different scheme devised by the Ministry of Health in 1958, 104 younger practitioners were allocated to thirty-one famous physicians with whom they studied as formal disciples. The intention was to extract their clinical knowledge from these famous physicians in order to make it more widely available to future generations.[8]

Discipleship in Chinese medicine (as in other Chinese arts and crafts) is founded on the pattern of the family and can be documented as far back as the second century B.C.[9] Sivin identifies in the handing down of "authentic, written medical revelations" within lineages of descent (from father to son or master to disciple) the hallmark of elite physicians at least until A.D. 500.[10] Changes in the social status of physicians from the late Song onward led to a steadily increasing influx of scholars from elite social classes. By the late imperial era this resulted in a distinction being made between hereditary physicians (shiyi 世医) and literati physicians (ruyi 儒医). The former were thought of as possessing empirical knowledge transmitted through family lines, whereas the latter studied the medical classics as part of their general education, translating their doctrines into medical practice. In practice, however, the line between these groups was never that clear. Many literati physicians came from medical families or studied with practicing physicians, and hereditary physicians also studied the medical classics.[11]

Social relations between master and disciple then as now are modeled on the filial relationship between father and son, one of the five cardinal relationships (wu lun 五伦) of Confucian ideology.[12] These relationships (some would say all relationships in Chinese society) embody a hierarchical relation of nonequals.[13] The father/master, as the senior element in the relationship, is accorded authority and a wide range of prerogatives over the son/disciple, which are circumscribed by rules of correct conduct (li 礼). Such rules in the old China were considered essential to the performance of filial duties and the harmony of the relationship.[14] This hierarchical ordering of social relations imposed by older ideologies of patrilineal descent has been closely linked, functionally and ideologically, to the practice of ancestor worship whereby a line was legitimized and maintained.[15] It also has crucially shaped Chinese preoccupations with status and face in a society whose members accept that power in institutions and organizations is by definition distributed unequally.[16]

The hierarchical structuring of discipleships and the mutual obligations this entails are clearly visible in the relationship between Professor Rong and his disciples, who walk behind the professor when accompanying him; are there for Professor Rong, at any time he requires, to assist his work or to carry out those jobs that are too menial for him; and subordinate their personal careers to that of their teacher's accumulation of status by contributing to a book that will be published under Professor Rong's name. Several disciples of famous Beijing physicians with whom I spoke emphasized that their teacher was very strict, and that they feared him because of that. Yet, such strictness was also considered an expression of care and concern. Whereas previously assertions of authority/expression of care may have included physical punishment such as beating, however, they are now limited to "not talking much and never smiling," "being stern," and "making demands that cannot be questioned."[17]

There is no uniform way by which one becomes a disciple of a famous physician, although famous physicians invariably have disciples. Before the establishment of Chinese medicine colleges in the 1950s apprenticeship might start at an early age either within one's own family or by moving into the household of the teacher. More often it consisted of a formal period of training usually lasting three to six years starting in a person's late teens. The beginning of such an apprenticeship was frequently marked by a formal initiation ceremony in which the disciple would acknowledge (bai 拜) the authority and status of his new teacher by kowtowing to him. The discipleship involved memorizing canonical works such as the *Shanghan lun* (with which Professor Rong, according to his students, started at age five), copying prescriptions during clinic hours, and participating in peripheral activities such as compounding medicines and boiling herbal decoctions.[18]

Today apprenticeship rarely begins before university training has been completed. Professor Rong's son, for instance, graduated from a provincial college of Chinese medicine, and Dr. Lu studied and now works at Beijing University of Chinese Medicine. The state controls not only the licensing of medical practitioners, but also access to positions of status and power within the Chinese medicine sector. Without appropriate professional qualifications such positions would be closed even to apprentices of famous physicians. Professor Rong himself, after all, is not only a practicing doctor, but also a member of the CCP and an emeritus professor at Beijing University of Chinese Medicine.

Disciples are admitted by their teacher on the basis of a variety of factors ranging from kinship ties and perceived merit to political pressure. According to Sivin, the extension of apprenticeship from strictly patrilineal transmission to a system allowing transmission also to the son-in-law or nonagnatic disciples signaled the transformation from a society in which birth alone determined livelihood to one based on flexible occupations. In the earlier system initiation and restriction of access to medical knowledge to a narrowly defined group of people functioned to mark off an elite stratum of physicians from those belonging to lower orders.[19] While such explanations of ancient relationships retain a certain validity, they demand important modifications in contemporary China.

Of crucial importance here are attempts by the state, which never managed to totally eliminate discipleships, to co-opt these into the state education system. In June 1990 the MOH in conjunction with the State Administration of Chinese Medicine and Pharmacology (Guojia zhongyiyao guanliju 国家中医药管理局) and the Ministry of Personnel (Renshibu 人事部) decided to institute a scheme whereby five hundred designated *ming laozhongyi* would train qualified physicians in state-approved and -supervised apprenticeships. After a brief selection process a ceremony was held in the Great Hall of the People in Beijing on 20 October 1990 allocating an initial 725 disciples to 462 physicians.[20]

The scheme, since institutionalized on a wider scale, blurs the boundaries between discipleship as an institution of learning based on personal relations and state-controlled education. More important, it can be seen as an instrument for the regularization of Chinese medical practice advanced by the Chinese state. Disciples are expected to publish their teacher's case records or use them as the foundation for more formal clinical studies. As I demonstrate in chapter 7, the rewriting of case records is not merely a vehicle for honoring medical ancestors but also involves transformations that subjugate diverse personal forms of knowing and practicing into officially approved kinds of "knowing practice." Given the importance of face and status in everyday life, recruiting subjects (both masters and disciples) is easy. Official entitlement to teach disciples considerably raises the status of *ming laozhongyi* above that of other physicians. For the apprentice, successful completion of discipleship is marked by an official certificate that confers some of the *mingqi* 名气, or fame, of the teacher onto the disciple.

Dr. Rong has no other disciples besides his son and Dr. Lu. Professor Xu, another famous professor of stature similar to Dr. Rong's, does from time to time admit short-term disciples under the system outlined above. Dr. Chao completed such a discipleship, and her accounts are the most detailed I was able to collect regarding contemporary discipleship. Dr. Chao graduated from the Beijing University of Chinese Medicine in 1991 and subsequently entered into a discipleship with Professor Xu in preference to postgraduate study at university. The following account of her discipleship is based on several interviews with Dr. Chao.

CASE 6.2. *Dr. Chao's Apprenticeship.* For Dr. Chao, becoming an apprentice was a process that stretched out over a period of several months. Dr. Chao first needed to establish a tentative relationship with Professor Xu. She succeeded in this because she was a close friend of one of his existing disciples, who made the first approach to her chosen teacher. She also was fortunate in that she knew one of Professor Xu's daughters, through whom she had been introduced to other members of the family. Further introductions and references supplied by these family members persuaded Professor Xu to grant an audience to Dr. Chao, who at the time was a recent graduate of the Beijing College of Chinese Medicine.

For this occasion Dr. Chao was formally invited to Professor Xu's home. A virtual relationship was thus transformed into an actual one. Dr. Chao managed, during the course of her interview, to strengthen a still extremely tenuous bond by the judicious use of other tactics. She had previously studied with another famous physician, which increased her credibility as a serious student in the eyes of Professor Xu. She also added to Professor Xu's face by suggesting that she wished to study with him in preference to postgraduate training at university. Furthermore, she had been involved in a research project that resonated with Professor Xu's own field of specialization. It is not uncommon for junior physicians to publish under the name of or at least jointly with their supervisor or superior. Dr. Chao explained to me that this benefits both parties. The student gains by association with a famous professor, and the professor increases his involvement with successful and potentially important research. According to Dr. Chao the implications of this joint interest were obvious to both actors when they met for the first time without the need to dwell explicitly on future cooperation. Finally, Dr. Chao was married to a Westerner. At present, many Chinese aspire, for themselves or for their sons and daughters, to study or work in the West. Dr. Chao's potential ability to facilitate such a move for a member of Professor Xu's own family did not go unnoticed.[21]

Following their first face-to-face meeting Professor Xu began to demand for Dr. Chao "to do this and that" (about which Dr. Chao did not want to talk in detail). Dr. Chao obeyed all his commands. After several months and further consultations between Professor Xu and his family and apprentices Dr. Chao was finally accepted as a disciple. The bond was affirmed with a formal banquet at a famous Beijing hotel for which Dr. Chao and another disciple admitted at the same time had to bear the cost. The banquet included a brief ceremony during which Dr. Chao had to acknowledge the now official filiation to her new teacher by means of three kowtows.

Thereafter she followed him in his clinics. She copied prescriptions for her teacher, prepared his tea, took care of his patients. There was little formal teaching, and Professor Xu would not tolerate any questions from his disciples during consultations. "You could see his prescriptions, then you would know what methods he used." Occasionally Professor Xu would demand a diagnosis from his disciples. If they answered contrary to what he expected, he would feel that they had not studied diligently and become very angry. He would tell them to consult a specific text to clarify their deficiencies.

Dr. Chao's official discipleship with Professor Xu lasted two years. Now she has very little direct contact with her teacher, but his influence continues to be strong. Morally, she finds it difficult to use any other method than that of her teacher. Personally, she feels that her apprenticeship has fundamentally changed her character. She has changed from being a headstrong woman with "bad manners," she told me, into a more mature person who can empathize with her patients. Learning about medical morality (*yide* 医德) from her teacher, including above all the practice of deference, was for Dr. Chao as important as learning clinical strategies.

Gradients of apprenticeship as well as their common denominators and their links to patterns of past tradition are discernible in the three discipleships we have encountered. The hierarchical ordering of discipleships is reflected in ritualized behavior (*li* 礼) that may demand of disciples to *koutou* during initiation or to pour tea for their teacher during consultations. *Li* demands that teachers be stern and strict on the outside and caring on the inside. It expresses *renqing* 人情, the observation of proper social forms of etiquette, yet can also be charged more deeply with *ganqing* 感情, a particular quality of emotionality that Chinese associate with long-standing relationships and often see as lacking abroad.[22]

In terms of both form and content, discipleships can thus be mapped according to the proximity of the relationships they entail. The relation between Professor Rong and his son is an extension of a preexisting father-son relationship and shares in its mutual obligations and symbolic connotations. Dr. Rong Jr. carries on a long-established family line going back apparently nine generations. He lives in the same household as his father and communicates with him in a southern dialect that remains unintelligible to Dr. Lu and his students.[23] Dr. Rong Jr. himself does not occupy a position in the university. He does, however, help his father with all consultations, including those for rich and influential patients carried out at the Rongs' home. Professor Rong's influence could easily secure an official appointment for his son. Why he has not done so, I do not know. One possibility is that the family may consider Dr. Rong Jr.'s cultivation of connections in Beijing to be of greater importance than teaching at a university. Or perhaps, given recent economic changes, a future in a privately run establishment and maybe even a move abroad may be viewed as more attractive options for his son's future.[24]

The relation between Professor Rong and his second disciple, Dr. Lu, is an extension of a bureaucratic relationship between superior and inferior. By way of this apprenticeship Professor Rong has successfully inserted his medical line into the bureaucratic organization of the state education system. As a professor in the same department of which Professor Rong himself is an emeritus professor, Dr. Lu is now the second link in a new chain of transmission. This chain has assimilated state education into the line's descent, but the lineage has had to accommodate itself to these new contexts too. Whereas for nine generations Professor Rong's family tradition has been transmitted through the male line according to classical ideologies of patrilineal descent, the realities of socialist education have opened up a space in this lineage allowing a woman to take up an important and visible position.[25]

A further notable difference between Professor Rong's two apprentices (and the relations they embody) manifests in their apparent division of labor. Dr. Lu sits in with her teacher only on certain days, for she also has teaching commitments. She is in charge of Professor Rong's archive of case histories and assists him in the writing of his books. If the Professor Rong–Dr. Rong Jr. line emphasizes clinical production (in which the accumulation of financial and cultural capital are intertwined), the Professor Rong–Dr. Lu line extends beyond the clinic to that of academic production (and its predominant accumulation of cultural capital).

Professor Rong thus is the node from which two lines branch off, never again to be located so close to each other as they are now. The link of both disciples to their master, however, defines what they are and can become. Already in her fifties, Professor Lu is known first and foremost as the disciple of Professor Rong. Dr. Rong Jr. likewise stands eternally in the shadow of his famous father. Whatever they themselves produce (in the clinic, in academe) will be linked with and reflect back on their teacher. This is so even for Professor Rong himself. Merely mentioning Professor Rong's name in Chinese medical circles invariably leads to stories about his even more famous father, who has been dead for nearly half a century but whose reputation still eclipses that of his now seventy-three-year-old son.

In contrast, the relationship between Professor Xu and Dr. Chao was from the outset temporary, even if its effects endure. In that sense, it has the character of a strategic alliance rather than a structural bond. Dr. Chao can legitimately claim to be Professor Xu's disciple, though that does not make her part of his line (in a narrow sense). Vice versa, Professor Xu might claim Dr. Chao as his disciple, either publicly (by providing a preface for one of her books, for instance, if she becomes a famous physician) or privately (if she can provide some personal favor). There is no pressure on either of them, however, to maintain a publicly visible relationship of enduring obligations.

The above examples show how master-disciple relationships of different grades of proximity, various degrees of longevity, and different functional characters are established on the basis of various socially effective relations: cognatic blood ties, bureaucratic hierarchies, and social networks. These grades of proximity express themselves, too, in the ways disciples learn from their teacher and later themselves become masters. For Dr. Chao, learning consisted largely of access to Professor Xu's method of prescribing. She was present while patients were treated but had to rely on interpretive methods to make explicit the diagnosis and treatment methods implicit in her teacher's formulas. On those rare occasions when his teaching became verbal, it was structured so as to test whether the student had succeeded in retracing her master's steps. Rather than receiving categorical instructions, the student was guided to a text that might help her in overcoming interpretive difficulties. While she was a disciple of Professor Xu, Dr. Chao was expected "to have his train of thought, exactly his train and no other." Now that bond has visibly thinned, but Dr. Chao admits to still being influenced by her master. It is an influence that, apparently, has as much to do with respect as with social pressure. "As a disciple of Professor Xu," she told me, "it was impossible for me to study different methods. If I wanted to do so, I had to do it secretly. Still now, I had better not let other people know."[26]

While they also rely on interpretive understanding, Dr. Rong's two disciples, in contrast, have ample opportunity to have their interpretations corrected in practice and to engage with their master in explicit discourse. Vice versa, the pressures and expectations brought to bear on them have increased with that proximity. Not only are they required to think like their teacher, he still checks on their every prescription even though both are middle-aged.

Discipleship in contemporary Chinese medicine thus seems to be geared toward turning disciples into copies of their masters. This may be seen as embodying classical concerns for the maintenance of a line (turning masters into ancestors and disciples into masters), but also as reflecting an often diagnosed aversion of conventional morality toward critical inquiry and innovation. Although undoubtedly of some merit, the implicit Orientalism of such an interpretation needs to be balanced by greater sensitivity to other aspects of filiality and learning within discipleships.

Given the general concerns of Chinese culture with issues of face and social standing, those ties that most closely involve one's own person and from which one can least easily dissociate oneself are those that must also be most closely controlled. No one would blame Professors Rong and Xu if one of their doctoral students or part-time apprentices failed to become an accomplished physician. Their own reputation and that of their line would suffer greatly, however, if their acknowledged heir failed to live up to expectations. What is at stake in the education of disciples, therefore, is not merely the transmission of knowledge but also prestige and the protection of status. Protecting what has been inherited through generations (protecting it, that is, from non-efficient change) seems an appropriate and highly moral strategy of education in a context in which it is precisely that inheritance (in terms of its clinical efficacy and its distinctive characteristics respective to other lines) that forms the foundation of present prestige and efficacy. Not surprisingly, much of the family tradition remains implicit (revealing itself only in the course of continued guided interpretation) or even secret.[27] This arrangement ensures that leakage to the outside is controlled while fortifying the position of the father/teacher as the embodiment and guardian of tradition.

Discipleship also embodies a very particular way in which the agency of physicians is perceived. A famous quote by the Han physician Guo Yu 郭玉 is still frequently invoked today when Chinese medicine physicians wish to express that medical practice is an art that refuses to be captured in words alone. Asked to explain to Emperor He (A.D. 89–105) how he had been able to cure a patient with a single needle, Guo Yu replied: "Medicine [yi 医] is attention [yi 意]. The regions of the skin are very finely divided. Following the flow of *qi* requires consummate skill. When inserting needles, an error of a hair's breadth will mean failure. A kind of spirit connects the physician's heart with his hand, and that is something I can know but cannot explain."[28]

The notion of *yi* 意 in Guo Yu's word play, translated in this context as attention, also carries the meaning of intention, idea, thought, or purpose, of an understanding that can be unfolded in practice but is not limited to representational knowledge. Later Chinese physicians used the concept of *yi* to point to those aspects of medicine "that can be apprehended but are difficult to explain in words" (*keyi yihui, nan yu yanchuan* 可以意会, 难于言传). *Yi* in this sense can refer to a physician's ability to grasp the ever-changing (*bian* 变) transformations of illness in clinical practice that lie beyond the regular (*chang* 常) manifestations described in books. It also signaled the difficulty of passing on those kinds of knowledge that, following Polyani, we refer to as implicit and link to craft through the medium of language.[29]

From this perspective, the endless copying of prescriptions for one's teacher, like the rote learning of classical texts and the memorization of formulas, must be understood as purposefully constructed situated learning through peripheral participation.[30] Such learning is designed to assimilate to one's own body/person the meaning, understanding, and intentions in practices like formula composition and pulse diagnosis that lie beyond words. This understanding will manifest, later on, in the sudden realization of an awakened mind that can penetrate below surface manifestations to the deeper patterns of a pathology, just as a scholar can grasp the subtle signification of a text that lies beyond the literal meaning of the written characters.[31]

Perceptions of agency and social relations within the education system developed by the socialist state since the 1950s differ in many respects from discipleship as discussed above. Whereas the latter expresses older forms of social organization, morality, particularism, and implicit (or even secret) knowledge, state education (henceforth referred to as studentship) self-consciously declares itself to be modern, universal, and scientific.[32] However, there are also points of crossover, contiguity, and propinquity that attest to the historical transformations that have shaped studentship both out of and against discipleship. I shall now explore these differences by examining the relation between Professor Rong and his students.

Studentship: The Influence of the Modern Socialist State

Professor Rong forms relations with students in two contexts: in a direct, immediate manner as lecturer, teacher, and supervisor; and in an indirect, mediated manner as the author of textbooks and the member of committees that determine what and how students learn Chinese medicine both in Beijing and at other colleges and universities throughout China. While disciples gain access to a master through networks of personal relationships, students are allocated to teachers via a state-controlled bureaucratic mechanism.

Students throughout China are admitted to academic courses on the basis of nationwide competitive examinations. Admission to undergraduate courses depends on the score obtained in a general university entrance exam. Admission to postgraduate courses is based on entrance exams for specific courses. All examinations are fiercely competitive. According to one of my informants, of more than a hundred acupuncture students who enrolled in his class at the Shanxi Chinese Medicine College in 1984, only three were studying for Ph.D. degrees ten years later.[33] Examinations are almost always written exams employing a mixed format of multiple choice and short-answer questions as well as the filling in of blanks in given sentences with standard phrases.[34]

Although a detailed analysis of state education in Chinese medicine is beyond the scope of this book, two observations relevant to my more immediate concerns can nevertheless be made. First, its emphasis on testing memorized knowledge establishes a clear link with patterns of examination in imperial China.[35] Second, these examinations should be regarded as being as much a cause as an expression of the standardization of classical medical knowledge that is characteristic of its contemporary transformation. Nationwide exams are meaningful only if the results are comparable. For that, the education system must produce roughly equivalent local contexts of learning, or at least transmit in these contexts a common core of testable knowledge. There are several important preconditions for the success of such an undertaking.

First, political control of education must be sufficiently centralized to arrange and supervise a process whereby previously diverse contexts of learning are progressively homogenized. In chapter 3 I documented the control exercised over Chinese medicine education by the state via the MOH and the MOE in terms of both its bureaucratic organization and its political connotations. We also saw there how, conversely, a breakdown of central control during the period of the Cultural Revolution was accompanied by the breakdown of centralized state education.

Second, teaching materials and curricula must transform personalized practices that accord a high value to implicit knowledge into shared, explicit, and highly formalized knowledge, a process examined in detail by Hsu.[36] We can take as an example the reaction of the editors of the *Great Encyclopedia* of *Chinese Medicine* to Guo Yu's statement, translated above, that medicine may be based on abilities that cannot always be put into words (*bu ke de yan* 不可得言). The editors of this important state project express their clear dismay at such particularistic views when they write that if "he [Guo Yu] also proposes that 'medicine embodies the idea of attention' and that the hows and whys of treatment 'cannot be put into words,' [then] these are aspects of his limited thinking."[37]

During the formative period of state education in the 1950s and early 1960s, when Chinese medicine along with the rest of society was to be modernized along socialist lines, older experts were recruited into the state system at the same time that younger physicians began to produce the first national textbooks. This dual task required the proponents of Chinese medicine to conceive of mechanisms by which Chinese medicine could be sufficiently modernized to satisfy the political demands of the day without surrendering in the process characteristics such as "holism" (*zhengti guannian* 整体观念) and "constant change" (*hengdong guannian* 恒动观念) that were thought to distinguish it from Western medicine. Professor Rong was actively involved in this process on many levels. The one most accessible to me was his contribution to the compilation of teaching materials.

Professor Rong's participation in this work began in the early 1950s in Jiangsu Province, where his family line originated. Lü Bingkui 吕炳奎, whose decisive influence on the shaping of Chinese medicine was briefly sketched in chapter 3, was also a native of Jiangsu, where he started his political career by organizing the education of Chinese medical physicians in the early 1950s. The courses Lü established at what was then the Jiangsu Province Chinese Medicine Teacher Improvement School (Jiangsusheng zhongyi shizi jinxiu xuexiao 江苏省中医师资进修学校) with the help of a group of young doctors later had a distinctive input into the development of the first Chinese medicine colleges. These doctors and their teachers soon occupied key positions at colleges in both Nanjing and Beijing. I have already described how Lü moved a core staff of young doctors drawn from his Jiangsu days to Beijing. Other famous physicians, such as Qin Bowei 秦伯未 from Shanghai, Pu Fuzhou 蒲辅周 from Chengdu, and Ren Yingqiu 任应秋 from Chongqing, were recruited to Beijing as well, though by means of different networks.[38] The key role played by these physicians in establishing Chinese medicine as an academic discipline is reflected nowhere more clearly than in the group's first major textbook, *Zhongyixue gailun* 中医学概论 (*Outline of Chinese Medicine*), a text compiled by the Nanjing Chinese Medicine College and published in 1958 in Beijing. Professor Rong was a member of the editorial committee. The manner in which the *Outline* divided up, systematized, and presented the entire field of Chinese medicine was extremely influential, though by no means the only way in which this was done.[39] The *Outline* has since been superseded by a series of more specialized textbooks, *Gaodeng yiyao yuanxiao jiaocai* 高等医药院校教材 (University and College Teaching Materials in Medicine and Pharmacology).[40] Professor Rong's own career mirrored this process of specialization. He became a professor at the Beijing Chinese Medicine College and in this role has been instrumental in the compilation and editing of all the editions of *Fangjixue* 方剂学 (*Formulas*), the standard textbook of the subject on which state examinations are based.[41]

An interesting observation in this context is that it would be impossible to reconstruct from the text of *Fangjixue* the manner in which Professor Rong himself prescribes to his patients. That is not to say that in his own practice Professor Rong does not draw on the formulas discussed in the text. But the manner in which Professor Rong selects, modifies, and combines these formulas in practice is nowhere explained in the very book that introduces them to undergraduate students. To understand the reason for this we must recall from chapter 5 that while standard additions and subtractions (*jiajian* 加减) exist for many formulas, these do not dictate practice. Rather, they are models from which the virtuosity of a physician—which is nowhere more visibly manifest than in the act of composing a prescription—develops. This virtuosity is referred to by Chinese doctors themselves with terms such as *ling* 灵 and *linghuo* 灵活. *Linghuo* is an adjective or adverb that translates as "agile," "quick," "nimble," "flexible," "elastic," "adaptable." Beyond these core meanings it carries connotations of being efficacious, effective, and sharp-witted, but also of an unmediated intelligence that comes from an ability to sense as well as reflect. A physician's *linghuo* characteristics are expressed emblematically in the composition of his or her prescription: in its suitability to the present context, its adaptable use of resources, its clever composition— and therefore in its spiritlike efficaciousness.[42]

Yet, it is precisely access to such virtuosity that is surrendered in *Fangjixue's* dissociation from local contexts of learning within the state education system. Students learn formulas in their second or third year of training, often from professional teachers with little clinical experience. Their knowledge of formulas is tested at the end of the semester in which they finish their course. When they move to the clinic in their fourth year, emphasis is placed, at least initially, on diagnosis rather than treatment. Only later are diagnoses again matched with formulas. This, of course, is an entirely different process of learning than one which from its outset centers on the clinic and in which a formula as often provides a diagnosis as follows from it.[43]

Certainly, almost all of the older physicians with whom I spoke lamented what they perceived as a communal loss of skills among younger physicians —a deficiency for which they partly blamed the separation of theory and practice within the state education system. Many younger physicians echoed these views. They complained to me about the lack of good teachers with clinical experience during preclinical semesters and lack of access to the very best physicians during their clinical training. Regarding formulas, it certainly was my own experience that most clinical interns and young physicians had forgotten most of the formulas they had once learned and that their manner of matching diagnoses with formulas was mechanical rather than nimble, flexible, and adaptable.

These issues cannot be dealt with exhaustively here. They return us, however, to a third point I wish to make concerning the state's attempt to standardize Chinese medical education: the homogenization of educational contexts demanded a similar homogenization of teacher-student relationships. This seems to have been carried out by means of a complex process that involved a distancing of social relations and an ongoing redefinition of mutual obligations between students and their teachers. Certain elements of established patterns of social relations were maintained, while in their entirety they were assimilated within a new social purpose. I shall unravel some of the complexities of this process with the help of excerpts from two interviews. The first is from a conversation with Dr. Chao, the disciple of Professor Xu.

> *V.S.:* It is said that relations (*guanxi* 关系) are very important in China. I want to know if *guanxi* is very important in studying Chinese medicine. *Dr. Chao:* You should know that studying Chinese medicine requires a relationship with the teacher. It is important. These old teachers have a distinct way of teaching. . . . They usually do not tell their knowledge to common students. Even to their Ph.D. students they grant access to only part of their experience. As an apprentice of his [Professor Xu] I respectfully requested that he teach me formally so he would regard me as his child and tell me everything. . . . These young teachers are different. When I studied in college as an undergraduate I had no special relations with my teachers. But studying as an undergraduate student, if you studied very hard and often asked questions, the teacher might like you. Then he might teach you more. On the other hand, some teachers are of bad quality. They request of students to give them presents or money and then they have a relationship.

The second excerpt is from an interview with Dr. Luo, a doctoral student of another famous Beijing *ming laozhongyi,* Professor Ding.

V.S.: Why is he [Professor Ding] so sought after as a supervisor?

Dr. Luo: One aspect is that he is very strict. We are afraid of him.

V.S.: Why do so many students still apply to study with him?

Dr. Luo: Although he is very strict to students, he will take care of them. For example, he will help them find jobs after graduation. Most students who come from outside Beijing want to stay in Beijing after graduation. This is their true purpose. They do not want to study. Professor Ding will try to help them. He hopes all his students get jobs. If not, he feels unsuccessful. . . . My teacher is very powerful and many people listen to him. He knows how to protect students, so students like him.

V.S.: Does his popularity also have to do with his clinical skills? What sort of results does he get in the clinic?

Dr. Luo: Not bad. He has many patients whom he sees in his clinic. He does not like the students to write the prescriptions for him. He wants his disciples to follow him to see patients and write down prescriptions. Students are different from disciples. A student should stay at school, study, and get a degree.

V.S.: How are students different from disciples?

Dr. Luo: They receive different treatment. He [Professor Ding] wants to hand down his ideas and experiences to his disciples, whereas students only need to study in school. He will instruct them in doing papers so they graduate and may become professors themselves.

These interviews seem to indicate that while certain categorical distinctions exist between studentship and discipleship, the two are related by way of historical contingency. Such contingency is embodied, literally, in Professors Rong, Xu, and Ding, who are all masters to disciples and teachers to students. It also surfaces in the stereotypical attributes expected of a good teacher in terms of demeanor and responsibility, which remain close to those previously expected of a master: sternness, strictness, and authority, on the one hand; obligation to care for students beyond merely imparting to them knowledge, on the other.[44] We have already noted how Professor Rong succeeded in inserting his line into the university infrastructure and how the state manages to influence access to and certification of certain types of discipleship. Further crossovers occur where students manage to construct particularistic ties to individual teachers.

The sheer number of students educated in university courses and the relatively short periods of time they are taught by the same teacher makes the forging of particularistic teacher-student ties during undergraduate training an exception.[45] Nevertheless, it does occur. While I was studying at the gynecology department of the Dongzhimen Hospital, one of the consultants was frequently accompanied by one of his final-year undergraduates. In his spare time, this student followed the consultant in the same manner described above for the disciples of Professors Rong and Xu: copying prescriptions; attending to patients; and, in the evenings, typing and editing his teacher's manuscripts. Another student recounted to me how being assigned for her internship to a small hospital in rural Sichuan proved advantageous. Owing to the small size of this institution (ten physicians and one student) all the staff lived in the same building and, according to my informant, had good relations. As a result, she was taken on as a personal student by the two senior physicians throughout the year of her internship.

Opportunities for developing particularistic ties become more frequent over the duration of one's education. Postgraduate students often select a course because they wish to study with a specific supervisor. Students benefit directly and indirectly from having a famous physician such as Professor Rong as their supervisor. Given the social organization of Chinese society and the influence of those placed in positions of power, a supervisor may be able to actively help with employment, promotions, research opportunities, housing, introductions, references, and even holidays. Having studied with a *ming laozhongyi* also, of course, adds to a student's face. A reciprocal pressure on physicians to show their standing by becoming supervisors is the reverse side of this coin. Unlike most other countries China certifies individuals rather than departments or programs to accept graduate students. The supervision of doctoral degrees, in particular, is reserved for eminent physicians. Status as a "doctoral supervisor" (*boshi daoshi* 博士导师) is therefore prominently displayed on the visiting cards of all those entitled to claim it, just as their students proudly present themselves as "doctoral candidates" (*boshisheng* 博士生).[46]

Once a particularistic teacher-student relationship has been established, it takes on some of the characteristics of master-disciple relationships. Physicians who had completed their postgraduate studies invariably mentioned to me how deeply their practice had been influenced by the style of their supervisor. Contexts and modalities of learning also frequently resemble those described for master-disciple relationships, as we saw with Professor Rong's doctoral students: the copying of prescriptions during clinical practice and the referral of students to source texts rather than the explicit resolution of questions. Even secret formulas (*mifang* 秘方), simultaneously functional emblems of knowledge and power and material representations of the bond between generations of practice, may be passed on by teachers to students. This may happen, for instance, if a teacher possesses such knowledge but occupies a rank in the state system that does not permit personal disciples.

One of the teachers of the previously mentioned student from Sichuan had been the apprentice of a locally famous physician in his own youth. According to my informant, "although he did not study in college, he inherited many secret formulas and experiences.[47] He wrote them all down and explained to me the theory of the treatment." Another student told me of a young teacher who possessed several secret formulas. At the time of her internship at a small Beijing neighborhood hospital this teacher's wife had died in a car accident. He had been very upset and the student had been very sympathetic. This established a bond between them based on *ganqing*. Later, he passed on his formulas to her. A very different case was that of a doctor in his mid-thirties who occupied a position of seniority in the state education sector far above those of comparable age and experience and was heir to one of the most respected acupuncture lines in north China. I met him instructing foreign students in the secret traditions of his line. He told me that in his opinion the very notion of secret knowledge was an anachronism at the end of the twentieth century. As an additional explanation it must be mentioned that trading in his line's secret knowledge had become a profitable business and facilitated extensive travel abroad. Thus, in addition to learning relationships facilitated by kinship(-like) ties, bureaucratic educational structures, or both, more spontaneous exchange relations are possible. These are mediated by factors extending from emotional bonds to financial transactions and have assumed a new social importance in post-Maoist China.

Guanxixue: Learning and the Art of Social Networking

Particularistic exchange relations, known locally as *guanxi* 关系, are established and cultivated by individuals from whatever resources of affiliation are at hand: kinship, friendship, neighborhood, membership in the same work-unit, bureaucratic filiation, classmates, surnames, or localities.[48] The role of *guanxi* ties in Chinese social life is so striking that some researchers identify an ability to form "pluralistic" identifications with others on the basis of shared attributes as a fundamental and unchanging aspect of Chinese social behavior throughout the ages.[49] Others interpret *guanxi* as local examples of universal "clientelist" relationships that are seen as "instrumental-personal ties" of "a somewhat casual and non-permanent alliance."[50]

More recently, anthropologists such as Kipnis, Yan, and Yang have moved away from stable portrayals of *guanxi*.[51] The ethnographies of these writers demonstrate that *guanxixue*, the art of establishing *guanxi* ties, is exhausted neither by accounts based on models of the universal rational human actor nor by those that posit the existence of unchanging cultural traditions. Both Yang and Yan point out that etic interpretations of *guanxi* negatively connoted in terms of the rational manipulation of social relationships for instrumental purposes fail to catch a much richer layer of emic perceptions. Not only are *guanxi* networks perceived by north Chinese villagers as the "objective foundation of the society in which they live," but *guanxi* also involves "sociability, morality, intentionality and personal affection."[52] With regard to the stability of cultural behavior patterns, all three ethnographers show that in establishing *guanxi* networks modern Chinese flexibly employ cultural resources in the pursuit of specifically contemporary ends. In the process, modes of relating to each other, definitions of bonding and the mutual obligations involved in establishing specific bonds, and the feelings associated with particular types of relation and what it means to be Chinese are continually redefined in relation to one another in the context of social practice.[53]

The ubiquity of *guanxixue* in contemporary China is evident in its infiltration already (against my best efforts) of my ethnography. We have encountered it in the networks along which Dr. Chao traveled in order to become a disciple of Professor Xu. It was via similar networks that I myself entered Professor Rong's surgery. We saw how his students expected Professor Ding to help them with jobs, housing, work permits, and so on. I described how patients related to Professor Rong through *guanxi* networks consulted him at his home, thereby avoiding the trouble of having to purchase appointment tickets the evening before and queuing again the next morning. His fame as a physician and his insertion into a wide range of different networks make Professor Rong an ideal example of the role of *guanxixue* in contemporary Chinese medicine.

Professor Rong began his career before liberation as a disciple of his father in Jiangsu Province. In 1947 he qualified as a state-registered physician by passing recently established state examinations. In 1951 he completed a one-year evening class in Western medicine at his local hospital. In 1956, at the age of thirty-three, Professor Rong became the leader of the Formula Teaching and Research Group at the Jiangsu Province Chinese Medicine Teacher Improvement School. By 1957 he had moved to Beijing, where he was appointed chairman of the Formula Teaching and Research Office at the newly established Beijing College of Chinese Medicine. He has since occupied or still occupies the following positions:

—*Within Beijing University of Chinese Medicine:* chairman of the Basic Theory [of Chinese medicine] Department and vice chairman of the university's Academic Committee.

—*Within the state administration of medicine:* vice president of the All-China Institute of Chinese Medicine, president of the Chinese Materia Medica Committee, president of the Research Committee on Formulas, visiting professor at the Chinese Academy of Chinese Medicine's Postgraduate Studies Department, member of the Chinese National Pharmacopoeia Committee and head of its Chinese medicine subcommittee, member of the MOH Drug Evaluation Committee and president of its Chinese medicine subcommittee, and member of the Academic Evaluation Subcommittee of the National Funding Agency for the Natural Sciences.

—*Within the state administration:* member of the Sixth and Seventh Chinese People's Political Consultative Conference and vice chairman of the Chinese People's Political Consultative Conference's Expert Committee on Medicine, Hygiene, and Health.[54]

I could not with the resources available to me trace all the mechanisms and associations that facilitated this illustrious career. Being in the right place at the right time (without which it is, of course, impossible to insert oneself into any network) played an undoubted role. As the son of a nationally renowned physician who had died early, Professor Rong occupied an ideal position to tie together the old and the new in the emergent Chinese medicine of the new China. Furthermore, Professor Rong was fortunate enough to belong to the group of people connected to Lü Bingkui that was to become such an important factor in the shaping of Chinese medicine both nationally and locally in Beijing. Finally, his move to the capital positioned Professor Rong closer to new centers of power within which useful *guanxi* ties could be established. Vice versa, with each new appointment Professor Rong occupied increasingly important "gatekeeper" positions that made it desirable for others to nurture his acquaintance.

We have already seen how establishing *guanxi* with a person of Professor Rong's standing is a crucial career move for Ph.D. students. I gathered much anecdotal evidence indicating that Professor Rong was popular because he helped his students in a manner that a good teacher is expected to do. He did his best to advance the careers of his students, and his personal networks reached far and wide. We also noted that Professor Rong counts among his patients politicians, businesspeople, and other members of the elite. My informants were in no doubt about the considerable influence exerted on the development of Chinese medicine via such personal networks. "You have to learn that in China policies change as people change," was a lesson my friends and teachers never tired of trying to impress on me. Historians of contemporary Chinese medicine, too, attach importance to personal relationships in the formulation of policy. The relationship between Mao Zedong and his friend and physician Li Dingming 李鼎铭 (1881–1947) is exemplary in this context. Li successfully treated Mao with Chinese medicine for an inflammation of his joints during the Long March in 1935 after Western medicine treatments had failed. Ma cites this event and the subsequent relationship between the two men as a small but distinctive contribution toward Mao Zedong's positive evaluation of Chinese medicine. More generally, Chen argues that social and political connections between scholar-physicians and the political and administrative elite, mediated by patronage, kinship ties, and personal relations that continued after the revolution, was a crucial factor in the survival of Chinese medicine both before and after 1949. While Chen's analysis is willfully tendentious in emphasizing such connections as a main reason for the survival of Chinese medicine, it is nevertheless useful for acknowledging their role.[55]

An important example of the direct influence exerted on the development of Chinese medicine by individuals connected to each other by personal networks (extending simultaneously across diachronic and synchronic time spaces) is the compilation of textbooks such as *Fangjixue*. As was stated previously, the content of these books is determined by MOH committees. According to informants who had worked on such committees, the more prestigious members exert an extraordinary amount of influence, allowing personal preferences to enter into official discourse.[56] The formulas discussed in *Fangjixue*, for instance, represent a selection of about 150 formulas out of a total of more than 100,000 in the classical literature. Similarly, the clinical patterns (*zheng* 证) on which teaching and increasingly research are based have entered textbooks and classification manuals via networks that have a clearly definable extension in time and space. The history of liver patterns provides a useful example.

> CASE 6.3. *The Problem of Liver* qi *and* yang *Depletion.* For reasons that are discussed in detail in chapter 7, pattern differentiation (*bianzheng* 辨证) occupies a central place in contemporary Chinese medical practice. Patterns relate sets of signs and symptoms to specified disease mechanisms, on the one hand, and to paradigmatic treatment strategies and formulas, on the other. The manifestation patterns one learns to recognize in school thus crucially delimit how physicians diagnose and treat in practice later. Considerable resources have been devoted by the MOH to

standardize pattern diagnosis in Chinese medicine in an effort to provide internationally recognized standards for the description of illness and the evaluation of outcomes. Clearly, therefore, whoever dominates discourse on pattern diagnosis dominates Chinese medical practice.

Visceral systems (zangfu 脏腑) patterns determined via the eight rubrics (ba gang 八纲) have been allocated a key position in this process. By using the eight rubrics a physician can distinguish among disorders of a particular visceral system such as the liver (gan) several distinct patterns. The first modern Chinese textbook, the Outline of Chinese Medicine, listed only four liver patterns: heat (re 热), cold (han 寒), repletion (shi 实), and depletion (xu 虚).[57] Contemporary textbooks such as Zhongyi zhenduanxue 中医诊断学 (Diagnostics of Chinese Medicine) further differentiate these basic patterns into eight subpatterns: (1) liver qi depression bind (ganqi yujie 肝气郁结), (2) upflaming liver fire (ganhuo shang yan 肝火上炎), (3) liver blood depletion (ganxuexu 肝血虚), (4) liver yin depletion (ganyinxu 肝阴虚), (5) upward hyperactive liver yang (ganyang shang kang 肝阳上亢), (6) liver wind stirring internally (ganfeng nei dong 肝风内动), (7) cold stagnating in the liver vessel (han zhi ganmai 寒滞肝脉), and (8) liver gall bladder damp-heat (gan dan shire 肝胆湿热).[58]

The differentiation of liver patterns contained in both the Outline and Diagnostics advances an implicit conclusion to a historical debate regarding liver disorders that remains unresolved to the present day.[59] Due to its particular physiological characteristics—in Chinese medicine the liver is said to be "yin in terms of its constitution but yang in terms of its function" (ti yin yong yang 体阴用阳)—classical authors such as Li Zhongzi 李中梓 (1588–1655) advanced the thesis that "the liver cannot be supplemented" (gan bu ke bu 肝不可补).[60] The idea here is that supplementation will invariably lead to an unbalanced exaggeration of the liver's yang functions. This notion runs counter to therapeutic formulas contained in some of the most ancient classics, which explicitly speak of supplementing liver depletion patterns.[61] To reconcile these diverging views authors such as the influential Ming physician Zhang Jiebin 张介宾 (1563–1640) explained that the "method of not supplementing the liver" (gan wu bu fa 肝无补法) referred only to liver qi (or yang) and not to liver blood (or yin).[62] During the Qing, various physicians provided extensive discussions of liver patterns of which Wang Qinlin's 王秦林 (1798–1862) "thirty methods to treat the liver" (zhi gan sanshi fa 治肝三十法) remain the most comprehensive to date.[63] The currently most influential systematization of liver treatments, however, derives from Ye Tianshi 叶天士 (1667–1746), who proposed a differentiation of liver patterns according to the three rubrics (*san gang bianzheng* 三纲辨证) of liver *qi*, liver fire, and liver wind, which gave predominance to liver repletion patterns and admitted depletion patterns only for liver *yin* and blood.[64]

The relation between Ye Tianshi's discussion and the patterns described in contemporary Chinese medicine textbooks is obvious. Of the eight patterns contained in *Diagnostics* three deal with disordered *qi*, one discusses wind, one fire, and two blood and *yin* depletion. The eighth (liver gall bladder damp heat) is a modern innovation influenced by biomedical reasoning.[65] These patterns are what students learn, what they are expected to know, and what dominates the contemporary literature. The recently published official *Classification and Codes of Diseases and Patterns of Traditional Chinese Medicine*, which researchers will have to use in applying for government funding, also reflects Ye's system. Apart from liver blood and *yin* depletion all other liver syndromes are repletion patterns organized according to the categories of *qi* (*yang*), fire (heat), and wind.[66] Liver *qi* and *yang* depletion and derivative patterns such as "liver *qi* sinking" (*ganqi xian* 肝气陷) are not discussed.

The above is quite astonishing given the fact that some of the most influential physicians of the last century, such as Tang Zonghai 唐宗海 (1862–1918) and Zhang Xichun 张锡纯 (1860–1933) wrote about these patterns and provided innovative treatment approaches.[67] Distinguished modern physicians like Qin Bowei and Pu Fuzhou also relied on these patterns in their treatments and discussed them in their writings.[68] Several doctors I met in Beijing used these patterns in clinical practice, among them Professor Yang Weiyi 杨维益, a professor at Beijing University of Chinese Medicine. In numerous articles published in Chinese medical journals Professor Yang and many other physicians have argued that more attention should be paid to liver *qi* and *yang* depletion patterns and that these patterns, too, should be included in the national curriculum.

So far, their struggle has had only limited success. Liver *qi* and liver *yang* depletion patterns are included in the national standards for clinical terminology published in 1997.[69] They are not mentioned, however, in the textbooks on diagnosis that form the basis for examinations at Chinese medical universities and colleges.[70] Because most students learn in order to pass exams, not a single undergraduate or postgraduate student I spoke with (admittedly not a representative sample) knew of liver *qi* or *yang* depletion patterns.

If Professor Yang and his colleagues have failed to change the national curriculum, it is not because of any deficiency in their arguments. Their writings, their links to the classical canons, the famous physicians (alive and dead) on whom they draw for support, the case histories and clinical studies they present to support their case—none of these seem any less convincing to me than the arguments that sustain the pattern differentiation taught in current textbooks.[71] The networks by which Professor Yang and his colleagues connect to the past and present of Chinese medicine, however, are different and, politically at least, less effective than those of their adversaries.

As head of the Chinese Medicine Diagnosis Teaching and Research Department (Zhongyi zhenduan jiaoyanshi 中医诊断教研室) at Beijing University of Chinese Medicine and Pharmacology, Professor Yang was appointed chief editor for the textbook on diagnosis that forms part of a series of teaching materials for tertiary-level Chinese medicine and pharmacology colleges and schools in north China (*Huabei diqu gaodeng zhongyiyao yuanxiao jiaocai* 华北地区高等中医药院校教材). Naturally, he used this position to include liver *qi* and *yang* depletion patterns. The textbooks on which national examinations are based, however, are edited by another group of physicians under the leadership of Professor Zhu Wenfeng 朱文锋 from Hunan University of Chinese Medicine. The committee obviously does not consider liver *qi* and *yang* depletion patterns important and has therefore excluded them from its textbook.[72]

In other cases the influence of particular networks on curriculum formulation appears less hegemonic. The pattern of "sinking downward of the great *qi*" (*daqi xia xian* 大气下陷), established by Zhang Xichun at the beginning of this century, is an example. I first learned of this pattern when I was studying with Professor Zhu, who diagnoses it almost daily in patients with cardiovascular disease. The pattern is not, however, taught in basic courses on diagnosis or internal medicine.[73] Nor is it included in official standards suggested for Chinese medical disease and diagnostic categories.[74] It is, however, discussed in textbooks that introduce the various schools of Chinese medical thought and which invariably include a chapter or lecture on Zhang Xichun.[75] *Sheng xian tang* 升陷汤 (Raise [What] Has Sunk Decoction), the representative prescription formulated by Zhang to treat this pattern, is cited in some but not all texts on elementary formulas. It is usually included as a variation of Li Gao's 李杲 famous *Buzhong yiqi tang* 补中益气汤 (Supplement the Middle and Benefit *Qi* Decoction)—a practice Zhang himself, who thought of his pattern as treating a more serious condition than that described by Li Gao, might not necessarily have approved of.[76]

Less powerful networks can also subvert hegemonic networks at local levels if they succeed in establishing subcultures. When I studied *wenbing* 温病 (Warm [Pathogen] Disorders) at Beijing, for instance, my teacher took great care to emphasize that his way of teaching the subject differed from that of official textbooks. He supplied us with photocopies of his own articles and a book written by Professor Zhao Shaoqin 赵绍琴 and his students in Beijing. This text organizes the subject in a substantially different way than do the standard textbooks edited by physicians from Nanjing and Anhui. My teacher also recounted several anecdotes about struggles at meetings of the committee charged with defining the content of *wenbing* courses between delegates from Beijing and the south. He indicated that the views of the chairman (a professor from Anhui), as was the norm, always prevailed. Depending on who teaches them, students of *wenbing* at Beijing now learn enough of the dominant southern interpretation to pass their exams but acquire this knowledge mediated through local interpretations.[77]

These examples all highlight *guanxi* networks that depend for their functioning on the reproduction of official hierarchies. Professor Rong occupies a central node in many such networks precisely because of his official positions. Other networks insinuate themselves across or even against the hierarchical structures of state and family. One evening I visited Dr. Cheng, a doctoral student of a famous Beijing professor, who was as usual engrossed in studying the work of classical medical authors. During our conversation that night Dr. Cheng showed me his collection of prescriptions by other well-known Beijing *laozhongyi*. I asked how he had acquired these. He was not one of their students, and in my experience doctors of such stature were normally quite particular about who had access to their clinical experience. My friend told me that he and some of his *tongxue* 同学 (students in the same year of a course) regularly exchanged and discussed the prescriptions of their supervisors. I later found that this is a common practice. The terms of the relationship between supervisor and student are obviously not scripted so as to avoid the trading of prescriptions. Yet, these prescriptions do not thereby pass into general circulation but remain restricted to specific *guanxi* networks.

Many other such lateral exchange networks exist as well, cutting across social domains, personal identities, time, and space. They connect by means of digital technology, financial transaction, ethics, and emotionality. And they blur the clinical with the economic and the political. Their composition is so varied and their modes of connection so heterogeneous that I can do no more than merely list some obvious and not-so-obvious examples.

Physicians connect within their work-units, at conferences and meetings, through medical journals, and nowadays on the Internet. While working within particular hospital departments I noticed repeatedly that physicians defined themselves against members of other departments or other hospitals. Different departments had secret formulas that were not known to outsiders. Physicians I met in Beijing who had graduated from medical schools elsewhere often maintained active links to their alma mater. Two graduate students at the China-Japan Friendship Hospital called in a former colleague who now worked in Shandong for help with their research rather than turning to physicians at other hospitals in Beijing. Networks thus are not only enabling, they are also restrictive. During my fieldwork, for example, I became involved in some translation work for one of my teachers. Before I left I wanted to introduce him to a Chinese friend who might have been able to continue this work. My attempt was blocked, however, by both my teacher and my friend, who had at that time begun studying with another well-known Beijing doctor. My teacher found it difficult to trust someone who was the student of someone else. My friend felt that if she worked for my teacher, she would be disrespectful to her own. Another friend who had no personal connections to well-known teachers was keen, however, for me to make an introduction.

Judith Farquhar repeatedly draws our attention to the mobilization of the experiences stored in the medical archive for daily clinical practice. What is less apparent from her account, though, is the sense of emotional attachment that can accompany and sustain the connection between contemporary physicians and their medical ancestors. When I discussed with my friends our "favorite practitioners," for instance, I could not help but notice the similarity between such talk and the attachments constructed at other times and in other places to pop stars, sporting heroes, or famous anthropologists. *Guanxi* networks thus extend to the past as much as the present and mobilize virtual as much as actual agents. They are stabilized, depending on circumstances, by rules of propriety not too dissimilar from those we encountered previously in kinship ties, but also by purely financial considerations.

Rules of hierarchical etiquette demand deference of the younger to the older, the junior to the senior partner in a relationship. While it is claimed in the West that such behavior is evidence of the authoritarian character of Chinese medicine and its qualitative difference from science,[78] I would argue that observation of these rules just as often facilitates information exchange and thereby the construction of novel syntheses. One of my teachers was a senior clinician already in his mid-fifties and a nationally renowned specialist in his area of expertise. He was very interested in the therapeutic approach of one of his hospital's *laozhongyi*, a man not generally given to sharing his experience with outsiders. This *laozhongyi* had heard of the clinical reputation of my teacher as well and perhaps saw benefits for himself in a relationship. Over time, they constructed a relationship that modeled itself on Confucian patterns of deference of younger to older brothers but provided a medium across which experience could travel. My teacher took care to use the respectful title *lao* (elder), to bow to his superior's clinical experience, and to remain the passive partner in any conversation. The older doctor would lecture about his approach but make enough space to benefit from his younger colleague's innovative thought.

Physicians also establish *guanxi* connections with various groups of laypersons (and vice versa). The boundaries between medicine, art, and philosophy are, as we have seen, highly permeable. Intellectuals and scholars can possess considerable medical knowledge, and some of the doctors with whom I studied were accomplished painters and calligraphers. The ensuing syntheses are both personally and practically efficient, as we saw in the case of Professor Zhu.[79]

The merging of the clinical and socioeconomic domains, on the other hand, becomes obvious in the course of daily practice. Patients use their *guanxi* to be introduced to a specific physician, or construct it spontaneously by playing on some joint identification. A common surname or home province is sufficient to put into play an emotional attachment that obliges a doctor to be just that little bit more attentive. Doctors, equally, are never too shy to seize an opportunity for widening their own *guanxi* networks. As one of my teachers—a man of the highest sophistication and moral integrity—advised me, being a physician in Beijing opened doors that those in the country did not even know existed.

It should be clear from these few examples that *guanxi* networks do not arise merely from the rational calculation of individuals; they draw on an ethics of relationship that implicates specific inflections of emotionality, selfhood, and morality. *Guanxixue* thus embodies patterns of agency that are developed and utilized by social actors in the stabilization of specific syntheses, yet that reciprocally also define these actors. *Guanxi* networks have increased in size and importance since the 1980s and now form alternative subjectivities to those enabled by older forms of kinship and bureaucratic forms of socialist social organization. This renewed importance of *guanxixue* has been facilitated by the reemergence of the individual as a social actor and a newly affirmed admissibility of older patterns of social behavior. Other factors, however, have worked to prevent social behavior/organization from sliding back toward prerevolutionary patterns: the bureaucratic organization of the socialist state remains in place, the cultural hegemony of modernization and scientification has been further amplified, and individual agency is increasingly defined in terms of economic goals.[80]

These changes are easily documented in the domain of Chinese medicine. There is considerable evidence, for instance, for the renewed importance attached to individual actors. Textbooks, even individual chapters of textbooks, are once again traceable as the work of individual authors who write in distinctive styles and put forward controversial opinions. The 1990s also witnessed the reentry into Chinese medicine of classical philosophy and a self-conscious "return to the sources" that is unashamedly concerned with reworking China's own tradition rather than learning from the West.[81] Modernization and the integration of Chinese medicine and Western medicine still remain national political goals, however, whose importance is emphasized by the economic and political benefits (real or imagined) seen to accrue from the internationalization of Chinese medicine. And while the state still controls education, it no longer can rely on the willingness of the practitioners it trains to care for the masses out of purely humanistic motivations, be they of a socialist or a traditionalist inflection. Increasingly what counts for doctors is personal fame, which translates into personal wealth. And if the former cannot be had, the latter will do on its own. Many young doctors are now leaving the profession for better-paid positions in private industry, one of the most common options being employment by pharmaceutical companies.

Professor Rong, like other physicians, has made the appropriate transitions. The following quote, taken from one of his books, admits to the modern, more individualistic mode of production in Chinese medicine.

> The editors of this book are professors and assistant professors who have been engaged in teaching and research of formulas for more than twenty years. [While] each has [already] achieved academic merits in this discipline, they all have striven to study assiduously in order to produce a teaching aid and reference text of high quality. For this purpose they have carried out an [especially] comprehensive selection and evaluation of sources. However, some of the most special and valuable literary sources of Chinese medicine formulas are scattered throughout the writings of the various schools of Chinese medicine. Therefore, shortcomings and omissions in selecting the content [of the present book] were difficult to avoid. If the viewpoints of individual [contributors] thus do not necessarily agree . . . then this can be of benefit for the teaching of *fangji*. And if debates arise out of the mistakes [of this work] this, too, can help to gradually lift [the discipline].

Plurality is admitted, even celebrated, here, and the diverse sources of tradition are emphasized. There is little reference to the West, though a language of progress remains in place. Professor Rong has accommodated on other levels, too. We have already encountered him as a successful entrepreneur in his surgery. The doctoral dissertations of his students double as pharmacological studies that will, in the future, be used to support the marketing of his patented formulas. In his capacity as chairman of government committees he is negotiating with the U.S. Food and Drug Administration about U.S. licences for classical pharmaceutical products. Several of his students are now living and working abroad, where they use his name to promote their own, yet also facilitate their teacher's transition into an internationally renowned physician and scholar.

In an environment where tradition again counts for something but only if it is suitably modernized, where the state still provides the basic structures of education and medical practice but individual status is newly important, where opportunities for jobs, housing, and promotion are always scarcer than the number of applicants, *guanxixue* emerges as a product of quite particular historical contradictions. Contemporary physicians of Chinese medicine have become what they are by passing through a state-controlled education system based on a vision of medicine as a social product. In practice they increasingly need to assert their own individuality or remain shackled to a system that cannot deliver on their aspirations. No wonder that they attempt to construct, in medical as well as social terms, their own lines of connection.

Chinese Medicine as a Field of Practice

A word of caution is nevertheless in order at this point. In attempting to limn the multifaceted and constantly evolving nature of Professor Rong's subjectivity, I have tended to fix (against my intentions) the background and contexts against and within which he acts. It is important, therefore, to read my case study in conjunction with others that make apparent the plurality of "discipleship," "studentship," and "*guanxixue*" as types of social relations that exist in multiple forms because they are—both historically and contemporarily—continually emergent.[82] Resisting the temptation to adduce yet more specifics that would render such multiplicity visible, I instead close this chapter by fleshing out the concepts of social topography and topology that were introduced in chapter 2 as a methodology for analyzing the spatiotemporal constitution of fields of practice.

The Chinese themselves have long ordered relationships spatially, both conceptually in thought and practically in ritual.[83] A metaphorical modeling of social relations in terms of networks, for instance, underpins both emic and etic discussions of *guanxixue*. Similarly conceived linear connections figure prominently in Chinese views of bodies physical, social, and aesthetic. We find them in conceptions of the *mai* or *mo* 脉, the vessels of Chinese functional anatomy that conduct different kinds of *qi*. *Mai* can also be the veins of calligraphy and the lines of mountains and hills.[84] Other connections reach back in time, such as the streams (*pai* 派) that connect contemporary physicians with their medical ancestors.[85] Networks, structuring and transmitting, thus fix actors in relationships of reciprocal obligation. From this perspective they appear as globally stable configurations that locally define agents through their positions.

As we saw above, however, the networks of Chinese medicine are anything but stable. Neither the medical streams described in chapter 2, nor the master-student relationships discussed here, nor even the socialist education system are static structures. Hence, as Hay argues regarding *mai* or *mo*, and Kipnis, Yan, and Yang point out in relation to *guanxixue*, the atemporal nature of structure is temporized once the dynamism of local agency and interaction is taken into account. It is through such agency, for instance, that studentship is transformed into particularistic personal ties for the exchange of money and favors or moved in the direction of ritually ordered master-disciple relationships. This tension between structural arrangement and dynamic emergence is captured well by de Certeau's distinction between place and space. Place is "the order (of whatever kind) in accord with which elements are distributed in relationships of coexistence." A space, on the other hand, is composed of "intersections of mobile elements." It "occurs as the effect produced by the operations that orient it, situate it, temporalise it. . . . In short, *space is a practised place*."[86] Which of these is foregrounded in description and analysis is a function not merely of specific networks but also of the interests and attentions of the participant observer (chapter 1).

The dynamic agencies that turn places into spaces are captured in Chinese thought by a logic of "dense centers and dispersed peripheries." Here, foci of agency as diverse as the visceral systems of function of Chinese functional anatomy, the emperor, and the main sacrificers (*zhuren* 主人) in rituals of ancestor worship unfold their agency onto phenomena.[87] Several philosophers and anthropologists have attempted to translate such logics into dynamic models of the Chinese self derived from and related to Confucian perceptions of the ritually ordered community. These models graphically depict foci from which radiate effects that disperse as they move progressively outward through successive zones of unfoldment. Efficacy thus ceases to be an abstract value and becomes instead a function both of the quality of an effect and of the proximity of the agents onto which it is unfolded.[88]

This assumption is supported by Professor Rong's relationships with his graduate students and disciples. We recognized that these relations were developed and affirmed through similar ritualized performances but that their intensity diminished with increasing social distance. We also noted that Professor Rong's status as master and teacher was not entirely determined by the structural order in which a specific relationship was embedded but also reflected his achievements within actual relations. Such achievements are continually threatened in the context of practice. Whether as a physician or as a teacher, Professor Rong is always onstage and must demonstrate anew in each consultation that he actually is a *ming laozhongyi*.[89]

The relational dynamics of unfolding agencies takes us once more, although from a different perspective, toward the emergent character of complex systems. In developing his focus-field model of the Confucian self the philosopher Ames points out that the individual foci or parts of a given system are neither necessarily all related to each other nor is each single local interaction connected to the system as a whole. As I argued in chapter 2, systems in which different foci of agency compete with each other can be conceived of as balancing on a dynamic center that need not correspond to a concrete or real center.[90] Plurality thus can be seen as a function of the overdetermination of global systems by the local unfolding of focal agencies.

This, however, is still only a partial explanation because it does not take into account the work accomplished by the structure of place itself. The constraints imposed on local agency by the structure of given networks is one example. As Latour shows, some nodes accrue more power than others by positioning themselves so that certain flows must pass through them.[91] I commented in chapter 1, for instance, on the special status of Beijing within the organization of Chinese medicine, and in chapter 3 on the role of the MOH. Professor Rong—residing in Beijing and the member of many MOH committees—is such a node of centrality, which accounts for his inclusion in many different social networks.

The network metaphor does not convey all the characteristics of the social topology of Chinese medicine either.[92] First, as we saw above, it suggests a stability that is never really there. In reading the ethnographies of authors such as Kipnis and Yang we come to know relational networks (*guanxiwang*) but also learn that what really matters is the art of *guanxixue*. This art is not merely a function of personal agency but requires deeper layers of association from which concrete networks can crystallize: speaking the same dialect, being classmates, coming from the same province. Networks thus represent one particular type of synthesis. They are conjunctive syntheses constructed through the conjunction of heterogeneous infrastructures. Connective syntheses, instead, are deeper, nonvolitional strata of fields of practice from which individual infrastructures differentiate themselves through their insertion into specific networks.[93]

Differences of shape and composition between various forms of social aggregation, too, get lost in the homogeneity of the network metaphor. Professor Rong's networks of discipleship are simple direct lines. The state education system, by comparison, is a vast and complex structure: dispersed, seemingly all-encompassing, implicating corporate as well as individual agents, human as well as nonhuman elements. It envelops the smaller lines of discipleships which can, at best, carve out for themselves a niche within the larger colossus. The interactions between such different shapes contribute, as we have seen, to the ongoing remolding of fields of practice and work against their solidification.

Time leaves a similar mark on fields of practice. De Certeau, with whose distinction of place and space we are now familiar, employs an archaeological metaphor to render this presence visible. He argues that although subsequent regimes of planning impose new regimes of order on given places, there invariably remain behind older structures, some fully functional and others in disrepair or sunken already beneath the surface. In the images they evoke and through the practices to which they refer they interrupt the cohesion of the present, guarantee complementarities, offer different futures.[94]

As I argued in chapter 2, both the past and the future define the arrangement of agents within fields of practice. Some students, for instance, would like social relations with their teachers to be more modern. They want them to be less an expression of status differentials and more of a joint effort between scientists striving for the same goals of truth and a better future (see chapter 8). Some physicians want to integrate more biomedical ideas and technologies into Chinese medicine (case 5.4). The government hopes for Chinese medicine to become a global power (chapter 3). Such desires constitute attempts to draw new elements into a given field of practice and to marginalize and exclude others. As we shall see in chapters 7 and 8, debates between proponents of different schools of thought are essentially struggles about the exclusion or inclusion of concepts, formulas, etiologies, techniques, and people from certain syntheses.

The simultaneous actualization of past, present, and future within fields of practice implies that synthesis extends not only to conjunctions of infrastructures in space but also to those in time. In the thinking of the philosopher Michel Serres time itself thus does not flow linearly but is an expression of topological mechanisms that filter time unevenly and thereby bring into conjunction infrastructures conventionally imagined to be precluded from interacting because of their distance from each other in space and/or time. Serres argues that if we apply the mathematics of topology to space-time rather than allowing only for the equidistances of metrical geometry and classical time, fields of practice reveal themselves as crumpled up and full of manifold possibilities. According to Serres, any object or circumstance is thus not homogeneous but "polychronic, multitemporal, and reveals a time that is gathered together, with multiple pleats."[95] Hence it is possible—and not at all odd—for physicians to formulate a prescription by drawing on Chinese medical literature from the Han and biomedical knowledge from the *New England Journal of Medicine* (cases 5.4 and 8.1), and possible, too, that networks of descent can stretch from ancestors in Qing southern China to a Beijing *laozhongyi* and on to his disciple in the United States, and that they circulate, simultaneously, knowledge, status, money, and favors (case 6.2).

Chinese medicine is thus revealed as a polychronous and multiply structured field of practice. I have concentrated on the humans who populate this field, yet nonhuman infrastructures have continuously made their presence felt: in the books and formulas that connect physicians and in the buildings and technologies that make their work possible. Integrating these elements into the field of Chinese medicine is a necessary task, though one I will postpone until chapter 8. First, I want to examine in greater detail how global fields of practice are constructed within local processes of synthesis.

7. BIANZHENG LUNZHI

The Emergent Pivot of Contemporary
Chinese Medicine

The present chapter examines the emergence of one of the defining practices of contemporary Chinese medicine: *bianzheng lunzhi* 辨证论治, or "pattern differentiation and treatment determination." This examination is motivated by a threefold objective. First, through tracing the evolution of *bianzheng lunzhi* as concept and practice over a period of fifty years I hope to add depth to the historical analysis of chapter 3. Second, by exposing the social construction of what is seen by both Chinese and Western scholar-physicians as "the pivot" of contemporary Chinese medicine, a stability that anchors an otherwise diverse medical system, I undercut from yet another angle notions regarding the historical unity of Chinese medicine. Third, examining the social construction of *bianzheng lunzhi* allows me to test from a different perspective the model of synthesis outlined in chapter 2.

This particular conjunction of goals has led me to embrace a narrative that focuses on *bianzheng lunzhi* as something created yet also creative. In that sense, *bianzheng lunzhi* shares essential characteristics with the human agents I have discussed in the previous chapters and those that populate the present one. Hence, although I examine the historical process of an emergence, I do not claim to have written its social history. I do not, for instance, analyze in any detail the political and institutional contexts in which the formation of *bianzheng lunzhi* occurred, nor do I claim to shed light on the minutiae of specific decision-making processes or the many motives that may have informed various agents. Furthermore, I specifically focus on perspectives from within the Chinese medicine community. The views and actions of the persons I introduce are exemplary but by no means exhaustive. A detailed analysis of the political, ideological, and socioeconomic context in which the emergence of *bianzheng lunzhi* occurred is undoubtedly necessary but is beyond both the scope and intention of my much more limited focus.[1]

I also must insist from the outset that *bianzheng lunzhi* does not denote a single definable practice.[2] Yet, in both China and the West the term calls forth a distinctly defined notion of practice by which it is collectively remembered. As one can make out movement only against a background of apparent stability, I shall begin my investigation by outlining the currently orthodox definitions of key terms that anchor the practice of *bianzheng lunzhi*.

Contemporary textbooks of Chinese medicine distinguish conceptually and practically between symptoms or signs (*zheng* 症, *zhengzhuang* 症状), patterns (*zheng* 证, *zhenghou* 证侯), and diseases (*bing* 病, *jibing* 疾病).[3] These are typically defined as follows:[4]

> —Diseases are disorders of structure or function of the human organism resulting from a loss of equilibrium between internal and external environments. Diseases have specific causes that produce regularly patterned pathologies by way of describable pathomechanisms. These pathologies and pathomechanisms express themselves externally in symptoms and signs.[5]
>
> —Symptoms and signs are the external manifestations of both diseases and patterns. They are experienced subjectively by the patient or determined diagnostically by the physician.[6]
>
> —Patterns describe typically occurring combinations of symptoms and signs. They reflect the temporal development of a disease through various stages (and thus the transformation of the disease itself) including deflections of the normal development of a disease by medical treatment and other factors such as constitution, climate, diet, and so on.

Modern physicians insist that treating patterns treats diseases because a pattern expresses four core aspects of disease development: its causation (*bingyin* 病因), location (*bingwei* 病位), pathomechanism (*bingji* 病机), and character (*bingxing* 病性). Each of these reflects the nature of disease not in some abstract generalized form but in its concrete and specific manifestation. As expressed by Kong Bohua 孔伯化 (1885–1955), one of "Beijing's four great and famous doctors" (*Beijing si da mingyi* 北京四大名医), Chinese medicine can understand the ill person only if it understands that person's disease; yet, it must simultaneously proceed from a consideration of the person as a whole. And precisely at this juncture between person and illness stand patterns.[7]

The above concepts have been analyzed from both historical and ethnographic perspectives by Chinese and Western scholars. Sivin and Farquhar, for instance, point out that Chinese medicine's concern for patterns makes for a medical practice organized around the unfolding of process rather than the manipulation of bounded structures.[8] Farquhar describes in detail how experienced physicians proceed, in practice, via "pattern differentiation" (*bian-*

zheng) to "treatment determination" (lunzhi). She concludes that bianzheng lunzhi constitutes the "pivot" and "privileged moment" of the clinical encounter in Chinese medicine.[9]

Most of the doctors I asked, and many of their patients, shared this sentiment. A modern teaching manual explains that bianzheng lunzhi is "a fundamental principle of discriminating and treating disease," that it constitutes a "special method of researching into and engaging with disease," and that it is one of the fundamental characteristics of the theoretical system of Chinese medicine."[10] It is important to note that bianzheng lunzhi is not seen merely as a concept but as a way of practicing medicine. This is stated eloquently by a reference manual for university lecturers: "Bianzheng lunzhi is the application of Chinese medicine theories, [therapeutic] strategies, prescriptions, and drugs within the realities of clinical practice. As such it is the theoretical principle that guides the clinical practice of Chinese internal medicine, but it is also a specific method for resolving concrete problems in diagnosis and therapy."[11]

As with many other aspects of contemporary Chinese medicine, the explicit or implicit reference point for discussions of bianzheng lunzhi seems to be Western medicine. "Chinese medicine differentiates patterns, Western medicine differentiates diseases" (Zhongyi bian zheng, xiyi bian bing 中医辨证, 西医辨病) is a maxim that was impressed on students and patients by their teachers and physicians in the course of many of the consultations I observed. It was often linked to another formulaic statement, encountered as frequently in lay as in professional discourse and cited already in chapter 4, that "Chinese medicine treats the root while Western medicine attends to manifestations" (Zhongyi zhi ben, xiyi zhi biao 中医治本, 西医治标). All my Chinese teachers informed me that Chinese medicine is superior to Western medicine because it understands illness as a process in which the same disease can express itself through different patterns. Thus, the same treatment might be described in the course of different diseases, while the same disease might require different treatments according to the pattern present (yibing tongzhi, tongbing yizhi 异病同治, 同病异治). And while scholarly analyses acknowledge that Chinese medicine also discriminates diseases and that Western medicine also recognizes syndromes, the conclusion reached is usually that the strength of Chinese medicine lies in pattern discrimination.[12] Hence, a textbook commissioned by the Academy of Chinese Medicine under the auspices of the MOH proclaims: "The one crucial and defining feature of the Chinese medicine diagnosis and treatment of illness is [its] discrimination of patterns and determination of treatments."[13]

Chinese medical historians depict the contemporary practice of *bianzheng lunzhi* as a continuation and progressive development of methods and theories that were already developed in the earliest medical classics. Usually, the theoretical foundations of *bianzheng lunzhi* are traced to the *Neijing* 内经, while Zhang Zhongjing's 张仲景 *Shanghan zabing lun* 伤寒杂病论 is credited with establishing its clinical practice.[14] These historical accounts often frame the development of pattern discrimination in terms of an evolutionary idiom that resonates with similar rewriting of history in other domains.[15] Having defined *bianzheng lunzhi* as Chinese medicine's most characteristic feature, a modern commentator states: "From the Song onward the therapeutic system of Chinese medicine gradually moved toward adopting '*bianzheng lunzhi*' as its nucleus. As throughout its history, so also in the future will this principle continue to manifest its unsurpassed superiority."[16] *Bianzheng lunzhi* thus appears to embody something of the very essence of Chinese medicine for physicians, patients, academics, and politicians alike. As I shall demonstrate, there is little evidence, however, to suggest that *bianzheng lunzhi* occupied this role prior to the 1950s. In fact, the very term is a recent invention whose significance transcends the purely clinical.[17] It links contemporary Chinese medicine not merely to its own past, but also to a universal natural dialectic (*ziran bianzhengfa* 自然辩证法). It not only guides medical practice but also attempts to elevate such practice to an "exemplar of correctly informed action."[18]

Not surprisingly, pattern diagnosis has been a focus for much debate throughout the last fifty years. While textbooks generally hide the constructed nature of the concept and practice, physicians and researchers continually destabilize it in their attempts to improve on it. And while most physicians see these developments as progressive and therefore implicitly positive, others identify modern transformations of *bianzheng lunzhi* as representative of a general loss of classical skills.

The Nonexistence of *Bianzheng lunzhi* before 1950

Prior to the 1950s *bianzheng lunzhi* did not exist. By this I do not mean that physicians did not know the concept or that they did not engage in practices that resemble what their contemporary colleagues would call *bianzheng lunzhi*. Rather, the place accorded to the concept in contemporary discourse, its conceptual coherence, and its naturalized history are the results of specific concerns faced by physicians from the 1950s onward.[19]

Most contemporary physicians and historians trace the practice of *bian-*

zheng lunzhi to Zhang Zhongjing's *Shanghan zabing lun*.[20] The therapeutic practice advocated in this text consists of several integrated steps.[21] First, different types of disease are defined according to various factors such as the location of pathogens in specific areas of the body (e.g., "greater *yang* disease" *taiyang bing* 太阳病), characteristic symptomatologies (e.g., "wasting thirst disease" *xiaoke bing* 消渴病), or certain kinds of body states (e.g., "postpartum diseases" *furen chanhou bing* 妇人产侯病).[22] These diseases are then broken down into more specific patterns characterized by a particular constellation of symptoms and signs. Patterns may or may not carry specific names. They are usually named after the prescriptions suggested for their treatment (e.g., *Xiao chaihu tang* 小柴胡汤 or Minor Bupleurum Decoction pattern).[23] Important guiding patterns are often further subdivided into more specific subpatterns each of which is associated with its own specific variation of a guiding formula. For instance, the wind stroke (*zhongfeng* 中风) pattern of the greater *yang* disease is characterized by such symptoms as sweating, body aches, fever, chills, and a superficial and relaxed pulse. It is treated with *Guizhi tang* 桂枝汤 (Cinnamon Twig Decoction).[24] If the same pattern is accompanied by coughing, it is treated with *Guizhi jia houpo xingzi tang* 桂枝加厚朴杏子汤 (Cinnamon Twig plus Magnolia Bark and Apricot Kernel Decoction).[25] If it is accompanied by neck stiffness it is treated with *Guizhi jia gegen tang* 桂枝加葛根汤 (Cinnamon Twig plus Kudzu Decoction).[26] Sometimes, however, as in the case of the Minor Bupleurum Decoction pattern, only a few of the many symptoms and signs defining the pattern need to be present to diagnose it. Certain additional symptoms may require changes to the original formula but do not thereby constitute a new formula or, by implication, a new pattern, although in other cases they do.[27]

The chapter headings of the *Shanghan zabing lun* generally use the term *bing* in relation to specific diseases and *zheng* with reference to the pulse (i.e., signs and symptoms interpreted by the physician). This nomenclature is by no means stringent, however, and allows for considerable flexibility. Diseases are sometimes subdivided into one or more other diseases.[28] At other times the composite term *bingzheng* (disease-patterns) is used.[29] Symptoms sometimes also flag diseases: "cough" (*kesou* 咳嗽), for instance, designates both a symptom and a disease.[30] At other times symptoms indicate specific disease locations such as "heart pain" (*xintong* 心痛).[31]

Zhang Zhongjing's differentiation and treatment of patterns and the relation of these patterns to diseases, symptoms, and signs thus show many of the characteristics by which modern authors define *bianzheng lunzhi*. We must note two important differences, however. First, where general principles of

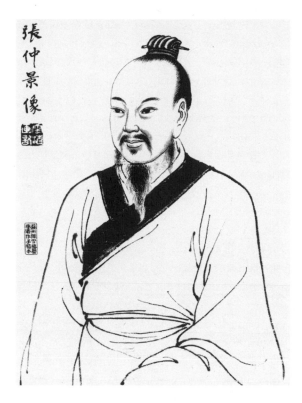

FIGURE 30. Zhang
Zhongjing (ca. 142–220)

illnesses and their treatment are elaborated in the source text, diseases rather
than patterns form the focus of these discussions.[32] Second, conceptual usage
and clinical practice are far less systematic than modern accounts would lead
us to believe. Current understanding of Zhang Zhongjing's thinking and imputations of underlying coherency are invariably based on interpretive efforts
of later commentators who disagree about many important issues.[33]

Zhang Zhongjing decisively influenced the development of various systems of pattern differentiation by later generations of physicians. Contemporary textbooks list six such systems, though physicians use many more in
practice.[34] Notwithstanding this influence, however, contemporary distinctions between symptoms, patterns, and diseases were never clearly defined
before the 1950s. Nor can the history of Chinese medicine in this field be
conceived of in terms of a steady and progressive development toward consistency.

For long periods, especially from the Han to the Tang, diseases rather
than patterns functioned as the most important diagnostic classifiers. The
Zhubing yuan hou lun 诸病源侯论 (*Treatise Regarding the Origin and Symp-*

toms of *All Diseases*) from the Sui dynasty is the most representative and influential example. The text is organized according to diseases (*bing*) such as wind disease (*fengbing* 风病), *qi* disease (*qibing* 气病), and miscellaneous childhood diseases (*xiaoer zabing* 小儿杂病), which are in turn subdivided into many different key symptoms (*hou* 候). In most instances these key symptoms correspond to what modern physicians would refer to as symptoms and signs. Only rarely do they correspond to modern patterns.[35] Later texts such as the *Qianjin yaofang* 千金要方 (*Important Formulas Worth a Thousand*) and the *Waitai biyao* 外台秘要 (*Arcane Essentials from the Imperial Library*) from the Tang dynasty draw heavily on the *Zhubing yuan hou lun* 诸病源侯论 for inspiration. The number of diseases discussed in each text varies enormously, however, at least partly because one text classifies as diseases what another would take to be different symptoms of the same disease.[36]

Starting in the Song dynasty, patterns reemerged as a focus of concern for literati physicians attempting to understand the root causes of disorders. Over the course of the following centuries pattern diagnosis became definitive of elite Chinese medicine, and the term *bianzheng* appears in the titles of many medical treatises from the late Ming onward.[37] Several influential authors, such as the Qing scholar Wang Ang 汪昂 (1615–1699), explicitly emphasized the practice of pattern differentiation as the key element of medical practice.[38] Others, such as the Ming scholar-physician Zhang Jiebin 张介宾 (1563–1640), used the terms *bianzheng* and *lunzhi* to organize their work, yet continued to refer to diseases when describing practice. In a statement often quoted today to show that pattern differentiation was always at the heart of Chinese medicine Zhang Jiebin wrote: "In all cases of diagnosing disease and administering treatment one must first carefully examine *yin* and *yang;* they are the guiding rubrics of the way of medicine" (*Fan zhenbing shizhi, bixu xian shen yinyang, nai wei yidao zhi gangling* 凡诊病施治, 必须先审阴阳, 乃为医道之纲领).[39] Some authors, such as the Qing physician Xu Dachun 徐大椿 (1693–1771), attempted to define more clearly the differences between diseases and patterns.[40] Xu is thus frequently cited today as an example that the ancients clearly made this distinction. Ren Yingqiu 任应秋, an eminent scholar of Chinese medical literature in Communist China, acknowledges Xu's contribution but thinks that Xu did not succeed and that he confused matters as much as he clarified them.[41]

Furthermore, no unequivocal or dominant nosological system ever emerged during the classical era. In practice, the emphasis on diagnosis and treatment of some diseases and patterns over others divided rather than unified physicians. For instance, the emergence of the *wenbing* (Warm [Pathogen]

Disorders) scholarly stream meant that while some physicians continued to label and treat externally contracted (*waigan* 外感) diseases on the basis of Zhang Zhongjing's *Shanghan lun*, others, particularly in the south, employed new labels and new theories while treating their patients on the basis of old prescriptions.[42] Some physicians employed what would today be classed as patterns as labels for diseases, while others openly questioned the necessity of patterns to guide treatment. Wu Youxing 吴有性 (1582–1652), for instance, argued that in pestilential illnesses one should treat each disease with only one type of medicine.[43]

Even texts that emphasized patterns as the key to therapy did not do so on the basis of precise and narrow definitions of the term. Lin Peiqin's 林佩琴 (1772–1839) *Leizheng zhicai* 类证治裁 (*Tailored Treatments According to Patterns*), a text often cited as a forerunner of contemporary pattern diagnosis, is a typical example. In the foreword the author states: "The difficulty of attending to life lies in knowing patterns. The difficulty in knowing patterns lies in differentiating patterns, to know whether they indicate *yin* or *yang*, repletion or depletion, [invasion by] the six pernicious influences or [damage by] the seven emotions, that is in surmising similarities among [what appears] different."[44] In discussing specific disorders Lin then presents different methods of making such distinctions drawn from different classical sources. The section on heart pain (*xintong* 心痛), for instance, includes a differentiation based on the possible cause of the pain in various organs of the body, a differentiation according to the presenting nature of the pain (hot or cold), and a differentiation according to etiological factors such as *qi*, blood (*xue* 血), and phlegm (*tan* 痰). While this represents a clinically useful method for matching different presentations of the same disorder to different methods of treatment, there is no apparent concern to systematically tie the various methods of differentiation into one overarching scheme.[45]

The situation was further complicated when Western medical knowledge penetrated Chinese medicine. Western medicine offered new ideas about diseases and their causes but also saddled Chinese physicians with the problem of situating their own methods of classifying and treating diseases within the apparently objective systems used by biomedicine. The political confrontation with Western medicine during the Republican era led to fundamental changes in all aspects of Chinese medicine, including systematization of the presentation of diseases, patterns, symptoms, and signs in the transmission of medical knowledge.[46] If we examine the works of individual authors, we still, however, find a considerable mixing of categories. Zhang Xichun's 张锡纯 influential *Yixue zhongzhong canxi lu* 医学衷中参西录 (*Records of the*

Assimilation of the Western to Chinese in Medicine), a collection of essays, articles, case notes, and case histories published between 1900 and 1934, is exemplary in this respect.[47] The 138 case histories collected in the third volume are systematically presented in a novel format. Each case history is analyzed in terms of its etiology (*bingyin* 病因), pattern of presentation (*zhenghou* 证侯), diagnosis (*zhenduan* 诊断), prescription (*chufang* 处方), analysis of prescription (*fangjie* 方解), and therapeutic outcomes (*xiaoguo* 效果). Interestingly, the category *zhenghou* 证侯 lists only the presenting symptoms, whereas "diagnosis" gives an explanation in terms of what would today be considered a differentiation of patterns and determination of treatment.[48]

In spite of his systematic presentation of data, however, Zhang does not distinguish clearly between diseases, patterns, and symptoms—or at least not in the manner such differentiation is advocated in modern texts. The titles of section headings (*men* 门) under which individual case histories are presented are drawn from a number of different sources. They include disease names from the Chinese tradition such as "jaundice" (*huangdan men* 黄疸门) and "dysentery" (*liji men* 痢疾门), but also entire specializations such as "gynecology" (*funuke* 妇女科). We find specific therapeutic orientations to the treatment of similar kinds of illness (*shanghan men, wenbing men*) and diseases characterized by specific symptoms such as "consumption with abnormal breathing and cough" (*xulao chuansou men* 虚劳喘嗽门). Zhang employs the term "disease" where many classical authors would have used "pattern," such as in "*qi* diseases" (*qibing men* 气病门) and "blood diseases" (*xuebing men* 血病门), and at least one category, *naochongxue men* 脑充血门, is influenced by Zhang's knowledge of Western medicine. *Naochongxue* denotes bleeding into the brain but is not a classical Chinese medical term. Western medical knowledge of the occurrence of such bleeding in the aftermath of strokes (known by means of pathological anatomy) greatly influenced Zhang Xichun's thinking and development of new therapies, which continue to be influential.[49]

Titles of individual case histories exhibit a similar mixing of categories. Thus we find diseases such as "jaundice" (*huangdan*),[50] symptoms such as "headache" (*toutong* 头痛), patterns such as "great *qi* sinking downward" (*daqi xiaxian* 大气下陷), disease patterns derived from assimilated Western medical knowledge such as "encephalemia headache" (*naochongxue touteng* 脑充血头痛), and even mixed Chinese and Western disease categories such as "cold damage with concurrent meningitis" (*shanghan jian naomoyan* 伤寒兼脑膜炎). Nor is any clearly discernible differentiation between diseases and patterns achieved within the main text itself. Under the heading "diagnosis" of the case "*shanghan* with concurrent meningitis" we read that "this is a pattern of the disease being replete and the pulse vacuous" (*ci nai bing shi mai xu zhi zheng* 此乃病实脉虚之证). In another case we learn that "here pattern and pulse correspond to each other" (*ji ci zheng mai xiang can* 即此证脉相参).[51]

I have cited Zhang Xichun at length because he constitutes as important a reference point in the prerevolutionary era as Zhang Zhongjing does for the origins of pattern differentiation at the end of the Han. Zhang Weiyao 张维耀, a contemporary Chinese scholar, lucidly sums up the development of pattern differentiation in the intervening two millennia: "One [thus] can see that all the way up to the Qing patterns, diseases, and symptoms and signs within Chinese medicine were not intrinsically different terminological constructs. Even though different historical periods and different authors may have endowed [these terms] with rigorous content, they later . . . stood side by side and [no one definition] was generally accepted. Thus prior to the 1950s 'patterns' are not the basic concept of Chinese medicine theory and therefore one can also say that *bianzheng lunzhi* was not [yet] established as a theoretical system."[52] Zhang's synopsis corroborates my own brief review. The question we now must answer is what happened in the 1950s that made it possible to establish conceptual (though not necessarily practical) consensus where previously there had existed undisciplined (though highly practicable) diversity.

The Emergence of *Bianzheng lunzhi* in Maoist China

Three novel elements appeared in the formulations of *bianzheng lunzhi* that began to circulate among Chinese medicine physicians in the 1950s: (1) the explicit and systematic usage of the term by a wide variety of authors, (2) the use of the term as a defining feature of Chinese medicine vis-à-vis Western medicine, and (3) the linkage of the term to the shifting Maoist vision regarding the function of medicine in society. I argue that the appearance of these elements demonstrates that *bianzheng lunzhi* became important because it accomplished, at least, the following: it allowed scholar-physicians to define the practice of Chinese medicine as being categorically different from Western medicine; it promised a solution to the problem of integration, if necessary, of the two medicines; it established a connection to the cultural heritage of the motherland that was politically correct (i.e., modern, systematic, and dialectical); and it facilitated the systematic teaching of Chinese medicine in newly emergent educational institutions.

IDEOLOGICAL DIMENSIONS

The ideological dimensions of *bianzheng lunzhi* are, perhaps, the most obvious. Given the historical pressures of the time, it was necessary for Chinese

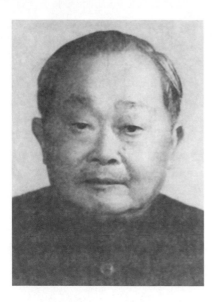 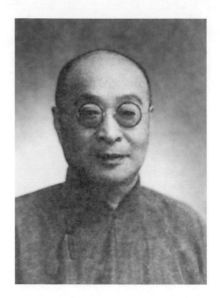

physicians in the 1950s struggling for the independence of their tradition to show that their practice, while possessing distinctly Chinese cultural roots, was capable of modernization and of contributing something unique to the contemporary world of medicine.

Shi Jinmo 施今墨 (1881–1969), one of "Beijing's four great and famous doctors," a leading activist in the defense of Chinese medicine during the Republican period, and a well-known advocate of medical syncretism, is identified by Zhang Weiyao 张维耀 as one of the first physicians to have explicitly thematized the pivotal role of pattern differentiation for contemporary Chinese medicine. The following quote (which I have been unable to date) appears in Shi's collected case records, his declared medical legacy published posthumously in 1982 by his student and disciple Zhu Chenyu 祝谌予 (1914–): "Approach patterns as you would approach a battle. Use drugs as you would use soldiers. One must clearly differentiate symptoms, carefully organize one's prescriptions, and flexibly employ one's drugs. If one does not know the principles of medicine, it becomes difficult to differentiate patterns. If pattern differentiation is unclear, one has no way to establish a method [of treatment] and merely piles up individual drugs in a disorganized fashion."[53]

Like the medical ancestors with whom he aligns himself in this quote by means of implicit references, Shi Jinmo accords pattern differentiation an important place in Chinese medicine.[54] As a practice it remains subordinated in his argument, however, to the knowledge of the principles of medicine (yili 医理); that is, to reflection. This is in line with Andrews's claim that Shi, like

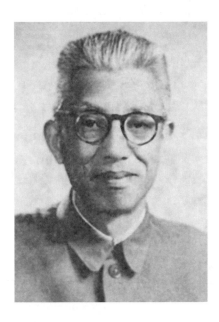

FIGURE 31. Jiang Chunhua (1908–1992)

FIGURE 32. Shi Jinmo (1881–1969)

FIGURE 33. Qin Bowei (1901–1970)

other leading Chinese medicine thinkers of his time, insisted on the relevance of theory to practice in response to those who had attacked the unscientific nature of Chinese medicine and who saw in it nothing more than a repository of empirically useful drugs, prescriptions, and treatments.[55]

Qin Bowei 秦伯未 (1901–1970), a student of Ding Ganren 丁甘仁 (1865–1926), and a leading physician, educator, and activist on behalf of Chinese medicine in Shanghai during the Republican period, was invited to Beijing in 1955 as a consultant to the MOH. Already a major scholar and educator before 1949, he subsequently became one of the leading architects of modern Chinese medicine.[56] In an article written in 1957 Qin echoes Shi Jinmo's sentiments about the relationship of theory to practice. Arguing against those who had already elevated *bianzheng lunzhi* to a pivotal position in Chinese medicine he states that *"bianzheng lunzhi* is a diagnostic and therapeutic law for treating disease in Chinese medicine [*shi zhongyi zhibing yizhong zhenliao guilu* 是中医治病一种诊疗规律]. It is not [however] the pinnacle of Chinese medical theories. *Bianzheng lunzhi* was produced by Chinese medical theory. Without the guidance of theory, there would be no such method [*faze* 法则]."[57] By 1961 Qin had subsumed under the rubric of pattern discrimination all aspects of medical practice: *"Bianzheng lunzhi* is a method [*faze* 法则] of Chinese medical therapeutics. Its vital essence is that [theoretical] principles, [treatment] techniques, prescriptions, and drugs are one integrated treatment system."[58]

Qin's reference to method is more than a hint, perhaps, in the direction of Engels's natural dialectics (*ziran bianzhengfa* 自然辩证法). The close relation "phonetically, substantively, and orthographically" between the classical medical term for pattern discrimination in diagnosis (*bianzheng* 辨证) and the modern Chinese term for dialectics (*bianzhengfa* 辩证法) was too obvious, certainly, for Chinese medical physicians to ignore.[59] It presented an opportunity to demonstrate that Chinese medicine was neither feudal nor outdated but enlightened, and to make it, as Farquhar notes, "ideologically unassailable."[60]

A less noted but equally important condition that facilitated the emergence of pattern differentiation in the intellectual climate of the 1950s was the fact that it resonated with dominant Pavlovian ideas of adjustment between external and internal environments. Rather than concentrating on specific organic functions in isolation, patterns could be interpreted as manifestations of the response of the total organism to an objective external environment.

The newly defined method of *bianzheng lunzhi* finally also put on an equal footing theoretical principles and treatment methods and thereby matched Maoist perceptions of praxis. In doing so it distanced Chinese medicine from Western idealism, established its roots in a presumed "naive materialism" of classical Chinese thinking, and moved it closer to the revolutionary unity of theory and practice.[61] This is clearly expressed by Qin Bowei: "One might thus say that theory guides practice, yet that theory is conversely [nothing but] a means [*fangfa* 方法]. '*Bianzheng lunzhi*' thus becomes the diagnostic and therapeutic rubric of Chinese medicine and as such is determined by the unity of theory and practice. . . . 'Patterns' (*zheng* 证) and 'treatments' (*zhi* 治) are given and regularized. 'Differentiating' [*bian* 辨] and 'determining' [*lun* 论] are flexible, demanding analysis and reflection."[62]

It is important to point out at this point that the Maoist influence on Chinese medicine involved transformations of subjectivity that cannot be explained as mere changes of belief or as paying lip service to political directives. I argue that in redefining Chinese medicine through *bianzheng lunzhi* the physicians who effected these redefinitions were themselves transformed. In the following extract from his autobiography Yue Meizhong 岳美中 (1900–1982), another influential Beijing *laozhongyi* of the postwar period, admits this with exemplary honesty.

After 1954 my studies and thinking underwent a further transformation. At the time, having studied medicine for thirty years, I had accumulated knowledge and experience through both textual studies and clinical practice. Nevertheless, I began studying *On Contradiction* and some other

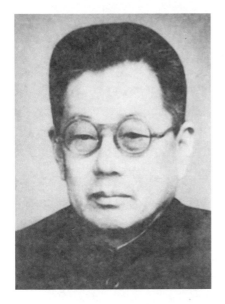 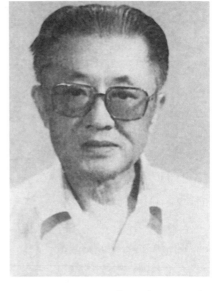

FIGURE 34. Yue Meizhong (1900–1982)   FIGURE 35. Fang Yaozhong (1921–1995)

works on materialist dialectics. Combining in my studies my personal scholarly approach with the methodological issues [of materialist dialectics] I engaged in [a process] of careful consideration and summing up. Basing oneself on the affirmation of past experience, yet feeling [my way through] to how one might employ dead methods in order to treat living people [truly] is to synthesize the old and the new, is to consider and deliberate [things] both foreign and Chinese.[63]

Yue did not come from a medical lineage but had studied medicine initially from Zhang Xichun's books and through a correspondence course. Like many of his contemporaries and their teachers before them he wanted to both continue and innovate tradition, "to study the ancients but not to get stuck in the old" (*shi gu er bu ni gu* 师古而不泥古). Dialectical practice seems to have offered itself to Yue as a method by which his goal could be achieved, though it required him to become a practical dialectician. Yue Meizhong was not alone.[64]

We have already encountered Shi Jinmo as an example of an earlier phase of transition. His student Zhu Chenyu is decidedly more dialectical. He emphasizes that in the development of Chinese medicine education equal importance should be attached to "inheriting" (*jicheng* 继承) and "carrying forward" (*fayang* 发扬). Zhu defines inheritance in education as the basis for any development and development as the purpose of any inheritance.[65] Fang Yaozhong

方药中 (1921–1995), another well-known Beijing *laozhongyi* and influential figure in the regularization of *bianzheng lunzhi*, similarly states in the foreword to a recently published collection of his essays that during the last fifty years his work has been guided by the terms "continuation" and "innovation" (*cheng qi* 承启).[66] It is interesting that in their teaching and biographical writings these *laozhongyi* expound the practice of *bianzheng* as both a defining characteristic of Chinese medicine *and* a fulcrum from which the modern development of Chinese medicine can proceed.

PRACTICAL DIMENSIONS

The need to find such a fulcrum was a main concern for physicians like Qin, Yue, Zhu, and Fang during the early 1950s. In the aftermath of liberation the survival of Chinese medicine as an independent practice was by no means assured. As we saw in chapter 3, the development of the medical sector at the time was driven by the slogan "unite Chinese and Western medicine [in the struggle against disease]" (*tuanjie zhongxiyi* 团结中西医). Considerable pressure was exerted on Chinese medicine throughout this period to modernize, systematize, and establish its scientific credentials. The main vehicle through which this was to be achieved was the Chinese medical improvement schools (*zhongyi jinxiu xuexiao* 中医进修学校), where even well-established physicians had to enroll in order to increase their theoretical and practical knowledge of Western medicine. Some physicians such as Fang Yaozhong and Tang Youzhi 唐由之 (1926–) were even seconded to study Western medicine full time.[67]

The future of the new China—including the future of its new medicine—was by definition bright. There was less certainty, however, as to how the bright future of medicine might be realized in practice. An urgency for quick results was often difficult to reconcile with longer-term ambitions for an entirely new medicine. Practical efforts to transform Chinese medicine by focusing on the use of single drugs or even chemical constituents of individual drugs instead of complicated prescriptions, by basing treatment on biomedical rather than Chinese medical diagnoses, and by emphasizing empiricism over outdated theories such as the five phases (*wu xing* 五行), though sometimes successful, did not translate into the hoped-for breakthroughs.[68] Writing in 1953, Fang Yaozhong described the sentiments in Chinese medicine circles at the time.

> Problems currently abound. Specifically, it appears that the work of uniting Chinese and Western medicine that has been initiated during the last three or four years is being carried out in a manner in which both part-

ners appear to be harmonious but are actually at odds with each other. With respect to Chinese medicine improvement courses, actually Chinese medical physicians are left after much advanced study depressed and irresolute. We know that the knowledge of the new learning by itself is also insufficient. With respect to our original knowledge of Chinese medicine we do not necessarily know how it might be linked to new things. And we lose trust if contrary outcomes put ourselves against our own previous experience. Thus, not knowing how to use the new, yet unable to progress by using the old, we are neither fish nor fowl, and we do not know from where to start.[69]

Clearly, what was needed was a method that allowed Chinese medical practitioners to hold on to their inheritance (if for no other reason than to be practically efficient) yet that also managed to be somehow modern and able to absorb whatever it could from biomedical science. Here *bianzheng lunzhi* offered itself for practical (rather than ideological) reasons and again was both a continuation and transformation of what had gone before. The wholesale enrollment of Chinese medicine practitioners in Western medicine classes certainly made them more open to working with biomedical disease concepts and modes of diagnosis. Yet, in working out differences and points of connection between the two traditions they could base their efforts on those carried out by the previous generation.[70]

Shi Jinmo and his student Zhu Chenyu are representative of these transformations. Shi Jinmo was an influential proponent of the standardization and scientization of Chinese medicine during the Nationalist period. In his practice he attempted to integrate Western and Chinese medicine by using, for instance, single Chinese pharmaceuticals to treat specific problems.[71] A proposition put to the newly established Central Institute of National Medicine (Zhongyang guoyiguan 中央国医馆) in 1932 by Shi and other leading physicians to adapt biomedical disease categories as guiding rubrics in the standardization of Chinese medicine was defeated, however, by widespread opposition from within the Chinese medical community. The general consensus then was that such a move would invalidate the autonomy of Chinese medicine and undercut its practical efficacy. Distinguishing Chinese medical pattern differentiation from Western medical disease diagnosis in order to facilitate their practical integration was thus also an attempt to find a novel solution to the modernization debates of the 1930s.[72]

Zhu Chenyu, Shi Jinmo's most influential disciple, studied Western medicine in Japan from 1939 to 1943 with the explicit encouragement of his teacher. As the first dean of the Beijing College of Chinese Medicine Shi was in a powerful position to disseminate the newly developed opposition between Western medicine's diagnosis of diseases and Chinese medicine's pattern discrimination. Historically, this opposition had been formulated in the 1930s by Yang Zemin 扬则民 (1893–1948), a scholar-physician from Zhejiang Province who was also the first to explicate the compatibility between Chinese medical thought and Western dialectics. In an essay entitled "Bianzheng yu shibing" 辨证与识病 (Differentiating patterns and knowing diseases) Yang had stated that "Chinese medicine emphasizes differentiating patterns. Western medicine emphasizes knowing diseases. The purpose of pattern differentiation is the therapeutic use of drugs, the purpose of knowing diseases is the discrimination of the location of a disease."[73]

Yang was labeled a reactionary after 1949, and this curtailed public acknowledgment of his influence and circulation of his ideas.[74] It was thus left to physicians like Zhu Chenyu to elaborate his distinction.[75] According to Zhu, Western medicine, rooted in experiment, physiology, and anatomy, provided better descriptions of diseases and their causes than Chinese medicine. Chinese medicine's pattern differentiation, on the other hand, permitted physicians to relate objective but decontextualized knowledge of diseases to the concrete specifications of each individual case and thereby to maintain a perspective on the functioning of the whole patient. Based on this opposition Zhu proposed the creation of a medicine that would assimilate Western knowledge of disease to the Chinese practice of pattern differentiation.[76]

The selfsame development of thesis, antithesis, and synthesis can be found also in the work of Fang Yaozhong, still a young physician in the 1950s, who contributed to the definition of *bianzheng* by tracing its basic principles to canonical texts such as the *Shanghan zabing lun*. Fang pointed out that in opposition to biomedical interests in the causation of specific disease entities, classical authors such as Zhang Zhongjing had concerned themselves with understanding disease as a process. Fang, too, therefore advocated a synthesis of Western disease and Chinese pattern discrimination.[77]

The practical value of such thinking was demonstrated by another leading physician of the time, Pu Fuzhou 蒲辅周 (1888–1975), in an episode that has since become one of the legends of contemporary Chinese medicine.[78] Pu Fuzhou was director of the Internal Medicine Section at the newly established Academy of Chinese Medicine in Beijing. During an outbreak of epidemic meningitis in Shijiazhuang in Hebei Province in 1956, physicians under his direction obtained very successful results by diagnosing a summerheat warm (*shuwen* 暑温) pattern using *Baihu tang* 白虎汤 (White Tiger Decoction) as the principal formula.[79] One year later, during a similar outbreak in the Beijing area, the same approach proved unsuccessful. Pu Fuzhou argued that the different climatic conditions of that outbreak (a damper environment caused by summer rains) necessitated an adjustment of the treatment strategy and the use of damp-draining and heat-clearing formulas like *San ren tang* 三仁汤 (Three-Nut Decoction).[80] Pu Fuzhou summarized his approach in a manner that underlines the resonance between Maoist and Chinese medical dialectics: "The knowledge arrived at by way of this practice is this: While this year's patients in terms of causation equally appeared to suffer from summerheat damp, due to the influence of climatic conditions this manifested in a specific transmuted pattern (*bianzheng* 变症). In the process of treating meningitis, we must pay attention to such specificity."[81] At the time, this achievement provided evidence to both Chinese medicine physicians and their political supporters of the value and clinical efficacy of pattern differentiation. Today, the episode has become one of the defining stories of contemporary Chinese medicine that is narrated time and again to students and foreigners and retold by physicians to one another in an affirmation of their own self-worth.[82]

DOCTRINAL DIMENSIONS

The systematization of Chinese medicine that becomes visible in the creation of *bianzheng lunzhi* as the pivot of modern practice involved several important labors. First, it necessitated for ideological reasons the definition of Chinese medicine as a medical practice whose knowledge embodied, albeit in primitive form, an understanding of process as an ongoing synthesis of oppositions. Pattern differentiation was employed as a prime example demonstrating how Chinese medicine approached the treatment of illness "dialectically." Rather than focusing on defined diseases, Chinese medicine understood illness as a process of emerging contradictions. The purpose of treatment was to resolve these contradictions flexibly and practically by treating changing symptom complexes. Chinese medicine thus became an expression of dialectics based on naive materialism, open to improvement under the guidance of the party and with the help of Western science.[83]

Second, systemization required symptoms and signs, patterns and diseases to be clearly separate both conceptually and practically. These, as I have shown, had previously overlapped but were now distinguished in the manner described at the beginning of this chapter. This separation—a separation that required imputing modern meanings into classical texts—appears fully elaborated for the first time in the *Outline of Chinese Medicine,* the first textbook of Chinese medicine, which was produced on behalf and under the supervision of the MOH between 1957 and 1958.[84] In truly dialectical fashion, these now-separated elements were combined again in the process of diagnosis. Only a few years later, this allowed Maoist physicians to argue that pattern discrimination was an advance over medicine based exclusively on theoryless symptomatology (empiricism) and exceedingly abstract and overtheoretical disease nosologies (biomedicine).[85]

Initially, this synthesis seems to have been driven by the political demands of the state and the resistance of the Western medicine physicians ordered to study Chinese medicine in the mid-1950s. As I discussed in chapter 3, many of the Western medical physicians ordered to study Chinese medicine in Beijing in 1955 were less than enthusiastic about this change in their careers. They found it particularly difficult to study from classical texts representing knowledge in a form quite different from the logic of Western science, as, indeed, did many of the students recruited to the newly established Chinese medical colleges. Furthermore, these Western medicine physicians needed a way by which they could assimilate Chinese medicine within the knowledge of disease they already possessed. The elaboration of patterns (which belonged exclusively to Chinese medicine) and their differentiation both from diseases (which belonged to Western medicine) and from symptoms and signs (which belonged to both medical systems) met this demand.[86]

Creating a more systematic Chinese medicine was thus not only a top-down process driven by political imperatives or the demands of modern educational institutions but also a response to pressure from below. This is demonstrated by the following quote from the foreword to *Zhongyi bianzheng shuyu de shentao* 中医辨证术语的深讨 (*An In-Depth Discussion of Chinese Medicine Pattern Terminology*). This book was a contribution to the systematization of pattern differentiation put forward by the Chongqing Research Class of Physicians of Western Medicine Seconded from Work to Study Chinese Medicine (Chongqingshi xiyi xuexi zhongyi lizhi yanjiuban 重庆市西医离职学习中医研究班) after graduating from their course.

> During the two and a half years in which we took leave from our jobs to study Chinese medicine we learned through personal experience that the essential characteristics of Chinese medical thinking and its theoretical principles lie in its naive dialectical materialist perspective. . . . Its method—pattern discrimination and application of treatment, which consists of applying Chinese medicine to the theoretical understanding as well as the treatment of disease—and also its principles should be followed in the process of general medical practice. . . . [However,] the use of pattern terminology in clinical contexts remains complicated and we Western medicine physicians studying Chinese medicine feel it is dif-

ficult to employ and not easy to come to terms with. We feel that the Chinese medicine reference materials in this area are equally unhandy. Hence, we have attempted the task of an initial systematization in this respect.[87]

Within the space of a few sentences, the Chongqing physicians indicate the multitude of factors that contributed to the formation of *bianzheng lunzhi*. We can see, for instance, that the ideologically correct connotations of pattern differentiation that assisted Chinese medical practitioners in establishing a niche for their tradition in the new China were used by the state as a tool for disciplining Western medicine physicians and their allies in the course of the political struggles outlined in chapter 3. The role of *bianzheng lunzhi* within the wider program of creating a new medicine is made clear. We also can see, however, that once the association between Chinese medicine and dialectical materialism, even if it was labeled "naive" (*pusu* 朴素), had been made, it became available to Chinese medicine physicians committed to the development of their own tradition rather than the Maoist vision of a new medicine, as a tool for effecting a quite different dialectical opposition — the working out of the opposition between Chinese medicine and Western medicine as an opposition between disease and pattern discrimination.

This opposition proved to be both externally and internally effective for those physicians who, like Zhu Chenyu, argued for the simultaneous preservation and development of Chinese medicine. Internally, it provided an effective argument against the use of Chinese medicine treatment and drugs on the sole basis of biomedical disease classifications. Only a diagnosis that incorporated pattern discrimination as its central element constituted Chinese medicine.[88] Externally, basing Chinese medicine on pattern differentiation helped to define it intellectually and practically as an independent discipline. It could never be assimilated by (disease-based) Western medicine without, in the process, destroying its very nature and, by implication, the root of its efficacy.[89]

Third, an overarching principle had to be found to which the many different and sometimes contrary methods of pattern discrimination developed in the course of Chinese medicine's long history could be assimilated. We saw that advocates of the *shanghan* and *wenbing* streams, for instance, frequently employed the same prescriptions but derived the rationale for their use from different principles of diagnostic classification. And not only did different practices and schools of classifying, understanding, and reacting to illness compete with each other, but entirely new diagnostic patterns were continuously added to the medical archive by innovative physicians.

The *Outline of Chinese Medicine* resolved this problem. Its authors employed a twofold strategy. On the one hand, they outlined a number of different subsystems in Chinese medicine by which the now clearly defined symptoms and signs could be organized into patterns.[90] On the other, they designated the "eight rubrics" (*ba gang* 八纲), a system made up of the four opposing pairs *yin/yang*, exterior/interior (*biao li* 表里), cold/heat (*han re* 寒热), and depletion/repletion (*xu shi* 虚实), as the basic matrix of Chinese medical diagnostics.[91] Although different methods of classifying symptoms into patterns (and Chinese medicine's historical plurality) were thus acknowledged, the authors claimed that the methods' overall spirit was identical and that "they all are methods of pattern differentiation under the directive [influence] of the theory of the eight rubrics."[92]

Bianzheng lunzhi thus provided the theoretical tool and practical method necessary for uniting physicians of different orientations without reducing (at this point, at least) historic diversity and thereby limiting practical efficacy. It permitted the theoretical systematization that was necessary to satisfy demands for the modernization of Chinese medicine, yet also managed to align Chinese medicine with the prevailing Maoist emphasis on practical knowledge. It allowed Chinese medicine physicians to distinguish themselves from Western medicine physicians and to assert their identity both as inheritors of tradition in general and as the students of particular teachers (thus being dually Chinese). It also, however, created a basis from which the old could be developed by assimilating it into the modern in the form of Western medicine's knowledge of "diseases."

DISPUTED ISSUES

Differences of opinion among leading scholar-physicians regarding pattern differentiation existed prior to the mid-1950s and did not disappear thereafter. Shi Jinmo for instance, whom modern Chinese commentators identify as an ancestor of the contemporary orthodoxy, had long argued that the number of core diagnostic rubrics should be extended from eight to ten by including the categories of *qi* and blood (*xue* 血). In typical Chinese style, he managed to contain this innovation without abolishing the eight rubrics completely, for "by using *yin* [and] *yang* as general rubrics, exterior/interior, depletion/repletion, cold/heat, *qi*/blood become the eight rubrics."[93]

The redefinitions outlined in the preceding section thus were not achieved without struggle. Until the mid-1960s Chinese medicine journals debated the value of the emerging opposition between Chinese medicine pattern differentiation and Western medicine disease differentiation. We can observe here two related processes. The first documents the crystallization of *bianzheng lunzhi* into a core element and defining feature of Chinese medicine. As the status of Chinese medicine became increasingly secure, some authors even went as far as asserting that *bianzheng lunzhi* "reflects an aspect of great superiority of Chinese medicine" (*zuowei zhongyixue de yi da youshi* 作为中医学的一大优势).[94]

The second process is one whereby this emergent consensus is challenged and tested. Qin Bowei, for instance, opposed the categorical separation between diseases, patterns, and symptoms proposed in the *Outline*. On the basis of lexicographical evidence he argued that the classical terms "evidence" (*zheng* 證), "symptom" (*zheng* 症), and "pattern" (*zheng* 証) were equivalent and were often used interchangeably. Differences between symptoms, patterns, and diseases thus were not natural but were rooted in practice. They were derived from whether a physician classified a headache, for instance, as a disease or a symptom, or whether he grouped it with other symptoms and signs (such as aversion to wind and a tight pulse) into a disease pattern such as "wind cold headache" (*fenghan touteng* 风寒头疼). Consequently, what was important about *bianzheng lunzhi* was not its distinction of diseases and patterns, it was learning how to synthesize on the basis of Chinese medical theory how specific symptoms are produced by specific causes and pathomechanisms and to derive appropriate treatments from such reasoning. Even at this stage, Qin Bowei and other leading physicians were concerned that medical education at that time was eliminating physicians' ability to do this, a stance they took, as we saw in chapter 3, at considerable personal risk.[95]

Another area of contention was the relation of diseases to patterns and, by implication, the relation of Western medicine to Chinese medicine. By defining Chinese medicine as predominantly concerned with patterns and Western medicine as treating diseases, physicians such as Shi Jinmo appeared to have realized their earlier objective—defeated in the 1930s—of abolishing the plurality of Chinese disease nosology and replacing it with the supposedly superior scientific rigor of Western disease classifications. This move did not go unopposed. Several leading scholars argued that disease differentiation on the basis of Chinese disease categories was theoretically and practically intertwined with pattern differentiation and must not therefore be abandoned.

For instance, all patterns of "phlegm-rheum disease" (*tanyinbing* 痰饮病), a disease first described in the *Jingui yaolue*, reflect disorders of the lung (*fei*), spleen (*pi*) and, ultimately, kidneys (*shen*). Therefore, by classifying a problem as a phlegm-rheum disease a physician is directed toward these organs in his formulation of therapeutic strategies. On the basis of her understanding of fluid physiology she will furthermore know that at some point in the course of treatment she will have to address the kidneys, even where this is not indicated by the currently presenting pattern. In the opinion of these physicians, Chinese medicine was never merely interested in a phenomenological understanding of disease as process but, like Western medicine, also searched for disease causes and attempted their eradication. They thus agreed with the basic premise of an integration of pattern and disease differentiation, but for both epistemological and practical reasons insisted that disease differentiation was carried out on the basis of Chinese medicine disease categories.[96]

Other authors, like the influential Ren Yingqiu 任应秋, attacked the assimilation of biomedical disease categories into Chinese medicine from precisely the opposite direction. He reasoned that although Chinese medicine historically distinguished between diseases and patterns, pattern differentiation had always been more important because nothing was outside the scope of *yin/yang* and the *ba gang*. Even if one did not yet understand the exact nature of a given disease, one could understand its manifestations by means of *yin/yang* and the *ba gang,* and therefore treat it. Ren argued that it was precisely this attribute that bestowed on Chinese medicine an important role in the revolutionary project of ensuring and protecting the health of workers and peasants.[97]

Yue Meizhong and Chen Keji 陈可冀 (1930–) offered another solution. In their contribution to a debate on the topic in the *Fuzhou Journal of Chinese Medicine and Pharmacology* they note that, in practice, pattern differentiation does not always yield the desired results. This problem can be overcome, they say, only by exploiting the dialectical contradiction between diseases as entities with distinct and stable characteristics and patterns as reflections of whole body processes. For this purpose it matters little whether diseases are defined in Chinese or Western medical terms.[98]

Differences also surfaced with respect to how pattern differentiation might best be systematized in a practically efficient and teachable manner. All the actors involved agreed on the importance of sorting out (*zhengli* 整理) and standardizing (*guifan* 规范) Chinese medicine in order to bring about its modernization. The explicit analyses and theoretical reflections on the practice of *bianzheng lunzhi* produced by many leading physicians of the time are one reflection of this process.[99] Another is the formulation of well-ordered therapeutic systems based on the principles of pattern differentiation. Various competing proposals were put forward during the 1950s and 1960s, though in the end it was the format of the *Outline* (privileged from the beginning as an official textbook composed by a collective that included many prominent physicians) that prevailed. (See Appendix A for a detailed presentation of four such systems.)

Bianzheng lunzhi during the Cultural Revolution

We saw in chapter 4 that during the Cultural Revolution the creation of a distinctly "new medicine"—neither classical nor Western but socialist, modern, *and* Chinese—was politically called for. It is more difficult to trace the uses of pattern differentiation in this period because most Chinese medicine journals ceased publication between the mid-1960s and 1970s and relatively few books were published. My analysis, therefore, awaits revision in the light of more detailed evidence from secondary sources and oral histories. A few preliminary observations can nevertheless be made. Most immediately obvious is a subtle terminological change that began to appear in the early 1960s. What had previously been known as *bianzheng lunzhi* became known instead by the slightly different term *bianzheng shizhi* 辨证施治 (differentiating patterns and applying treatment) in several key publications.

Just as the terms *bianzheng* and *lunzhi* were taken from the discussions of previous generations of physicians, so too was the term *shizhi*. It appears, for instance, in the passage by the Ming dynasty scholar-physician Zhang Jiebin quoted above. Its systematic contemporary usage, however, seems to stem from attempts at systematizing the teaching of internal medicine (*neike* 内科) at Chinese medicine improvement classes (*zhongyi xinxiuban* 中医进修班) organized by the Shanghai Department of Health during the late 1950s and early 1960s.[100] When the first national textbook for internal medicine, edited by the Shanghai College of Chinese Medicine, was published in 1964, it, too, adopted *bianzheng shizhi* as the heading for all sections discussing clinical practice.[101] In 1971 a book entitled *Bianzheng shizhi gangyao* 辨症施治纲要 (*Differentiating Symptoms and Applying Treatment: An Outline*) was published by the Revolutionary Committee of the Beijing Chinese Medicine Hospital, and in 1972 the Shanghai College of Chinese Medicine used *Differentiating Symptoms and Applying Treatment* as the title of an important textbook on therapeutics.[102] Although by no means universally accepted, the term replaces *bianzheng lunzhi* in essays written by Qin Bowei (who came from Shanghai) from 1964 onward, though not in those by Ren Yingqiu (who came from Chongqing) from the same period.[103] After dominating throughout the 1960s and 1970s, *bianzheng shizhi* gradually disappeared again after the end of the Cultural Revolution, when usage of *bianzheng lunzhi* emerged as the norm once more.[104]

It was difficult to ascertain from my informants what precisely this terminological shift was meant to signify. Some said they had never thought about it. Others indicated that the two terms mean more or less the same thing. A more differentiated analysis was that *lunzhi* refers to the discursive, standardized, and generalized treatment of disease patterns, whereas *shizhi* indicates the detailed, individualized, and specific treatment of single patients. One of Qin Bowei's students told me that while in his lectures Qin continued to use *lunzhi* throughout the 1960s, he replaced it with *shizhi* in his written work after 1963 in order to emphasize the connection of diagnostic reflection to clinical work rather than to theory.

In the attempt to replace *lunzhi* (which carries connotations of discussions, discourse, and theoretical reflections) with *shizhi* (which expresses a sense of executing or using something), one thus may sense an intention to move Chinese medicine further away from its associations with elite culture and speculative philosophy toward a practice more suited to the concrete needs of the clinic. This thesis can be supported by examining an essay discussing the place of Zhang Zhongjing in the history of Chinese medicine written by Zhang Cigong 章次公 (1903–1959) and published in the influential *Zhongyi zazhi* 中医杂志 (*Journal of Chinese Medicine*) in 1955.[105]

Zhang was a prominent Shanghai physician committed to the radical modernization of Chinese medicine who was then an adviser to the MOH based at the Academy of Chinese Medicine in Beijing. One of his teachers had been Zhang Taiyan 章太炎 (1869–1936), a prominent intellectual and nationalist revolutionary, whose views regarding the development of Chinese medicine he adopted. These held that the empirical spirit that characterized early Chinese medicine had increasingly been watered down from the Song dynasty onward by a proclivity to metaphysical speculation imported into medicine by literati physicians. Recovering the empiricism of ancient Chinese medicine, embodied in particular by Zhang Zhongjing's *Shanghan lun* model of pattern diagnosis and treatment, was thus a move directed at two audiences at once. It demonstrated the scientific nature at the very heart of Chinese medicine while opening it up to assimilation into the new medicine of China. "Applying" treatment carries none of the metaphysical baggage associated with "discussing" or "determining" it, not least because the term *lunzhi* was popular with many literati physicians in late imperial China. Hence, it is not at all surprising that Zhang should replace it with *shizhi* in his own essay.[106]

Though motivated, perhaps, by similar purposes, not all advocates of this shift cared as deeply about the subtleties of classical medicine as Qin Bowei, Ren Yingqiu, and Zhang Cigong. This impression is supported by a detailed examination of the 1972 Shanghai text mentioned above. While following broadly the approach of the *Outline, Differentiating Symptoms* emphasizes most strongly those aspects of clinical reality resonating with the political buzzwords of the time: dialectics, contradiction (*maodun* 矛盾), struggle (*douzheng* 斗争) (between the correct and the evil), and the interplay between general principles (*yuanze* 原则) and flexible (*linghuo* 灵活) practices. Also, following Mao's maxim to separate out those elements of traditional culture that contained revolutionary elements from those that were degenerate, the modernization of Chinese medicine was accelerated by means of systematization, simplification, revision, and terminological adaptations, all of which moved Chinese medicine in the direction of Western medicine. The Shanghai text presents basic theory, for instance, in chapters entitled "Physiology and Pathology" (*Shengli yu bingli* 生理与病理) and "Diseases and Their Aetiology" (*Jibing yu bingyin* 疾病与病因). The principal rubrics of pattern differentiation are pared down from eight to four (*yin, yang,* repletion, and depletion), and Chinese medicine and Western medicine concepts are frequently used together.

The text also contains few signs of historic diversity, and, indeed, every effort was made to reduce it. Where the *Outline* merely systematized by subsuming different methods of pattern differentiation under the one roof of the "eight rubrics," *Differentiating Symptoms* is far more explicitly revolutionary. Concerning the differentiation and treatment of "externally contracted heat diseases" (*waigan rebing* 外感热病), for example, it states: "This chapter smashes the boundaries between the *shanghan* six stages and the *wenbing* [four aspects] *wei, qi, ying, xue* [methods of diagnosis] by synthesizing their content and by using the concepts of repletion and depletion as sole rubrics. . . . In this way it not only gets rid of the sectarian views of *shanghan* and *wenbing* theories, but also fits in even [better] with the realities of the clinic."[107]

A similar reductionism extends to the general practice of pattern differentiation and is most evident in the case histories intended to illustrate the practical application of theoretical principles. These case histories are divided into three sections: (1) the development of the disease (*bingshi* 病史, lit. "disease history"), which gives a brief etiological account and lists presenting signs and symptoms; (2) the prescription (*chufang* 处方), which indicates the drugs used; and (3) an analysis of symptom patterns (*bianzheng fenxi* 辨症分析), which provides the rationale by which diagnosed patterns are linked to the prescription. Instead of a detailed discussion and differential explication of symptoms and signs (as found, for instance, in the modern case histories of Zhang Xichun,

Yue Meizhong, Pu Fuzhou, and Shi Jinmo), analysis is limited to a listing of standardized disease mechanisms such as static blood (yuxue 瘀血) and stomach qi depletion (weiqixu 胃气虚) that serves as a link between symptom complexes and prescriptions.[108]

On other levels, too, previous syntheses were given new emphases and integrated into new practices. Whereas knowledge of biomedical diseases had previously been advocated as one tool among many in the formulation of a Chinese medicine treatment, Western medicine disease categories were now suggested as primary diagnostic signposts. Each biomedical disease was to be subdivided into several distinct Chinese medicine patterns, now frequently referred to as "types" (xing 型) rather than "patterns." For each "type" specific treatments were then suggested.[109] Thus, whereas pattern differentiation was conceived of as a complex of the subjective (the differentiating) and the given (the patterns), the language of types tried to move the process further toward the objective and the technical valued in biomedicine. This model, referred to as "distinguishing types and applying treatment" (fenxing shizhi 分型施治)," seems to have been proposed initially by Chen Ziyin 沈自尹—one of the Western medicine physicians who studied Chinese medicine in the 1950s—in 1973.[110] Its advocates did not succeed, however, in establishing it as a standard within Chinese medical circles.

In 1980, when discussion became possible once again, the method of distinguishing types and applying treatment emerged as a hotly debated issue in journals of both Chinese and Western medicine. The debate was initiated by physicians like Yue Meizhong who had been active in establishing pattern differentiation at the core of contemporary practice. These physicians argued that differentiating types rather than patterns constituted an inferior method of practice. It was of some benefit in guiding physicians toward an initial understanding of pathological process, and appropriate when little formal training was possible. It was not a subtle enough method, though, to allow an understanding of multiply interconnected factors such as constitution, temperament, pathogen penetration, and climatic and seasonal influences that contributed to a given manifestation of symptoms and signs. Applying fixed prescriptions to types of illness was thus a simplification of all that Chinese medicine stood for—"the use of dead formulas for the treatment of living disorders."[111]

A second group of physicians countered such arguments by pointing to clinical outcomes as demonstrated by various studies. They also argued that the method was helpful in developing the dialectical materialism inherent in Chinese medicine by ridding it of its subjective elements. A third group argued that the method of treatment according to types could be traced back as far as the *Neijing*, thus establishing it as an integral aspect of Chinese medicine. The problems pointed out by Yue Meizhong and others were therefore aspects not of the method as such but of an insufficient grounding in Chinese medicine by the people who used it.[112]

Through his evocative use of language Yue Meizhong signaled that this debate was not merely about diagnostic preferences but about the heart and soul of Chinese medicine. For Yue the practice of Chinese medicine as a consummate skill (*shulian* 熟练) consisted of an ongoing effort aimed at "understanding the present through reviewing the past" (*wengu zhixin* 温故知新). He describes this effort as a "smelting" (*duanlian* 锻炼), in which past knowledge is constantly refined in an ongoing process of training (another meaning of *duanlian*) that consists of wide reading and self-reflective clinical practice. Developing as a physician is thus as much about the cultivation of the self as it is about that of medicine. Merely matching formulas with symptoms and signs classified as types represents a vulgarization (*yongsuhua* 庸俗化) of Chinese medicine, which kills it off precisely because it fails to grasp it as a practice.[113]

While Yue Meizhong and his allies succeeded in establishing the dominant position of pattern differentiation on the level of discourse, clinical medicine is moving more and more in the direction of type differentiation even if the types are often labeled as patterns. Type distinction also has been adopted as an organizing framework for many textbooks and research into the integration of Chinese and Western medicine, the area that almost all of my informants saw as the cutting edge of Chinese medicine in contemporary China. Chen Ziyin's own research is frequently portrayed today as the epitome for the potential of such an integrated approach. Chen was one of those young graduates of Western medicine trained in Chinese medicine in the 1950s. One of his teachers was Jiang Chunhua 姜春华 (1908–1992), another luminary *laozhongyi* and the first professor of Chinese medicine appointed in Shanghai. Jiang wrote commentaries on classical texts but also participated in innovative research carried out in Shanghai during the 1960s that attempted to establish correspondences between Western pathophysiology and Chinese medical patterns.[114]

The most significant of these efforts was the demonstration by Chen and his collaborators that patients diagnosed as suffering from kidney *yang* depletion (*shenyangxu* 肾阳虚) showed consistently low urine levels of 17-hydroxicorticosteroid, which led them to propose a correlation between that pattern and adrenal insufficiency. Thirty years and many studies later, the aspirations of the 1960s have not been fulfilled. There exists a large body of piecemeal studies, but no general synthesis was ever achieved.[115] Not that this would perturb the average practitioner. In an effort to teach me the importance of flexibility, one of my teachers, a graduate of the first course for Western medical physicians taught at the Beijing Academy of Chinese Medicine and a contemporary of Chen Ziyin, told me the following insider joke with reference to the work of the latter. "The integration of Chinese and Western medicine works for kidney *yang* depletion. But that does not mean it has to work for kidney *yin* depletion, too."

Bianzheng lunzhi in Post-Maoist China

Toward the end of the Cultural Revolution the drive toward reductionist uniformity and a fully integrated Chinese medicine and Western medicine was slowed by a reemergent plurality (see chapter 3). Throughout the next decades lively discussions took place in Chinese medicine journals concerning the nature of pattern differentiation and its relevance for the identity of Chinese medicine. We find more detailed dissections of symptoms, signs, and patterns; more examinations of Chinese medical dialectics; more debates concerning the role of disease differentiation in Chinese medicine; more comparisons between Chinese medicine diagnosis based on pattern differentiation and Western medicine diagnosis based on disease differentiation; and more attempts at their practical and theoretical integration. By the 1990s these discussions had become increasingly more sophisticated and had begun to challenge simple distinctions between symptoms, patterns, and disease and between Western medicine and Chinese medicine.[116] Overall, however, and in particular in the main textbooks, the syntheses produced in the 1950s and 1960s were reaffirmed and elaborated, establishing the orthodoxy cited in the introduction to this chapter.[117]

Bianzheng lunzhi is thus remembered today as the defining feature of Chinese medicine. Its complex history has been rewritten so that for patients and practitioners alike, comparisons between Chinese medicine and Western medicine now *naturally* evoke the opposition between pattern and disease differentiation. Nevertheless, lines of friction can still be made out within this apparent consensus betraying its historical construction. The most significant conflict is that between those who seek to develop patterns and their treatment into an increasingly objectifiable science and those who continue to emphasize practice and experience as the mainstay of Chinese medicine. This opposition is not merely one between tradition and modernity (both, of course, contemporarily defined) but also, simultaneously and cutting across the former, one between Maoist and post-Maoist visions of development.

As we saw above, dialectics and a particularly Maoist emphasis on practice that aligned well with classical concepts of Chinese medicine were the initial epistemic guiding lights for the construction of *bianzheng lunzhi*. In the area of reform and opening up, the Dengist emphasis on science and technology—mediated directly through official state policy and working indirectly through the increasing popular valorization of things modern and Western—led to a search for more up-to-date modes of legitimation that would hold firm under the inspection of foreign eyes. Systems theory, informatics, and cybernetics thus became the "three theories" (*san lun* 三论) to which more philosophically oriented physicians—encouraged by their superiors in the state administration—increasingly turned for inspiration and legitimation.[118]

In the area of clinical research, the same factors resulted in an accelerated importation of biomedical thinking and research methods into the Chinese medical field. Much effort has been devoted to transform patterns into objective entities by a younger generation of physicians less rooted in the medical classics but able to employ statistics and electron microscopes. The most telling example of this trend is the creation of animal models of specific patterns created to test treatments and prescriptions in a manner that closely resembles Western medical research. The first such model, a model of *yang* depletion (*yangxu* 阳虚), was developed in the early 1960s by Kuang Ankun 矿安昆. By 1984 more than fifteen such models had been officially recognized by the MOH. These models have since become essential aspects of Chinese medicine research even if their value remains disputed within the profession. Certain formulas that have demonstrated their clinical usefulness during hundreds of years of practice show no effect in treating animal models, while new formulas developed on the basis of animal models stubbornly refuse to work in clinical practice.[119]

One can furthermore observe a clear interest on behalf of Chinese medicine as a state institution to naturalize *bianzheng lunzhi* for reasons of bureaucratic control. This interest is realized on many levels. The determination of course curricula and the compilation of teaching materials are two examples that have already been discussed (in chapters 3 and 6). Two further examples are the production of encyclopedic collections of Chinese medicine patterns and efforts to standardize a diagnosis, of which I shall discuss here only the latter.[120]

In 1987 an MOH-sponsored study group published *Zhongyi bingming zhenduan guifan chugao* 中医病名诊断规范初稿 (*Standards for Disease Names and Diagnostic Categories in Chinese Medicine: A First Draft*).[121] In their fore-word the authors argue that the standardization of disease names is a difficult task but necessary for the systematization of Chinese medicine in general and for the standardization of diagnostics in particular. No further explanation is given, though the project is described as a continuation of Shi Jinmo's propos-als made in the 1930s. We saw previously that at the time such efforts had been motivated by the desire to reshape Chinese medicine (conceptually and pro-fessionally) in order to ensure its continued existence. In the 1980s this was no longer necessary. Chinese medicine survived not because it had become an independent profession but because it had been co-opted by the state. Stan-dardization thus takes on an entirely different character today. A hegemonic scientism that sees in standardization an important aspect of modernity in-formed Shi Jinmo and Qin Bowei as much as it does their modern heirs. What has changed is the agency desiring to implement such systematization and the mechanisms by which it is mediated. Unlike in the 1930s, standardiza-tion is no longer promoted by individual Chinese medicine physicians but imposed on them from above.

As of 1 January 1995, all institutions engaged in Chinese medicine teach-ing and research had to adopt national standards regarding the diagnosis and therapeutic efficacy of 406 specifically defined diseases and patterns. A year later, classifications and codes of diseases and patterns in Chinese medicine (*zhongyi bingzheng fenlei yu daima* 中医病证分类与代码) modeled on the *International Manual for the Classification of Diseases* were brought into effect. This was followed in 1997 by the publication of official standards re-garding clinical terminology in Chinese medical diagnosis and treatment (*zhongyi linchuang zhenliao shuyu* 中医临床诊疗术语), covering diseases, pat-terns, and treatment methods. The explicit purpose of these standards is to facilitate the administration of disease records and their statistical analysis by the state as well as to coordinate teaching and scientific research. It is also intended that this classification will be adapted as a model for future interna-tional standards in Chinese medicine and will promote economic as well as scholarly exchanges.[122]

These national standard codes on diseases and patterns employ Chinese medicine disease names rather than Western medicine disease names as their primary classifiers. Each disease is subdivided into several patterns accord-ing to standardized disease mechanisms. The disease "infertility" (*buyuzheng* 不育症), for instance, is divided into five subpatterns: (1) desertion and deple-tion of kidney *yang* (*shenyang kui xu* 肾阳亏虚), (2) desertion and depletion of kidney *yin* (*shenyin kui xu* 肾阴亏虚), (3) internal obstruction of phlegm damp (*tanshi nei zu* 痰湿内阻), (4) depressed and stagnant liver *qi* (*ganqi yuzhi*, 肝气郁滞), and (5) stasis [of blood] in the uterus (*yuzhi baogong* 瘀滞胞宫).[123] These disease mechanisms are essentially the same as those used in *Differentiating Symptoms*. On this level, therefore, standardization as an instrument of orchestrated medical pluralism continues not only in spirit but also in practice as the reductionism of previous periods.

One encounters both open and implied criticisms among the rank and file of Chinese medicine physicians regarding such simplification and the development of Chinese medicine over recent decades. Here, too, *bianzheng lunzhi* provides a useful point of orientation. The following comment, taken from Yue Meizhong's autobiography, summarizes what many of China's *laozhongyi* seem to think of the simplification—even if they themselves laid the foundations for the contemporary transformations. Yue writes regarding diagnosis: "Regarding symptoms one must analyze the [particular] synthesis between 'disease' and 'pattern' [they represent]. One must seek out the intrinsic character of [each specific] illness. One cannot [in this endeavor] limit oneself to a superficial [analysis in terms of] hot, cold, repletion, and depletion. . . . If one encounters a severe illness or a complicated pattern one must be even more particular. With meticulous care and great artistry one must [penetrate] in each case to the precise disease mechanism."[124] Similar sentiments can be found in the writings of Zhu Chenyu, Fang Yaozhong, and others, and I picked them up from talking with Lü Bingkui and other experienced physicians whom I questioned on the subject. *Bianzheng lunzhi*, as they kept impressing on me, is not about matching patterns with prescriptions but about a synthetic understanding of how concrete symptoms are linked to each other within particular disease mechanisms. This, as they also stressed, requires the continued engagement with both patients and classical texts, not merely the memorization of symptom patterns and matching formulas.[125]

Experience (*jingyan* 经验) has thus been revived as an important key word in contemporary Chinese medicine. Maintaining important semantic associations with Maoist ideas of praxis, the language of *jingyan* expresses resistance to what is perceived by many of its users as a dangerous narrowing of *bianzheng lunzhi* and of Chinese medicine itself.[126] Emphasizing experience (and thus a perception of *bianzheng lunzhi* as a process of individualized skill over and above its value as diagnostic technology) has motivated *laozhongyi* to publish their biographies, case histories, and clinical experiences and to organize supplements and even alternatives to state education. The downside (at least in the opinion of many younger doctors) of the accompanying valorization of *ming laozhongyi* has been an increase, once more, of the pursuit of personal status rather than shared goals, and hence of interprofessional rivalry and division.[127]

Lü Bingkui, who was in charge of producing the original *Outline*, was instrumental in the founding in 1984 of the Pure Chinese Medicine Correspondence University (Guangming zhongyi hanshou daxue 光明中医函授大学), a correspondence-based college which by 1992 had graduated more than twenty thousand students. The project was actively supported by leading bureaucrats and physicians, including Health Minister Cui Yueli 崔月犁 and the Beijing professors Liu Duzhou 刘渡舟, Zhao Shaoqin 赵绍琴, and Cao Xiping 曹希平. The establishment of Guangming University originally had a dual purpose. It was to increase the number of practicing Chinese medicine physicians, particularly in the countryside, which in Lü's opinion had fallen to dangerously low levels; and it was to promote higher standards in Chinese medicine. In 1993 the university widened its brief and began teaching regular students as an alternative to state education. The emblematic disenchantment of the octogenarian Lü with state Chinese medicine is perhaps nowhere expressed more unambiguously than in an address given to the first class of undergraduates at Guangming. Holding on to both the Maoist vision of Chinese medicine as a great treasure-house that needs developing and the modernist vision of Chinese medicine as a science, Lü explicates a view of development dangerously gone astray when he notes that "there are not many capable graduates of [regular] Chinese medicine colleges who have studied traditional Chinese medicine really well. [What they have studied] is a Westernized Chinese medicine, and Chinese medicine colleges are rapidly changing into Western medicine colleges. This is very dangerous. . . . [Admittedly], at present this university does not yet resemble a real university, but you can lead the way. The first step is to establish a proper university and then also a hospital. [If in this way] we manage to truly hand down Chinese medical science, its [future] development will be bright and great."[128]

I shall not attempt to examine the complex problem addressed by Lü Bingkui—considered, in any case, by most contemporary physicians I know as not much more than the residue of a bygone era—of whether or not Chinese medicine as a practice has undergone a notable decline over the last fifty years. Too many conceptual, methodological, and practical problems converge in any attempt to take sides in this debate. Besides the difficulties of defining what would count as "progress" and "decline," the sorting out of fact from rhetoric, and the careful analysis of how precisely issues of authority, status, and power (of the state versus physicians, individually and collectively; of older versus younger physicians) are intertwined with clinical practice and research, such investigations would also require complex studies examining the development of individual physicians over time.

Bianzheng lunzhi as a Process

Now, as in the past, Chinese medicine is continually changing and developing, even—or perhaps especially—at its very core. In chapter 2 I suggested that such change can be modeled as an emerging and disappearing of infrastructural alignments within fields of practice that are themselves transformed in the process. Simplified as it is, my narrative is still replete with examples of such transformations.

Supported initially by the state as an instrument in the course of creating a new national medicine that would be based on dialectical materialism and reflect China's unique contribution to world culture, *bianzheng lunzhi* was quickly appropriated by Chinese medicine physicians hoping for the independent survival of their tradition. However, even as the vision of *bianzheng lunzhi* as the pivot of a distinctive Chinese medicine has been established, some of the very people who contributed to the emergence of this orthodoxy are suddenly found amongst its fiercest critics. They see their tradition as threatened by young doctors who no longer know how to practice pattern diagnosis, by researchers trying to objectify what was previously never completely expressible in words, and by the state, which employs *bianzheng lunzhi* as a tool to effect the bureaucratic systematization necessary to integrate Chinese medicine into national and international health care networks.

Once a new infrastructure or element of practice has been synthesized and made available for integration into other practices, the agencies that controlled its original production invariably cede control over its further use. Naturally, infrastructures vary in their adaptability to new use contexts. While some accommodate easily, others offer enormous resistance and demand accommodations from other elements in participating syntheses. The final outcome of any such integration and the reshaping of infrastructural agencies it demands cannot be predicted but emerges itself as a consequence of the operation of the mangle of practice.

The creation of *bianzheng lunzhi* as the pivot of contemporary Chinese medicine repeatedly confirms this observation. Chinese medicine physicians used pattern differentiation to delimit their own practice from Western medicine while simultaneously allowing for its modernization. This restructuring required simultaneous realignments between various elements within Chinese medicine's field of practice, from the reshaping of doctrine to the reorganization of social networks. As a result of this process *bianzheng lunzhi* became a focus of centrality similar to the human foci analyzed in the preceding chapter. To be integrated into the syntheses of contemporary medicine—for new ideas to become accepted and old ones not to be forgotten—today requires translation into the discourse of *bianzheng lunzhi*. I will demonstrate this important point with a final case study that takes us back to the physician Zhang Xichun, whose case records I introduced earlier as examples of medical practice prior to the modern synthesis of *bianzheng lunzhi*.

CASE 7.1. *Re-presenting Zhang Xichun.* In 1999 the World of Learning Press (Xueyuan chubanshe 学苑出版社) published a volume of Zhang Xichun's case histories edited and annotated by Liu Yue 刘越, a contemporary Beijing *laozhongyi*. Liu is an expert on Zhang Xichun and has used his methods in clinical practice for many years. Liu Yue's own case histories and clinical essays were published by the same printing house seven months earlier. Of the sixteen essays in that volume, four also deal with Zhang Xichun.[129] As his engagement with Zhang Xichun distinctively shaped Liu Yue's own practice, it behooves him to popularize his teacher's works among younger physicians. In a context in which the influence of previous generations of physicians depends on their integration into contemporary networks of affiliation and synthesis, the continual affirmation of such links between past and present needs to be considered as at once socially and clinically effective.[130]

Examining Liu Yue's own cases, we find that they follow mainstream discourse on *bianzheng lunzhi* by dividing disorders into several patterns and discussing their treatment. In his theoretical discussions Liu Yue is less conventional, however. In one essay he suggests, for instance, extending the key rubrics (*gang* 纲) for the analysis of patterns from eight to ten by including ascending (*sheng* 升) and directing downward (*jiang* 降) of *qi*. Regulating ascending and directing downward was a key aspect of Zhang Xichun's own therapeutic approach (see cases 5.2 and 5.4), and Liu readily acknowledges his influence. In another essay Liu Yue opposes the orthodox opposition between Western medicine as treating diseases and Chinese medicine as treating patterns. Rather than opposing pattern and disease differentiation, he says, they should be seen as complementary methods of treating illness within a historically evolving Chinese medicine.[131]

Liu Yue's second book re-presents case notes dispersed throughout Zhang Xichun's voluminous writings as formal case histories. For this purpose Liu first systematically rearranges Zhang's own words under

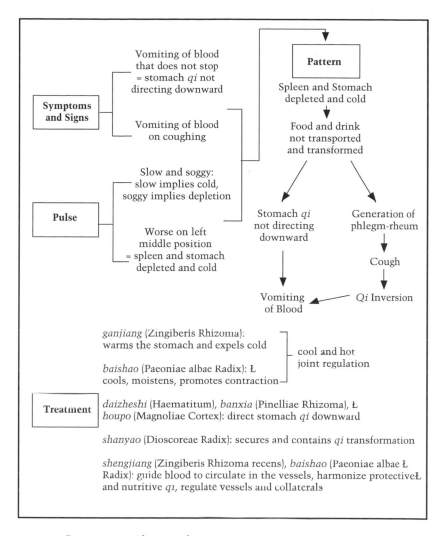

FIGURE 36. Representing Zhang Xichun

three distinct headings: (1) "Diagnosis of Symptoms and Signs" (*zheng zhen* 症诊), (2) "Treatment of Patterns" (*zheng zhi* 证治), and (3) "Prescription" (*fang* 方). In a fourth section entitled "Notes" (*an* 按) the content of each case history is then re-presented once more in the form of a diagram. These diagrams allow Liu to portray Zhang's clinical agency as a process that logically proceeds from the synthesis of symptoms, signs, and pulse (*zheng* 症, *mai* 脉) into one or more patterns (*zheng* 证) to the treatment of these patterns (*zhi* 治) by a given formula. These diagrams are apparently considered so self-explanatory that they are only occasionally supplemented by further written explanations of Zhang's reasoning.[132]

Quite obviously, Liu Yue has engaged profoundly with the work of Zhang Xichun. He also appears to be an independent thinker not afraid to go against mainstream opinion, as his attempts to innovate pattern differentiation demonstrate. In my opinion, Liu's editing of Zhang Xichun's case histories therefore makes sense only as an attempt to supply something essential that is perceived to be missing in the original. This missing piece is the logic of *bianzheng lunzhi*. Unless this logic is made obvious to modern readers of Zhang Xichun, he risks becoming a marginal presence in the contemporary field of medical practice, remembered and celebrated as the composer of several famous formulas but not widely read or deeply understood. By translating Zhang's medicine into the modern idiom Liu Yue therefore reconnects it to one of the core tools of contemporary practice. In this way he makes Zhang more easily accessible to a younger generation of physicians for whom treatment based on pattern differentiation simply *is* Chinese medicine. At the same time, however, Liu also extends backward in time the logic of *bianzheng lunzhi*, thereby affirming its pivotal function in contemporary practice. In that sense, the present is revealed not only as a whirlpool of simultaneous emerging and disappearing, but also as one in which past and future are continuously reconnected to each other in the syntheses that configure a field of practice.

Yet, *bianzheng lunzhi*—accepting for a moment the socially constructed and collectively remembered unity of the concept—is itself continually tested by such assimilation into ever new syntheses. On the level of doctrine, this manifests in ongoing critique and in attempts to modify, extend, or revise its position vis-à-vis other practices such as treatment based on disease differentiation or the analysis of types. On the level of clinical practice (as evidence presented in chapters 2 and 5 demonstrates) *bianzheng lunzhi* remains but one of a number of diagnostic and therapeutic strategies employed by physicians. Professor Zhu, for instance, also treats patients on the bases of biomedical disease classifications (case 5.3) and of novel hybrids that assimilate Western pathological anatomy into Chinese processual pathology (case 5.4). In these contexts clinical outcomes clearly matter more than the doctrinal integrity of Chinese medicine.

Even where *bianzheng lunzhi* forms the core of actual practice, physicians have different ideas about how it should be carried out. Professor Zhu's skills at pattern differentiation (case 5.2) were so unlike what his students had learned in college that some had considerable difficulty following his reasoning. Physicians also continually deviate from the ideal typical model of *bianzheng lunzhi* outlined at the beginning of this chapter. Rather than proceeding from pattern (*zheng* 证) to prescription (*fang* 方) via clearly formulated treatment strategies (*zhifa* 治法), they may match a patient's presentation to the indications of a formula and determine from its doctrinal indications the name of the pattern. This widely used method of prescribing is known as *bian-fang* 辨方 (differentiation via formulas), though when pressed physicians using it insist that they are also practicing *bianzheng* (differentiation via patterns).[133]

The current solution appears to be to assimilate all kinds of diagnostic practices into the model of pattern differentiation—even the differentiation of types that many scholar-physicians genuinely concerned about the integrity of their tradition think of as an abomination.[134] Not surprisingly, the creation of the hegemonic discourse in which Chinese medicine and *bianzheng lun-zhi* have come to stand for each other continually threatens to fall apart and needs to be reasserted.[135] After all, in Chinese medicine, as in biomedicine or nuclear physics, nothing is given or essential. *Bianzheng lunzhi* continually emerges and disappears as an object, discourse, and practice. In doing so it structures the field of Chinese medical practice even as it is itself continually reconstructed.

8. CREATING KNOWLEDGE
The Origins of Plurality

The emergence of *bianzheng lunzhi* described in chapter 7 took place over a period of several decades and involved a large number of participating agents. In the present chapter I shift my focus toward a synthetic process on a much smaller scale: the development of a novel nosology and acumoxa treatment for cerebrovascular accident–induced speech impediments (*zhongfeng hou yanyu zhang'ai* 中风后言语障碍). This examination serves a threefold purpose. First, it explores the process of synthesis in contemporary Chinese medicine from yet another angle and thereby deepens our understanding of it. Second, the scaling down of the space and time dimensions of this case study (compared with those of previous chapters) allows me to observe with greater acuity the interaction between different infrastructures. Third, the need of the main actor in my study, a young acupuncturist, to enroll various machines and tests into his research helps to illustrate the input of nonhuman agency into synthetic processes in Chinese medicine.

The case study discussed here is based on research undertaken between 1993 and 1996 by Dr. Lin, who at the time was a doctoral candidate at the Beijing University of Chinese Medicine. In describing and analyzing Dr. Lin's research I have drawn on three types of source material: his published Ph.D. dissertation, fieldwork observations carried out from February to December 1994 and during March and April 1996, and an ongoing dialogue with Dr. Lin since 1994. Dr. Lin fully collaborated with me during all stages of my research, from the initial data collection through several revisions of my manuscript. I do not claim, however, to represent Dr. Lin's own understanding of what he did. While my constructionist analysis has made him see his research from a very different perspective—a perspective he finds interesting and valuable— he still favors a naturalistic account. He asserts that the redefinition of disease categories he has accomplished equates to a more objective description of disease process in Chinese medicine and that his treatment protocols are therefore definitively more advanced than previous ones. Nor do I claim that my study is representative of innovation in contemporary Chinese medicine. Based on my reading of modern Chinese sources, my contact with other researchers, and the reception of Dr. Lin's published papers I do, however, believe that it is not marginal either.

It is beyond the scope of this ethnography to detail all the manifold and complicated processes of synthesis that resulted in Dr. Lin's final dissertation. There were simply too many potential infrastructures involved (ranging from unconscious desires to the political background of research financing) and no way to test the input of each. In addition, the very act of translating multiple simultaneously occurring events into linear narrative turns a knot of many strands (none of which necessarily holds the entire knot together) into a thread with a definite beginning and end. Nevertheless, some generalizable understanding of synthesis can be derived even from the analysis of more narrowly defined aspects of the overall process.

Through focusing on the transactions through which Dr. Lin's dissertation emerged—paying particular attention to the interaction between the various infrastructures he had to recruit in the process—I explore three distinct aspects of his research: how Dr. Lin came to formulate his precise research topic, how he succeeded in developing a novel nosology, and, finally, how he translated this innovation into therapy. My goal is not to evaluate whether or not Dr. Lin did good or bad science or good or bad Chinese medicine. I am interested only in documenting synthesis as a process of interaction between various agencies in order to observe how agencies affect each other and how such interactions emerge within (but also reshape) a particular field of practice. I shall begin by placing Dr. Lin's study into its sociocultural and historical context.

Research on Cerebrovascular Accidents in Acumoxa Therapy

In contemporary China, cerebrovascular accidents (CVA) and CVA-related disorders constitute one of the most important groups of disorders treated by acumoxa therapy (zhenjiu 针灸). A combination of general and specific factors contribute to the relative predominance of these disorders in acumoxa departments. First, CVAs and CVA-related disorders constitute one of the largest categories of morbidity in contemporary China. Second, biomedical treatment of these disorders remains palliative. Third, given the division of contemporary Chinese medicine into distinct specialities—reproduced in the course of training and reinforced by the organization of hospitals and outpatient clinics—acumoxa therapists have had to carve out for themselves a unique niche in the health care marketplace. This niche is constituted by disorders that are difficult to treat by both Western medicine and Chinese pharmacotherapy and that match acumoxa's particular affinity to channels and collaterals (*jingluo* 经络).[1] Disorders of the skeletomuscular and nervous systems such as CVAs and CVA-related disorders, Bell's palsy, and pain not arising from internal organ disorders fit this match.

As in other Chinese medical specialities, doctrinal understanding and treatment of CVA-induced speech impediments is heterogeneous and contested. At present, most physicians equate the biomedically defined disease category CVA with the classical Chinese category *zhongfeng* 中风, or "wind stroke." The situation is complicated, however, by the existence of two different orthodox doctrines regarding the origin of wind stroke disorders. The first and historically older of these doctrines thinks of wind stroke as contraction from the outside (*waigan* 外感) of wind pathogen (*fengxie* 风邪), which lodges in the body's channels and collaterals (*jingluo*) and visceral systems of function (*zangfu* 脏腑). Physicians in the Jin-Yuan period revised this doctrine by arguing for the existence of a second type of wind stroke disorder in which pathogenic wind was generated internally (*neisheng* 内生). Symptomatically, this disorder resembles wind stroke and is therefore commonly known as *leizhongfeng* 类中风, or "windlike stroke." Its very different etiology necessitates, however, an entirely different treatment approach. While treatment of wind stroke is primarily aimed at dispelling wind (*qufeng* 驱风) and concomitant obstructions from the channels and collaterals, treatment of windlike stroke is aimed primarily at extinguishing internal wind (*xifeng* 熄风). Most physicians nowadays believe that CVAs correspond to windlike stroke disorders, though at least one prominent acupuncturist with whom I studied argued that more attention should be paid to wind stroke.

The influence of biomedicine has provided both new problems and new mechanisms for the resolution of old debates. Neither of the two Chinese disease categories pays much attention to brain or blood circulation, concentrating instead on the obstruction of channels and collaterals by wind (*feng* 风), phlegm (*tan* 痰), and cold (*han* 寒). How precisely this should be related to Western medicine's location of CVA pathology in the brain and nervous system has been an issue ever since these ideas first became known in Chinese medical circles. Problems arise partly from the fact that Chinese medicine classifies the brain (*nao* 脑) as an extraordinary visceral system (*qiheng zhi fu* 奇恒之腑) attached to the kidneys (*shen* 肾) and attributes the function of consciousness to the heart (*xin* 心). Not only does this rather secondary function of the brain not accord with its importance in Western physiology, it is also difficult to establish one-to-one correspondences between the two systems.

While the dispute remains unresolved, clinicians have been integrating bio-medical theories of CVAs into Chinese medical treatment approaches for at least a century.[2]

Contemporary Chinese medical research concerning CVAs and their sequelae thus address three interrelated issues: (1) the resolution of histori-cal debates and the promotion of standardization, (2) the objective documen-tation of pathologies and treatment mechanisms, and (3) the objective docu-mentation of treatment effects. As far as I can make out, for researchers such as Dr. Li, use of the term "objective" (keguande 客观的) in this context refers to the documentation of data by means of nonhuman inscription devices.[3] In official discourse the development (fazhan 发展) of Chinese medicine is usually given as the natural purpose of such documenting. In private conver-sations with physicians such as Dr. Lin, I perceived the translation of Chinese medicine into an idiom intelligible to a biomedical audience as an equally important goal. Dr. Lin and many of his colleagues repeatedly and explic-itly pointed out to me that the main target audience of Chinese medicine research is not the Chinese medicine community itself but biomedical physi-cians and a national and international public no longer or not yet convinced of the value of Chinese medicine. It is to satisfy the perceived needs of this audi-ence that the state (which today has important political and economic inter-ests at stake in the promotion of Chinese medicine) and the Chinese medical elite demand that researchers effect translations that express through num-bers, statistics, graphs, ultrasound, and CT scans what physicians communi-cated to each other in the past by means of cryptic case histories, allusions to canonical texts, pulse descriptions, and sketches of tongue coatings.[4]

It was against this background that Dr. Lin carried out his study. Its aims were to sort out the heterogeneous nosology of CVA-related speech impedi-ments in Chinese medicine, to offer treatment protocols reflecting this nosol-ogy, and to document the efficacy of these treatment protocols in terms of both clinical outcomes and physiological effects. As we shall see, Dr. Lin solved all three problems by importing into Chinese medicine biomedical theories regarding the production of speech and its pathology.

Defining a Research Topic

Dr. Lin enrolled as a Ph.D. student at Beijing University of Chinese Medicine in the 1993–94 academic year. It took him about a year to define precisely his research topic and program. A complex process led to this decision.

Dr. Lin comes from a small town in northeastern China. He completed his undergraduate training and a subsequent master's degree in acumoxa at a provincial college of Chinese medicine. He is sincerely interested in his chosen career and, unlike many other physicians of his generation, sees it as an exciting profession rather than a job he ended up doing for one reason or another. Further study as a doctoral student—a process that as we saw in chapter 6 affords contact with master practitioners—constituted a natural avenue through which he could develop his knowledge. Dr. Lin also considered that a doctoral degree would provide him with a strategic advantage in an increasingly competitive society. Dr. Lin is married and has a daughter. Like almost everyone else around him, he wants his family to live in a metropolitan area. Applying for a place at Beijing University of Chinese Medicine to study for a doctorate was the first step for him and his family to obtain a residence permit for Beijing. It thus afforded him with an opportunity to realize these diverse aspirations, even if it meant living apart from his wife and young daughter for the three years of his studies.[5]

During his early training Dr. Lin had gained considerable experience in the treatment of CVA-related disorders. There also were many such patients at the Beijing hospital where he worked during his doctoral studies. As clinical research depends on both the availability of a particular patient population and physicians with expertise in a given field, CVA-related disorders thus naturally suggested themselves to Dr. Lin as a potential field of research. When applying for a place at Beijing University of Chinese Medicine—a process that consists of a written test and a formal interview with the prospective supervisor—he therefore selected a supervisor whose expertise broadly matched his own. This supervisor was Professor Liao. Already in his seventies, Professor Liao is one of Beijing's most respected acupuncturists. He is an experienced physician of considerable influence whose clinical skill in the treatment of CVA-related disorders is widely acknowledged by both his peers and his large clientele.

As I pointed out in chapter 6, the status of doctoral supervisor (boshi daoshi 博士导师) at universities of Chinese medicine is a mark of distinction to those so designated. Due to their often advanced age, however, many doctoral supervisors do not possess the necessary knowledge in areas such as research methodology or statistics required to guide their students through a doctoral degree in a modern educational system. Doctoral candidates are therefore assigned an assistant supervisor (fudaoshi 副导师) who possesses this knowledge. For Dr. Lin this was Professor Ding, a man in his fifties and the chief physician in his hospital's acupuncture department. Unlike Professor Liao, Professor Ding is not a renowned clinician. He is himself actively involved in acupuncture research, however, and familiar with modern research methodologies. Professor Liao's research at the time involved exploring the functions of the hand lesser *yin* heart vessel (*shou shaoyin xin jing* 手少阴心经) in acumoxa.

Professor Liao's research, like almost all other research presently carried out at Chinese medicine universities and colleges, was funded by the Chinese government and administered by the State Administration of Chinese Medicine and Pharmacology (Guojia zhongyiyao guanliju 国家中医药管理局). Within the general remit of each five-year plan the government, in consultation with various committees such as the People's Consultative Conference and the Academy of Chinese Medicine, determines overall research priorities. Individual physicians compete for a share of funds allocated to specific research goals and can filter these grants into smaller projects at the local level. Presently, the state attaches most importance to applied and clinical research. Research projects in these areas are consequently easier to fund than theoretical studies. Professor Ding's research was funded in this way and constituted a very small part of a nationwide research project into channels and collaterals.[6]

Via the same mechanisms the state defines outline criteria for Ph.D. research and provides basic funding for it. Outline criteria for Ph.D. research specify the standards that doctoral research must meet to be passed by a graduation committee, which consists of both internal and external examiners. In Dr. Lin's case the committee comprised ten academics and physicians: three physicians from the Chinese medicine hospital at which Dr. Lin carried out his research, three academics from Beijing University of Chinese Medicine as the institution awarding the degree, and four experts, including biomedical physicians, from other hospitals and universities in Beijing. Funding consists of a small budget (RMB 1000–1500) allocated to each research student. This amount is insufficient, however, to carry out the kind of research students, supervisors, and universities aspire to; that is, research comparable to that carried out at Western medicine universities. One way to obtain access to additional funds is to attach one's own studies to a larger research program.

In deciding on his research topic and program during the first year of his doctoral degree, Dr. Lin—according to his own testimony—was influenced by a number of factors. First, he made an assessment of his own skills, knowledge, and expertise within the field of acumoxa therapy. Although he perceived (and still perceives) of these as continually evolving, basing his research within a field of practice with which he was already intimately familiar seemed obviously advantageous.

Second, Dr. Lin had to take into account the skills and expertise of his supervisor, Professor Liao, who had to approve of the chosen topic and research plan. For academic reasons, it was unlikely that Professor Liao would grant permission for a research topic outside his own area of expertise. Morally, too, Dr. Lin felt obliged to show due respect to his supervisor's sense of honor (*gei ta mianzi* 给他面子) by locating his own research in relation to Professor Liao's practice. Not doing so, furthermore, would considerably impede Dr. Lin's chances of learning from Professor Liao. As we saw in case 2.1 and throughout chapter 6, such learning is mediated by forms of affiliation in which students honor their teachers in return for access to personal knowledge. Finally, as we also saw in chapter 6, teacher-student relationships can have considerable implications for the future career development of a physician.

Third, Dr. Lin did not see his doctoral research as an isolated event but placed it within the wider context of his career development. In working out his research program Dr. Lin decided that his research should constitute a study that was at the leading edge of Chinese medical research in terms of both methodology and content. Ideally, this would involve clinical experimentation utilizing the most advanced technology and a clinical study that comprised a control group. His research should also lead to results that could easily be translated into publications; even better if those publications shaped the development of Chinese medicine. This implied devising a research program that reflected official research priorities in terms of both form and content and that produced genuinely new and clinically useful knowledge. Finally, Dr. Lin wanted to locate his research in a field in which biomedicine was not very effective. If he could demonstrate the efficacy of acumoxa therapy in such an area, it would be advantageous for Chinese medicine at large and also might facilitate his own career. In his more ambitious moments, Dr. Lin dreamed of designing and carrying out a study that would attract interest from prestigious national or even foreign institutions with the prospect of future work in such settings.

For all these reasons Dr. Lin decided on the acumoxa treatment of CVA-induced speech impediments as his basic field of interest. This combined his own background knowledge with an area of clinical specialization in which Professor Liao is widely respected. Yet, inasmuch as Professor Liao's reputation rests on the treatment of all kinds of CVA-related disorders it allowed Dr. Lin enough space to establish his own position. In Dr. Lin's opinion specializing in the acumoxa treatment of CVA-induced speech impediments also fulfilled two of his other criteria. There existed no systematic approach to its treatment in Chinese medicine, whereas Western medicine offered much theory to be exploited but not, on the whole, much in terms of therapy. CVA-induced speech impediments, furthermore, constituted a common problem among patients in the acupuncture department of Dr. Lin's hospital, suggesting to him that it would not be difficult to enroll sufficient numbers of them in his study. Finally, as speech in Chinese medicine functionally relates to the heart, and the hand lesser *yin* heart vessel (*shou shaoyin xin jing*) connects with the tongue, examining CVA-induced speech impediments also tied in with the research interests of his other assistant supervisor, Professor Ding. Not only would Dr. Lin thus succeed in acknowledging both his supervisors, he also kept open the possibility of attaining funds for his own project via Professor Ding.

Designing and Carrying out the Research Project

Once Dr. Lin had chosen the general field in which to locate his study, his next goal consisted in designing a project that promised to realize his ambitions. Besides accommodating to the various demands exerted by the infrastructures outlined above, that also implied taking into account factors such as time, access to research equipment, anticipating the demands of the various audiences to which his study addressed itself, and enrolling patients as subjects.

For reasons outlined above, Dr. Lin envisioned his research project as centering on a clinical study that would examine the efficacy of a specific treatment protocol. This would be supported by clinical experiments, which would objectify clinical efficacy by exposing its physiological mechanisms. Even at the outset of his research there was no doubt at all in Dr. Lin's mind that his treatment protocol (which at this point did not yet exist) would show statistically significant effects. Did not his own work in the clinic and that of his teachers and peers demonstrate daily that acumoxa can help patients with CVA-related disorders? Dr. Lin was also convinced, however, that efficacy can be continuously improved upon and that research is an effective way to design ever-better treatment protocols.

At this early stage, it was also clear that in order to achieve his goals, Dr. Lin would have to enroll into his study a number of instruments, or "inscription devices," not indigenous to Chinese medicine. The first of these were computed tomography (CT) and magnetic resonance imaging (MRI) scanners, which were necessary in order to establish objectively that the patients recruited for the clinical part of Dr. Lin's study had suffered a CVA. As a consequence, Dr. Lin had to redefine the semantic content of the Chinese nosological category wind stroke. In classical Chinese medicine the terms *zhongfeng* (wind stroke) and *leizhongfeng* (windlike stroke) include what biomedicine would label acute infectious diseases and certain types of paralysis as well as CVAS. Dr. Lin (following widely accepted contemporary practice) equated both types of wind stroke, however, with "cerebral infarction" (*nao gengsai* 脑梗塞) or "cerebral hemorrhage" (*naochuxue* 脑出血). Only patients who had suffered either of these (as demonstrated by CT or MRI) were therefore subsequently admitted as subjects.[7]

A second type of device needed was one that would allow Dr. Lin to measure and statistically evaluate therapeutic outcomes in the treatment of CVA-induced speech disorders. The one tool Dr. Lin was able to find for this purpose was a test known as the Aphasia Battery of Chinese, or ABC (Hanyu shiyuzheng jianchafa 旱语失语证检查法). This diagnostic test measures (in numerical terms) various aspects of neurological functioning involved in speech such as speaking, memorizing, and comprehending. It was developed in 1993 by Professor Gao Surong 高素荣 of Beijing Medical University (Beijing yike daxue 北京医科大学) on the basis of earlier Chinese-language tests that had in turn been modeled on tests developed in the United States.[8]

The choice of this inscription device had important implications for the subsequent development of Dr. Lin's research. If he wanted to use the test, he had to integrate into his study the biomedical distinction between *dysphasia* (dysfunction of speech due to a lesion of the language areas of the brain) and *dysarthria* (dysfunction of speech due to damage to the motor control systems for the muscles responsible for speech production) on which the ABC is based.[9] While this had always been an option—simply because Dr. Lin knew of this distinction while Chinese medicine prior to the publication of his thesis did not—enrollment of the test made it a necessity.

Having decided on use of the ABC as a measuring device, Dr. Lin went to the Beijing Medical University in order to learn how to administer the test. There he met Professor Gao, the inventor of the ABC. Professor Gao was interested to learn of Dr. Lin's research, partly because he and his colleagues were frustrated by the fact that they had little to offer to their patients in terms of therapy. Professor Gao subsequently became a major influence on Dr. Lin's research.

Including the ABC in the study had yet another important consequence. In order to finish his study within the two years that he had still available at the time, Dr. Lin decided to focus on the treatment of dysphasia patients only and to drop all patients suffering from dysarthria from his study. This meant that he would have to evaluate just one treatment protocol rather than two. The choice in favor of dysphasia was influenced partly by the fact that, as outlined above, the function of speech in Chinese medicine can be related to the heart. As we know, Dr. Lin's assistant supervisor was engaged in research on the hand lesser *yin* heart vessel and Dr. Lin was keen to keep alive the connection between his own research and that of Professor Ding.

Next Dr. Lin needed to devise a treatment protocol. Given that the dysphasia/dysarthria distinction is not indigenous to Chinese medicine, there existed no readily available protocols either in the literature or in the clinical repertoire of his teachers. In order to fulfill what Dr. Lin perceived of as moral obligations of filiality to his teachers and in order to locate his own research firmly within the Chinese medical tradition, his treatment protocol had to be visibly related to these sources. Yet, it simultaneously should also be both effective and new. Dr. Lin met these criteria by selecting seven acupoints as his basic protocol: *shenting* 神庭 (GV-24, spirit court), *benshen* 本神 (GB-13, root spirit), *sishencong* 四神聪 (alert spirit quartet, a nonchannel point), *tongli* 通里 (HT-5, connecting *li*), *xinshu* 心俞 (BL-15, heart transport), *shendao* 神道 (GV-11, spirit path), and *shesanzhen* 舌三针 (tongue three needles, a nonchannel point).

The first three of these points (*shenting*, GV-24; *benshen*, GB-13; and *sishencong*) were points frequently used by Professor Liao in the treatment of CVAS. Using his supervisor's treatment protocols in his own practice, Dr. Lin had rejected some other points as not being specifically effective in the treatment of aphasia. Out of those points that appeared to have a definite effect he chose the above three because they were all located on the skull and thereby resonated with the biomedical location of CVA lesions in the brain.

A second group of the acupoints Dr. Lin chose (*tongli* [HT-5], *xinshu* [BL-15], and *shendao* [GV-11]) is functionally related to the heart and thereby to speech. From the perspective of channels and collaterals, *tongli* (HT-5) is the network point (*luoxue* 洛穴) of the hand lesser *yin* heart vessel (*shou shaoyin xin jing*). In acumoxa theory this point is said to open and regulate the associated vessel, which as we know connects with both the tongue and Professor Ding's research. The point is furthermore cited in the contemporary acumoxa literature as the most frequently used point to treat inability to speak. *Xinshu* 心俞 (BL-15) and *shendao* 神道 (GV-11) were cited as an effective combination in the treatment of *zhongfeng buyu* 中风不语 ("wind stroke with inability to speak") by the Tang dynasty physician Sun Simiao 孙思邈, who, as we shall see shortly, provided the major anchor for Dr. Lin's protocol in the classical literature.

The acupoint *shesanzhen* (tongue three needles), finally, was included following an encounter with a practitioner of Manchu medicine to whom Dr. Lin had been directed by one of his patients. The practitioner was renowned locally for the treatment of CVA-induced speech disorders, which he treated by a form of bloody needling of the tongue body. Dr. Lin was impressed by the results but reckoned that few patients in his clinic would consent to this form of needling. A search of the Chinese medical archive revealed, however, that points on or near the tongue were sometimes used to treat the sequelae of CVAs. Dr. Lin therefore decided to include *shesanzhen*, a point at the root of the tongue, in his protocol. In order to mirror the bloody needling Dr. Lin decided that this point should be needled quite deeply.

Like the choice of his topic and research program, Dr. Lin's basic treatment protocol thus reveals itself as a complex synthesis. Ostensibly it had been assembled by Dr. Lin's agency—that is, his personal experience, desires, and idiosyncratic reasoning. Accepting this would ignore, however, the various kinds of agency exerted on Dr. Lin by the infrastructures he sought to enroll into his study. These infrastructures were extremely heterogeneous, extending from his supervisor's expectations to university regulations, from the rules governing statistics and other aspects of research methodology to the pathophysiology implicit in the ABC, from patient expectations to the physiological response of their bodies, from modern transformation of classical acumoxa to Manchu medicine. Most of these agencies operated indirectly—that is, they manifested within Dr. Lin as emotive feelings of moral obligation, rational cost-benefit calculations, experientially based efficacy evaluations, and the anticipation of patient reaction. This does not mean, however, that agency was located only in Dr. Lin and not also within patients, teachers, test batteries, and machines. Rather, the mental, emotional, and physical reactions that manifested as Dr. Lin's actions were themselves syntheses of enormous complexity. They were directed, undoubtedly, by his own desires but equally resulted from accommodations to the agency of all these other infrastructures. This is confirmed by examining how Dr. Lin succeeded in translating the biomedical distinction between dysphasia and dysathria into Chinese medicine.

Developing a New Nosology

The translation of the biomedical distinction between dysphasia and dysathria into Chinese medicine is accomplished in the first part of Dr. Lin's dissertation, which is entitled "Theoretical Research" (*lilun yanjiu* 理论研究) and has two main objectives: to standardize the Chinese medicine classification of stroke-induced speech impediments and to relate these to classical and modern discussions of their treatment by acumoxa therapy. According to Dr. Lin the contemporary literature on CVA-related speech impediments is disabled by a heterogeneous confusion of disease classifications. Dr. Lin argues that this heterogeneity makes it difficult to evaluate and compare different studies. He therefore proposes a new nosology at which he arrives via a number of intermediate steps.

The first of these consists in a meticulous etymological and semantic analysis of technical terms. Table 4 lists the different terms for CVA-related speech impediments Dr. Lin found in a comprehensive literature search through the archive of Chinese medicine. With the exception of *zhongfeng shiyu* (widely employed in contemporary writing and derived from *shiyuzheng* 失语证, the modern Chinese equivalent of the biomedical term "aphasia") all of these are classical terms. Dr. Lin rejects the terms *yin* 喑 or 瘖 (loss of voice) and *yin fei* 瘖痱 (loss of speech and use of limbs) because they are no longer in common usage and would be difficult to popularize again. Furthermore, as the name implies, *yin fei* encompasses pathologies that go beyond pure loss of speech. He discards *fengyi* 风懿 or 风癔 (wind choke) because in Chinese medical usage the term refers only to serious cases of stroke-induced speech disorders and because its constituent radicals do not readily convey the intended meaning of the term. The expression *sheqiang buneng yan* 舌强不能言 is unsuitable because it encompasses only dysarthric and not dysphasic pathologies. *Zhongfeng shiyin* 中风失喑 (lit. "wind stroke with loss of voice") is a double negation and therefore logically unsound. The modern *zhongfeng shiyu* 中风失语 (wind stroke with loss of speech), finally, is rejected as a problematic borrowing from Western medicine. Dr. Lin therefore proposes to adopt the term *zhongfeng buyu* 中风不语 (wind stroke with inability to speak) as the Chinese medicine disease name for CVA-related speech impediments because it concisely expresses etiology (*zhongfeng*) and pathology (*buyu*); is easy to read, write, and understand; and is manifestly different from the biomedical *shiyuzheng* (aphasia).

It may appear that the disease category *zhongfeng buyu*—classical but newly synthesized and therefore modern—has been constituted by Dr. Lin's hermeneutic agency. This would unduly discount, however, the role played by other infrastructures—none of them controlled by Dr. Lin—in this synthetic production, from the semantic range of classical medical terms to their material reality as written ideograms, from the anticipated effort expected of prospective users to the logical relations between signifier and signified, from the desire to be modern that Dr. Lin shares with many Chinese to the desire to establish an identity for Chinese medicine that distinguishes it from Western

TABLE 4. Classical and Modern Terms for CVA-Related Speech Impediments

Term	Source
yin 喑 or 瘖 Loss of voice	*Suwen* 23 (1992: 340), and *Lingshu* 42 (1989: 307).
yin fei 瘖痱 Loss of speech and use of limbs	*Suwen* 49 (1992: 623) has *yin fei* 瘖非.
sheqiang buneng yan 舌强不能言 Stiff tongue so that one cannot speak	*Zhubing yuan hou lun* 诸病源候论 (*On the Origins and Symptoms of Disorders*) 1.4 (1992: 8) has "*feng she qiang bu de yu*" 风舌强不得语.
fengyi 风懿 or 风癔 Wind choke	*Zhubing yuan hou lun* 1.2 (1992: 6) has *fengyi* 风癔. *Qianjin yaofang* 千金要方 (*Important Formulas Worth a Thousand*) 8.6 (1993: 133) has *fengyi* 风懿.
zhongfeng shiyin 中风失喑 Wind stroke with loss of voice	*Zhubing yuan hou lun* 1.5 (1992: 8) has *feng shiyin* 风失喑. *Qianjin yaofang* 8.6 (1993: 134) has both *zhongfeng shiyin* 中风失喑 and *zhongfeng shiyin* 中风失瘖.
zhongfeng buyu 中风不语 Wind stroke with inability to speak	This term stems from *Yixue xinwu* 医学心悟 (*The Awakening of the Mind in Medical Studies*) 1.27 (1990 [1732]: 58) by Cheng Guopeng 程国彭 (1662–1735), which has a chapter entitled *Zhongfeng buyu bian* 中风不语辨 (Differentiating wind stroke with inability to speak).
zhongfeng shiyu 中风失语 Wind stroke with loss of speech	Widely employed in contemporary writing and derived from *shiyuzheng* 失语证, the modern Chinese equivalent of the biomedical term "aphasia."

medicine that he shares only with his colleagues. An antithetical proposition, that Dr. Lin's terminology is not of his own making but was forced on him by some preexisting system or episteme, seems to me equally implausible because there exists no apparent linguistic, aesthetic, or practical necessity that enforces this particular innovation. In fact, Dr. Lin's suggestions oppose what appears to be a very practicable pluralism. The apparent popularity of the neologism *zhongfeng shiyu* is proof, furthermore, that Dr. Lin's *zhongfeng buyu* is not the only possible manner in which classical nosologies might be modernized.[10]

I propose, therefore, that Dr. Lin's synthesis makes sense only within the particular environment of orchestrated pluralism in which it emerged. In this environment the autonomy of Chinese medicine is newly asserted (*zhongfeng buyu* rather than *zhongfeng shiyu*), while Chinese medicine as a practice is simultaneously opened up to influence from agencies located outside the Chinese medical community (the Chinese state, Western medicine physicians, the international scientific community). It is important to note, however, that these outside factors do not control Dr. Lin's synthesis but merely make available additional infrastructures that demand inclusion in the transforming field of contemporary Chinese medicine.

My analysis receives further confirmation from the subsequent unfolding of Dr. Lin's argument. Having proposed a general term by which to relabel cva-related speech impediments, Dr. Lin suggests that two distinct symptom patterns belonging to the disease category *zhongfeng buyu* can be distinguished by a detailed exegesis of classical texts. The first describes a dysfunction of voice production, which manifests in symptoms such as difficult pronunciation, unclear sounds, and disorders of speech tempo and rhythm. It is accompanied by signs such as paralysis of the tongue, contraction of the root of the tongue, and wry mouth. The second pattern is marked by a functional disordering of the expressive or analytic aspects of linguistic communication. It manifests in symptoms such as difficulties of expression, mistakes in word use, and inability to respond correctly to questions.

Dr. Lin, therefore, suggests using the two terms *sheyin* 舌瘖 (lit. "tongue loss of voice") and *yuse* 语涩 (difficult speech), taken from Sun Simiao, to differentiate between these two patterns. He claims that both terms not only communicate appropriately the symptomatic and pathological characteristics between the two patterns but also match the biomedical distinction between dysarthria and aphasia. The term *sheyin* conveys the meaning of dysarthria as a disorder of speech production by referring to the tongue (*she*) as the locus of the disorder and to loss of voice (*yin*) as its predominant symptom. The term *yuse* corresponds to aphasia because its first component, *yu*, refers to language rather than sound, while the second component, *se*, expresses the precise quality of its dysfunction. Dr. Lin's final nosological system is summarized in figure 37.

Dr. Lin has to admit that although he can produce evidence that classical authors distinguished symptomatologically between the two patterns he labels *sheyin* and *yuse,* there is no evidence that they employed them practically, either as a matrix for diagnosis or as a basis for therapy.[11] This, indeed, is his innovation. The final step in his theoretical discussion, therefore, consists in defining treatment principles that match his new nosological system. These principles are summarized in table 5.

It is important to point out that while the emergence of Dr. Lin's treatment protocol and nosological system are discussed as separate events here, they evolved concomitantly in real-time practice. This observation is important not merely to emphasize the complexity of the synthesis I am describing but also to stress the input of actual acumoxa practice and the many concepts that govern it into this process. That social factors contributed to the synthesis of both Dr. Lin's treatment protocol and his nosological system does not imply that bodily reactions and their capture by acumoxa therapy fall by the wayside.

The centrality of the heart visceral system in Dr. Lin's understanding of *yuse* pathology, for instance, is based entirely on classical medical doctrine and is not determined by the biomedical concepts that underpin his differentiation. These latter concepts do, however, force him to clearly separate the *yuse* pattern from that of *sheyin,* both conceptually and practically. This

TABLE 5. Dr. Lin's Differential Diagnosis and Acumoxa
Treatment of *zhongfeng buyu*

sheyin 舌瘖	The disease is located in the kidneys (*shen* 肾) and spleen (*pi* 脾), in acute cases also in the liver (*gan* 肝). The pathology affects, apart from the channels associated with kidneys and spleen, the *yang* channels of the hand, the governing vessel (*dumai* 督脉), and the conception vessel (*renmai* 仁脉). The treatment method consists of expelling stasis, transforming phlegm and freeing the collaterals (*quyu huatan tongluo* 祛瘀化痰通络), selecting points from these channels, and in acute cases also local points on the head and liver channel points.
yuse 语涩	The disease is located in the heart (*xin* 心), in acute cases also in the liver (*gan* 肝). The treatment method consists of clearing the heart; awakening the spirit and opening the portals (*qingxin xingshen kaiqiao* 清心醒神开窍); selecting holistically points relating to the head, tongue, and heart; and in acute cases also *jing*[a] 井 and liver channel points.

[a] *Jing* or "well" is a term used to designate a group of points in acumoxa therapy, where the flow of *qi* in the channels is thought to originate. They are often used in the treatment of CVAS.

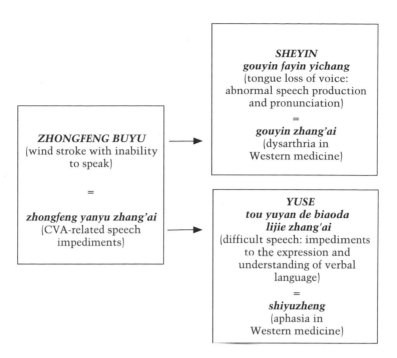

FIGURE 37. Dr. Lin's nosology of *zhongfeng buyu*

leads to the definitive separation between a heart pathology in the *yuse* pattern and a kidney-spleen pathology in the *sheyin* pattern,[12] a differentiation absent, for instance, in the treatment protocols of his supervisor Professor Liao and Sun Simiao. Hence, when designing his treatment protocol, Dr. Lin could not simply import Professor Liao's treatment strategies. Rather, he had to select those acupoints that both fitted into his theoretical model and appeared to be effective in clinical practice. The acupoint *yamen* (GV-16, Mute's Gate; also known as *yinmen* 瘖门, Loss-of-Voice Gate), which Professor Liao uses in all cases of CVA-related speech disorders, for instance, was excluded from Dr. Lin's protocol. According to Dr. Lin he found through repeated usage in practice that the point was of very little use in the treatment of the *yuse* pattern, though it did appear to be beneficial in the treatment of the *sheyin* pattern. The experience confirmed that his new differentiation constituted a definite development of Chinese medicine and empowered him to drop the point from his treatment protocol.

If Dr. Lin had merely wished to demonstrate his modernity or to systematize Chinese medicine, he could have embraced the popular *zhongfeng shiyu* or simply adopted the biomedical disease categories dysarthria (*gouyin zhang'ai* 构音障碍) and aphasia (*shiyuzheng* 失语证). Nothing in the text of the final dissertation or my conversations with Dr. Lin leads me to conclude that he wanted to demonstrate that Chinese medicine arrived at important discoveries prior to the West. Dr. Lin is also not, to my knowledge, a principled advocate of integrated Chinese and Western medicine. Educated in the late 1980s and 1990s, he belongs to a generation of physicians no longer enchanted by the dream of a "new medicine." He favors development but is equally determined not to forsake the roots of his own medical tradition.

No a priori structural or psychological factors (other than that as a Ph.D. candidate he was obliged to produce new knowledge) forced Dr. Lin to restructure the classical nosologies. On the contrary, this restructuring presented him with the problem of having to accommodate the treatment strategies of his medical ancestors to his novel synthesis, and vice versa. We thus arrive by a different route at a restatement of my previous argument: while Dr. Lin's synthesis appears to have been constructed by his experience and thinking, neither he nor anyone else ever fully controlled it. Rather, Dr. Lin's nosology and treatment protocols emerged performatively out of his need to enroll many different infrastructures into his research, a process that came to a stop when all participating infrastructural agencies were balanced with each other to form a pattern that was "just so."

What do I mean by "just so"? When I observed Dr. Lin administering the ABC test in October 1994, he explained to me in detail the biomedical differentiation between dysarthria and aphasia and told me that it was one of his goals to introduce this distinction to Chinese medicine. When I asked why he did not wish to go further and base his nosology on the specific brain area damaged in individual patients, he responded that this was too complicated. Given modern treatment techniques such as scalp acupuncture (in which needles are inserted over specific brain regions), such a nosology would have had undoubted therapeutic uses and cannot be ruled out on practical grounds. It would, however, not have been stable—or "just so"—given the many other infrastructures that demanded inclusion into Dr. Lin's synthesis.

To understand this, we must recall Dr. Lin's dependence on the ABC test as an instrument for measuring numerically changes in patients' symptomatology. Tests like the ABC are aphasia tests. In order to use the ABC Dr. Lin was forced to narrow his patient population to aphasics whose CVA etiology was confirmed by means of CT or MRI scans. He then began treating them on the basis of a treatment protocol that was assembled within a second interrelated process of synthesis, translating treatment outcomes into changes of numerical values produced by the ABC. This treatment protocol was derived partly from the clinical experiences of Dr. Lin's teachers and medical ancestors, which predated the existence of the *sheyin/yuse* distinction. These older treatment protocols consisted of body needling and were derived from classical physiological concepts. Scalp acupuncture might have allowed for a more specific reflection of pathophysiology in therapy, but it would also have meant moving acupuncture practice away from the bonds that tied Dr. Lin to the ideas and practices embodied in his teacher. Table 5 showed us, instead, that it was possible to effect a synthesis between the treatment strategies of Chinese medicine embodied in Dr. Lin's teachers and the nosology demanded by the ABC. In his dissertation Dr. Lin provides precise information regarding the site of the CVA for all of his subjects, though he does not integrate these data into his theoretical redefinitions. Why? In his words, because it was "too complicated"; in mine, because it was unnecessary. Dr. Lin's synthesis succeeded in accommodating to all the agencies brought to bear on it. Why destabilize it by introducing further elements?

The fact that I have chosen to use Dr. Lin as an example does not therefore imply that I attribute a distinct quality to his agency. It is crucial for the synthesis described, but not, therefore, more free. As soon as we adopt a different perspective, Dr. Lin appears less as an agent and more as a tool. Viewed from the perspective of the ABC test, Dr. Lin succumbs to the test's power and widens its ecological niche. Should his model be adopted by other practitioners, it will from now on be the ABC and no longer the individual diagnostic skills of individual physicians that decides whether patients are labeled *yuse* or *sheyin*, and therefore what treatment they are likely to receive. From the perspective of Professor Liao, Dr. Lin showed his filial respect by demonstrating to the world the power of Professor Liao's treatments and thereby added to his reputation. From the perspective of the state, Dr. Lin is nothing more than an instrument for the implementation of long-term strategic goals. Yet, none of these different agents controlled the emerging synthesis any more than Dr. Lin did himself. Even as his research program got under way, it would have been difficult to predict what synthesis precisely would emerge at its end. For what is at stake in the process of synthesis is not merely a controllable alignment of forces in the pursuit of predetermined goals but the transformation of each participating infrastructure and the entire field of practice in which they are located.[13]

Synthesis as Transformation

My case study has already provided ample evidence to corroborate this assertion. If, for instance, we examine contemporary acumoxa textbooks and the manner in which the subject is taught in undergraduate courses, we find there the same emphasis on pattern differentiation described in chapter 7. Dr. Lin's differentiation of CVA-related speech disorders established an entirely different mode of diagnosis and therapy, one closer to the biomedical notion of disease than to the modern Chinese medical definition of pattern. Seen from this angle, Dr. Lin's research reshapes not merely a very small area of clinical practice but also opens up the entire field of Chinese medicine to a much more fundamental restructuring. Such restructuring implies the importation of new infrastructures (such as the ABC) into this field, where they are aligned with existing notions about visceral systems of function, with ideas about pathology and illness, with needling techniques and patient demands.

Like all syntheses, Dr. Lin's nosology is itself unstable even as it destabilizes previous alignments between infrastructures in this field. Destabilization threatens from three directions at once: (1) from the future, through new developments within biomedicine, further refinements to the ABC, or the emergence of new and different tests that might render Dr. Lin's research obsolete; (2) from the past, in the continuous availability of other concepts and treatment strategies from the Chinese medical archive; (3) and from the present—even within the synthesis effected by Dr. Lin as a result of its constructed nature. During a conversation I had with Dr. Lin in the course of preparing my manuscript it emerged, for instance, that in practice certain patients suffering from *sheyin* apparently also show signs of *yuse*, and vice versa. When I questioned him about what this meant for his nosology, he opined that it did not necessarily undercut it but rather presented opportunities for further research. He did, however, admit that the point at which his own research had come to rest was, if not arbitrary, then at least governed by factors such as time, money, and the need to tie everything together, and that having to admit this gave weight to my constructive explanation.

The instability of all synthesis was defined in chapter 2 as the reason why plurality constitutes an essential rather than a derived aspect of all cultural process. It has emerged at various points throughout this discussion of Dr. Lin's research: in the tenuous connection between biomedical knowledge and technology that can be disassembled and partially assimilated into the field of Chinese medicine; in the unstable connection between the different acupoints in Professor Liao's treatment protocols that was ruptured by Dr. Lin's new diagnostic system; in the precarious relation between medical interventions and patient demands, as in the Manchu physician's efficacious practice that needed restructuring before it could be integrated into Dr. Lin's hospital-based practice. It is particularly obvious in some of the transformations that occurred within Dr. Lin himself in the course of his research.

Like all of his contemporaries, Dr. Lin has to chart a difficult course between allegiance to the stability (real or imagined) of the tradition that roots his practice and its ongoing development, which continuously transforms it. Dr. Lin is neither a rigid conservative nor a radical modernizer. During our initial encounters, shortly after we had both arrived in Beijing, Dr. Lin was enticed by the prospect of studying with a renowned *laozhongyi.* He devoted much effort to constructing ties of affiliation with his teacher and was successful to a certain extent. Whenever Dr. Lin speaks of Professor Liao he does so with affection, emphasizing what he has learned from him and how he has benefited from their relation. The same is true of his relationship with assistant supervisor Professor Ding. Professor Ding did, in fact, offer to support Dr. Lin's research financially out of his own research budget, though as it turned out Dr. Lin did not need the money.

Yet, Dr. Lin often expressed to me his frustration with the closed world of Chinese medicine, where the transfer of information and knowledge remains closely tied up with personal relations. This feeling was thrown into particular relief by Dr. Lin's encounter with Professor Gao at Beijing Medical University. Dr. Lin had no previous relation to Professor Gao, yet the latter spontaneously offered him support (personal as well as institutional) for the remainder of his project. Professor Gao made valuable suggestions regarding the design of clinical experiments and arranged for the use of advanced technologies at Beijing Medical University. What impressed Dr. Lin most about this help was that it was apparently motivated above all by a desire to advance knowledge. Ever since, Dr. Lin has emphasized to me the value of openness and sharing that he perceives to be at the heart of Western science and culture and of which Professor Gao has become a representative for him. Accepting these values has had a definite influence on the personal development of Dr. Lin.

Plurality and Synthesis

Clearly, the entire topic of plurality and synthesis in Chinese medicine is deserving of more detailed investigation both on the macrolevel of institutional practices and arrangements and on the microlevel of individual treatment episodes and specific knowledge claims. What is important here is the observation that it is not only conceptually possible (though it is still, perhaps, unconventional) to impute agency to nonhumans, but that such imputations facilitate explanation in different domains of understanding. Human and nonhuman agencies are obviously not equivalent, and differences exist with respect to their complexity and efficacy. Yet, as my case study of Dr. Lin indicates and as is confirmed by research in a wide variety of other domains, these agencies meet not just occasionally but all the time.

I argued in chapter 1 that from its inception anthropology has been informed by the idea that human behavior is guided by rules and norms residing in the mind. I argued that this perception is an important obstacle in our attempts to come to terms with plurality. We can now see how an alternative approach might be formulated.[14] In this new vision synthesis is not the achievement of meanings imposed onto the world by human subjects or, alternatively, of biosociocultural systems that structure human agency, but of environmentally extended systems, in which humans participate, that are established locally through interactions of various infrastructures. There is in this vision no room for a unitary subject. Rather, the syntheses that constitute being human are always hybrids of the natural (body, environment), the technological (tools, machines), and the sociocultural (language, concepts, practices). And it is within the ontology of these syntheses as a coming-into-being that plurality is grounded.

This assertion may be clarified by visualizing syntheses as having both an inside and an outside. The "outside" is the surface of the emergence of synthesis as a global state at which is produced a surplus that transcends what is given by participating infrastructures. The "inside" is the event horizon of local interactions between infrastructures at which synthesis is (re-)produced via a process of resistance and accommodation. The stability of syntheses (the possibility of the present repeating the past, of timelessness, of reversibility) is forestalled on two levels: reproduction and production. First, on the level of reproduction. In my model the transmission, persistence, and change of traditions is conceived to be an effect of local interactions. Learning, from the perspective of emergent synthesis, is not an internalization of totalities but a shaping of subjectivities, selves, and human/machine *collectifs* in local contexts of learning. In these contexts individual human performance is disciplined by the tools, machines, and other infrastructural agents with which humans interact, while tools, machines, and other infrastructures are similarly reshaped by the activities of humans. This interaction allows for the persistence of tradition over time as well as its gradual or sudden change.[15]

The stability of syntheses is also disrupted on the level of production. Emergence adds a surplus to the total environment. This something extra introduces new infrastructures (whether in terms of behaviors, concepts, technologies, or material things) that are available for and, indeed, demand by their own agency the inclusion into ongoing syntheses. These new infrastructures (emergent by intention or nonintention) threaten to disrupt, potentially at least, the reproduction of existing syntheses. Furthermore, the destabilization of one synthesis will affect others that are dependent on its productions. Syntheses produce effects as long as they are held together, as long as connections are maintained locally, as long as there is something passed between infrastructures. There is in my model no sense, however, of persistent effects or predetermined developments. Syntheses persist but eventually adjust, transform, or break up.[16]

Synthesis is thus a process that is grounded as much in the past (its present organization resulting from the interactive stabilization of agencies unfolded by participating infrastructures) as it is in the future (its future organization motivated by the agencies presently unfolded by participating infrastructures). If agency itself, however, is an emergent property of synthetic production, then we can know only after something has stabilized in a particular way that it has done so. And it is in this uncertainty that plurality is grounded. Walter Benjamin has captured within one beautiful and haunting image, the image of the *origin*, this ontological givenness of plurality within the emergence and disappearing of any synthesis: "Origin [*Ursprung*] although a thoroughly historical category, nonetheless has nothing to do with beginnings. . . . The term origin does not mean the process of becoming of that which has emerged, but much more, that which emerges out of the process of becoming and disappearing. The origin stands in the flow of becoming as a whirlpool . . . ; its rhythm is apparent only to a double insight."[17]

Our ability to grasp this impermanence of being bestows a final important advantage on our ability to adopt a pluralist perspective. Anthropologists have repeatedly drawn our attention to the short-term value of narrow conceptions of science implicated in dismantling the richness of other kinds of knowledge.[18] Another facet of the same short-termism is the homogenization of these other kinds of knowledge themselves. The political mechanisms contributing to such homogenization are manifold and cannot be discussed here. They are accelerated, however, by romanticized perceptions of stable traditional healing systems prevalent not only among anthropologists but also among advocates of so-called alternative medicines.[19] Such romanticizing—and the homogenizing comparisons between biomedicine and traditional medicines with which it is associated—impedes our capacity to render visible the fragmentation of all medical practices and to challenge the regimes that benefit from hiding their synthetic nature. Above all, it makes it more difficult to discern the diverse and not always predictable alignments between different medical practices—alignments that already exist in many forms in contemporary China and that will become ever more obvious and important in the rapidly transforming landscapes of medicine in the West.

PART III
ANTHROPOLOGICAL
INTERVENTIONS

9. THE FUTURE OF CHINESE MEDICINE

My ethnography demonstrates plurality to be an intrinsic aspect of contemporary Chinese medicine. It extends from health care policy and institutional organization to diagnostics, therapeutics, and even the subjectivities of individual physicians. Using this analysis to develop a general, if still rather basic, model of medicine in society has also shown that such plurality is not a distinguishing characteristic of Chinese medicine.[1] Plurality turns out to be nothing else than a term denoting the way things always are—forever changing and transforming origins in the whirlpool of their simultaneously present pasts and futures.

Even if this statement appears rather self-evident, I believe that it significantly deepens our understanding of contemporary Chinese medicine and of medical practice at large because it links the description of plurality to a comprehension of social dynamics that is no longer haunted by a delusive search for essences. There simply are no fixed borders between medical traditions or between different regions of a cultural space. Nor is there only one direction in which medicine can develop. Instead, Maoist philosophies of practical dialectics were seen to be infiltrating the treasure-house of Chinese medicine, biomedical concepts of physiology and cybernetics met with the health care of workers and peasants, while century-old tools of clinical practice reshaped modern biomedical physiology.

Plurality as Process and Transformation

I do not mean to imply that the ongoing transformation of Chinese medicine lacks structure, that it cannot be mapped out or compared with other, similar processes. One distinctive aspect of plurality in contemporary Chinese medicine, for instance, is that it openly admits into its syntheses infrastructures from many different periods. On the contents page of the March 1992 edition of the *Beijing zhongyi xueyuan xuebao* 北京中医学院学报 (*Journal of the Beijing College of Chinese Medicine*) we therefore find within a single field of practice the legendary culture heroes Fu Xi 伏羲 and Yu 禹, medical classics from the Han dynasty and their successive interpretations, modern *laozhongyi* narrating their clinical experiences, rats poisoned by the logic of biomedical research paradigms but treated with traditional pharmaceuticals, and contemporary interpretations of older diagnostic practices.[2]

Structurally, the centrality of some infrastructures gives them power over others. Mao Zedong's exalted position within the CCP leadership during the 1950s, for instance, meant that his ideas regarding the development of the medical sector were effectively translated into policies that shaped Chinese medicine. Yet, the resistance of the various infrastructures to which Mao Zedong's ideas had to relate themselves in order to become effective meant that his ideas also had to accommodate.[3] As we saw in chapter 3, true to his principles, Mao learned from experience and adjusted his policies numerous times.

Likewise, the hegemonic position of *bianzheng lunzhi* within contemporary Chinese medicine requires that all other doctrines and practices be aligned to it. The case records of previous generations of physicians are rewritten, and young physicians learn to write elaborate case histories that analyze patterns, even if at the bedside biomedical drugs are what matters. But *bianzheng lunzhi* itself—and with it Chinese medicine—is also significantly transformed in the process. I have shown this already on numerous occasions in chapter 7 but want to do so once more with the aid of a final case study.

CASE 9.1. *Creating Chinese Emergency Medicine.* Chinese emergency medicine (*zhongyi jizhen* 中医急诊) is a newly emerging field of practice in contemporary China. During the Eighth Five-Year Plan it was officially recognized as one of the thirty-eight subjects taught at Chinese medicine universities and colleges. The first national textbook was published in 1997, and the first course in the subject at Beijing University of Chinese Medicine was offered during the 1998–99 academic year. In this brief case study I examine the manner in which emergency medicine configures itself as an intrinsic aspect of Chinese medicine. I show that it does so by accommodating to the hegemonic discourse of *bianzheng lunzhi* discussed in chapter 7, but that in doing so it also contributes to the ongoing reshaping of the practices constituted by that discourse.

The third chapter of the national textbook *Zhongyi jizhenxue* 中医急

诊学 (*Chinese Emergency Medicine*)—according to which the subject is taught and examined—defines the relation of the discipline to the practice of pattern differentiation as one of subjugation: "Diagnosis and pattern differentiation in Chinese emergency medicine must accord with the theoretical system of Chinese medical diagnosis and pattern differentiation." However, the authors also underline the need to shun traditional strategies of learning and practice such as "awakening the mind" (*xinwu* 心悟), that is, guiding it toward sudden illumination. Instead, objective data analysis based on integrating the four methods of examination (*si zhen* 四诊) with modern biomedical technology (e.g., CT scans, ECGs) is defined as the only acceptable foundation of medical practice.[4]

The main part of the book is devoted to the diagnosis and treatment of twenty-eight emergency disorders ranging from high fever, poisoning, and bites to ectopic pregnancy and angina. Some of these disorders are derived from traditional nosological categories such as (summer)heat stroke (*zhongshu* 中暑) and abandonment patterns (*tuozheng* 脱证). Others, however, have been newly invented. By this I mean that these disorders exist neither in current biomedical disease classifications nor in traditional Chinese medical texts. Two strategies of such invention can be distinguished. The first turns what were previously viewed as symptoms—such as "convulsions" (*chouchu* 抽搐) or "stirring palpitations" (*xindongji* 心动悸)—into distinct disorders. The second creates entirely new disorders such as "acute spleen heart pain" (*jixing pixin tong* 急性脾心痛) and "kidney debilitation" (*shenshuai* 肾衰). These disorders are constructed from biomedical precedents that are anchored—with some effort and much imagination—within the existing field of Chinese medicine.

The creation of the disorder "kidney debilitation" (*shenshuai* 肾衰) exemplifies this process. The name "kidney debilitation" is extracted from a passage of the Tang dynasty text *Qianjin yaofang* 千金要方 (*Important Formulas Worth a Thousand*) that describes the symptoms and signs of kidney *qi* weakness: "The kidneys resonate with the bones, the bones and kidneys correspond to each other, . . . when its [the kidney's] *qi* is debilitated (*qi qi shuai* 其气衰), the hair falls out, the teeth become desiccated, the back and waist are drawn toward each other and become painful." The symptomatology of the disorder, which is presented next, does not, however, follow this historical precedent. Instead, clearly resembling the biomedical presentation of uremia, it is described as being characterized by "little urine, rough and stertorous breathing which smells of urine, headache, nausea, edema, bleeding, fatigue, apathetic appearance, somnolence, vexation and restlessness, if severe also clouding of consciousness and tremors."

In a final step, these symptoms and signs are linked to another text passage from the Chinese medical archive, the *Zhongding guang wenre lun* 重订广温热论 (*Newly Revised Expanded Discussion of Warm [Pathogen] Heat [Disorders]*). This text, which is itself the product of an early-twentieth-century revision of a late-nineteenth-century rewriting of an eighteenth-century text, contains a passage discussing the pathology of "urine poison entering the blood" (*niaodu ru xue* 尿毒入血).[5] "When urine poison enters the blood, then after the blood poison has attacked above there will be headache and dizziness, clouding of visual acuity, tinnitus and deafness, nausea and vomiting, stertorous breathing with a foul odor, intermittent occurrence of sudden withdrawal and epilepsy or clouding of consciousness and tetanic inversion, loss of consciousness, picking at bedclothes and groping in the air. The tongue coating takes on a rotten [appearance] and is interspersed with black dots."[6] This quote has no relation whatsoever with the first one from the *Qianjin yaofang* other than that both were written by physicians of Chinese medicine. It does, however, succeed in linking the biomedical presentation of uremia, previously defined as kidney debilitation, to similar descriptions from within the Chinese medical tradition. Through a succession of mimetic movements the authors of *Zhongyi jizhenxue* thereby manage to disassociate a constellation of symptoms and signs commonly encountered in emergency wards—where for reasons discussed in chapter 3 they are generally grasped through the gaze of Western medicine—from the stranglehold of that gaze. What was previously uremia is now kidney debilitation and as such becomes available for treatment as a distinctly Chinese medical problem.

Such treatment is discussed by the authors of *Chinese Emergency Medicine* under a number of different headings ranging from "Discussion of Treatment Options" (*lunzhi* 论治) and "Adapting Treatment Methods to Deviations from the Norm" (*quanbianfa* 权变法) to "Transmutations of the Disorder and Return to the Normal State" (*zhuan gui* 传归) and "Care during Convalescence" (*tiaohu* 调护). The section "Treatment Options" includes strategies for both "First Aid Treatment" (*jijiu chuli* 急救处理) and "Treatment Based on Pattern Differentiation" (*bianzheng zhiliao* 辨证治疗). First aid treatments range from intravenous infusions and injections to enemas and acupuncture. The drugs used are drawn exclusively from the pharmacopoeia of Chinese medicine. They are administered, however, according to an understanding of each disorder as a distinct nosological entity. Contrary to the logic of *bianzheng lunzhi* this allows each condition to be treated by a repertoire of more or less standard interventions.

Such treatment does not, however, reflect the basic doctrinal premises of contemporary Chinese medicine. A section on *bianzheng lunzhi*, which discusses the application of treatment once an acute crisis has been managed, is therefore also required. This section divides each disorder into several patterns and suggests formulas for their treatment. For this purpose, each pattern is further subdivided into discussions on "Pattern Presentation" (*zhenghou*), "Treatment Method" (*zhifa* 治法), and "Formulas and Drugs" (*fang yao* 方药). All of the patterns as well as the formulas and drugs suggested for their treatment are drawn from classical sources.

Treatment of emergency conditions is, of course, not a new aspect of Chinese medicine. As the medical literature attests, Chinese physicians have always treated acute and serious disorders. Recuperation of these ancient methods by means of detailed textual analysis in the context of biomedical knowledge constitutes at least one other option by means of which modern Chinese emergency medicine might be reconfigured. A typical example of this approach is Fu Youfeng's 符有丰 research into the original indications of Li Gao's 李杲 (1180–1251) classical formula *Buzhong yiqi tang* (Supplement the Middle and Benefit *Qi* Decoction). While modern physicians generally employ the formula for the treatment of chronic conditions (see case 5.2), Fu argues that its original indication must have been pulmonary plague.[7]

If such research is not carried out more widely, this is perhaps because the synthesis achieved in *Chinese Emergency Medicine* is more successful in accommodating to the agency of all the diverse infrastructures that have an interest in its construction. In contemporary China these include the facilities of modern urban hospitals but also the ideological and practical resources necessary to legitimize—and if possible extend—Chinese medicine's autonomy within a plural health care system. Chinese medicine as an institution is now strong enough, it appears, to attempt a colonization of what is widely regarded as the exclusive domain of Western medicine. Clearly, such interests are not served by subsuming the indication of Chinese medical formulas to biomedical disease categories. Yet, the pattern differentiation that informed classical treatment of emergency conditions is also not suited to modern contexts because of the different pathologies treated in modern Chinese emergency wards and the different means by which these conditions are grasped.[8]

The reshaping of the field of Chinese medicine attempted by the authors of *Chinese Emergency Medicine* can therefore not be explained as driven by clinical factors alone. Rather, it represents a complex alignment of infrastructures that reshapes Chinese medicine in the light of modern biomedicine without thereby detaching it from its classical roots. Yet, and this must be made equally clear, this importation of classical patterns and formulas into the newly constituted field of emergency Chinese medicine is not achieved without loss. In their original use contexts, the patterns used by the authors of *Chinese Emergency Medicine* constitute precisely defined stages in the development of a specific type of problem; for example, a cold damage (*shanghan* 伤寒) disorder analyzed via six-channel (*liu jing* 六经) pattern differentiation or a warm pathogen disorder treated via a four-aspect (*wei qi ying xue* 卫气营血) differentiation. Within these contexts patterns are made intelligible—and thus usable—through understanding their position within a larger frame of reference. Assimilated into the context of emergency medicine, each pattern is transformed instead into a subtype of a newly created disorder. Without the guarantee that students have a prior grasp of these original frames of reference, the intelligibility of such "old patterns in new contexts," and therefore the practical efficacy of treatment, is by no means assured. Hence, what is gained in the process of asserting and extending the institutional standing of contemporary Chinese medicine is lost in loosening the very connections that have nurtured its practice in the past.

The Future of Chinese Medicine

I have chosen this brief case study not because it is representative of all innovation in contemporary Chinese medicine,[9] but rather because it summarizes in a practical manner everything I have labored to say in this book about synthesis as a process of simultaneous emerging and disappearing and about Chinese medicine in contemporary China. Regarding the former, it affirms that Chinese medicine is not a system in the conventional structural sense of the term but an ongoing process. Regarding the latter, it adduces not only the continued vitality of Chinese medicine as a living tradition but also the agencies that currently nourish, constrain, and seek to transform it. After a century of struggle against domination by Western medicine, of modernization and revolution, Chinese medicine now stands at the threshold of emergence as a truly global medicine.[10]

Such globalization encompasses various processes. Within China, it refers to attempts to infiltrate territory that was once the sole domain of biomedical power and technology. It refers to the standardization of teaching, practice, and bureaucratic control necessary for such a process to succeed. Globalization also, of course, refers to the dispersion of Chinese medicine throughout the world, where it is now practiced in an increasing number of different settings. Such globalization is a remarkable achievement given the worldwide hegemony of biomedicine during the last century. Yet, it is also associated with tremendous risks.

In this final section I move from description to intervention by outlining some of these risks. I shall do so by linking the globalization of Chinese medicine currently in progress to similar processes in other domains. For this purpose I draw on James Scott's examination of modernist schemes to improve the human condition.[11] Inasmuch as the transformations of Chinese medicine described in this book have been guided to a large extent by this very goal, Scott's analysis provides a fitting point of departure for my conclusion.

The various modernization projects analyzed by Scott range from scientific forestry developed in nineteenth-century Prussia to Soviet collectivization in the 1920s, from the design of Brasilia in the 1950s to the "villagization" of Tanzania in the 1970s and 1980s, and further to World Bank sponsored development projects throughout the developing world. According to Scott, all these different schemes are characterized by an absolute faith in science and technology as tools by which the human condition can be improved. Central to the realization of this vision, wherever it emerged, has been the state, for only the massive powers of the modern nation-state can transform the local resistance invariably encountered by global schemes aimed at the transformation of nature-culture.

In order to make a plurality of local agencies legible and thereby controllable, modern nation-states enforced various kinds of "state simplifications." Simplification in this context refers to processes of normalization that have in common the creation of normalized individuals and contexts: from the demand for fixed surnames and the creation of land registries to the objectifications implicit in modern biomedical practice. Only on the basis of the uniformities constructed by means of such a "heroic constriction of vision" did it become possible to implement the various state-sponsored and state-controlled schemes for the improvement of society. Yet, the very heroism that empowered these visions is shown by Scott to be also the root of their potential failure, a failure that, as modernity wore on, became the norm rather than remaining an exception.

Prussian scientific forestry serves as an example. In creating "a perfectly legible forest planted with same-aged, single-species, uniform trees growing in straight lines in a rectangular flat space cleared of all underbrush and poachers," agronomists improved profitability at the cost of natural diversity. "Failing to see the real forest for the commercial trees," they also failed to see that left to its own devices nature favors untidy mixed-species environments. Forest death in Germany a hundred years later remains as the enduring legacy of the Prussian vision of progress.

From this and many similar examples of social and natural engineering based on "thin simplifications" supported by a "visual aesthetic of progress" in which only the linear and uniform "looked modern," Scott deduces an opposition between the global homogeneity and hubris of "high modernism" and traditional skills characterized by plasticity, diversity, adaptability, and stochastic reasoning. Scott calls these skill *mētis*, after the ability that enabled Ulysses to survive his many irregular adventures. Such *mētis* is built on local knowledge and experience aptly captured by the Chinese recipe instruction, "Heat the oil until it is almost smoking." Unless the cook has once experienced the smoke of burnt oil he can never know the "almost."

It does not take much imagination to sense a close affinity between the concept of *mētis* elaborated by Scott and various conceptions of efficacy in classical Chinese thought.[12] The flexibility of practice consistently demanded by senior physicians (chapters 5 and 7) and the grounding of medicine in personal experience we have repeatedly encountered in this ethnography (chapters 5, 6, and 7) are practical instantiations of these doctrines. Yet things are not as simple as Scott would have them appear. Deference to the authority of canonical texts or living masters continually threatens to disable the plasticity of such knowledge. This certainly is one reason why physicians of Chinese medicine like Dr. Lin (chapter 8) look toward the West for inspiration. And even Scott, whose sympathies clearly lie with the *mētis* of small networks, has to admit to the benefits derived from the global perspectives of modernization in public health and medicine.

The model of synthesis I propose in this book helps us to undercut the categorical distinctions implicit in Scott's opposition between tradition and modernity that so easily lead us in the direction of false generalizations. It demonstrates, instead, that all agency must invariably encounter resistance and that such resistance will sooner or later demand accommodation. Hence, the benefits of any global vision of efficacy—whether those of overly rigid traditional doctrine or those of medicine blind to the pluralities of local contexts—are necessarily extracted at a price. The side effects that are accepted as the invariable accompaniment of biomedical treatment and the emergence of antibiotic-resistant bacteria that threatens the foundations of modern medical practice are therefore as much rooted in the simplifications imposed by biomedical reductionism as are its successes. Yet biomedicine itself is, of course, also immensely plural, varied, and diverse. It offers models and interventions both complex and simplistic and therefore also succeeds in finding answers to problems it has itself created.

Traditionally, Chinese medicine has favored the construction of small local syntheses, a vision that finds its contemporary expression in individualized treatment on the basis of pattern differentiation. This does not imply that Chinese medicine never fails. In fact, as the case records of even the most famous physicians demonstrate, it frequently does. Such failure, however, is always a limited local event corrected by adjusting the local alignment of infrastructures. The traditional adage "follow the ancients without getting stuck in the old" (*shun gu er bu ni gu* 順古而不泥古), like the modern slogan "inheriting and carrying forward" (*jicheng fayang* 继承发扬), therefore clearly resonates with Scott's recipe for sustainable development: take small steps, favor reversibility, plan on surprises.

Mētis and its Chinese equivalents—and I cannot overemphasize this— are not, however, essential elements of Chinese medicine. Throughout its history physicians and scholars have striven for global systematization and synthesis. Today, too, powerful forces inside and outside Chinese medicine are working toward the regularization of its practice and the repression of local knowledge. Such regularization is widely informed by the same utopian vision of progress that Scott examines, a vision reflecting a conception of efficacy so narrowly focused that it can accord no value to plurality and diversity. In the course of its ongoing globalization Chinese medicine will therefore have to engage—even more than it has to date—with this vision and its powerful protagonists. The following quote, taken from a survey conducted by the *Journal of the American Medical Association* regarding the future of alternative or complementary medicines, forcefully underlines this point.

By 2020, [ ] interventions [currently deemed elements of complementary and alternative medicines] will have been incorporated into conventional medical education and practice. . . . The biological and pharmacological basis for effectiveness of selected herbal and nutritional supplements will be clarified, leading to their standardization and to the rational design of yet more potent congeners. Advances in neurobiology will elucidate mechanisms underlying ancient practices such as acupuncture and meditation, as well as the phenomenon of "the placebo effect." . . . The field of integrative medicine will be seen as providing novel insights and tools for human health, and not as a source of intellectual and philosophical tension that insinuates itself between and among practitioners of the healing arts and their patients.[13]

To date, historians and anthropologists have focused on the loss of internal coherence resulting from the transition to modernity as the main danger to the survival of Chinese medicine. Its advocates in China and the West, on the other hand, appear to believe that Chinese medicine embodies a kind of knowledge that is categorically different from biomedicine and therefore intrinsically immune to the social and economic factors that drive modernization. I eschew the essentialism implicit in both views. As my ethnography has demonstrated, such essentialism does not facilitate our understanding of Chinese medicine's actual plurality. In fact, it constructs Chinese medicine in such a manner as to make it vulnerable to invasion by precisely those discourses of efficacy that are inimical to its hitherto multiple points of view and to the models of agency that have guided its development.

Deliberating the future of Chinese medicine thus is not a question of whether or not its essence can be preserved or whether it can be transplanted into a different culture. Rather, it is a question of what course of development to steer: increasing systematization, regularization, and integration into extended global syntheses and fields of practice leading to its eventual assimilation into an "integrative medicine" or a self-conscious embracing of diversity conjoined to a piecemeal assimilation into local networks of nature-culture around the world?

It should be clear by now where my personal sympathies lie. Plurality, as I have labored to show, is the essential factor in the origin not merely of nature but also of society. Repression of such plurality—even or especially where it is carried out in the name of science—is only ever driven by two forces: ignorance and the desire for power. This desire takes many forms and must not be seen as intrinsically negative. After all, the wish to control and manage disease lies at the heart of all medical practice, Chinese or Western, ancient or modern. It is important, however, to realize that such desire is never pure but rather is born out of the synthesis of many agencies and is tied to many synthetic networks; that these networks and syntheses reflect in their construction distinct alignments of power between patients, healers, industry, and the state; and that they embody different evaluations of risk, different ethics, and different aesthetics.

Intervening in the future of Chinese medicine from the perspective of the social sciences means uncovering these connections and asking the questions that arise as a result: What, ultimately, is gained from restraining Chinese medicine by means of a rationality blind to its own irrational constitution, and gained for whom? What would be lost by embracing its different aesthetics of practice? Why not entertain the notion that the plurality of agents that impinge on human health may best be engaged by means of a similar plurality in the domain of medicine? The answer to these questions will not be provided by any single agent. Pondering the future of Chinese medicine in terms of the model elaborated here may allow us to see more clearly, however, what is at stake.

Four Attempts at Systematizing Pattern
Differentiation and Treatment Determination

This appendix summarizes four attempts at systematizing "pattern differentiation and treatment determination" (*bianzheng lunzhi* 辨证论治):

1. A model proposed by the Nanjing College of Chinese Medicine (Nanjing zhongyi xueyuan 南京中医学院) in the *Zhongyixue gailun* 中医学概论 (*Outline of Chinese Medicine*), published in 1958.[1]

2. A model regarding the systematization of patterns put forward by the Chongqing Research Class of Physicians of Western Medicine Seconded from Work to Study Chinese Medicine (Chongqingshi xiyilizhi xuexi zhongyi yanjiuban 重庆市西医离职学习中医研究班) published in 1959.[2]

3. A model proposed by Qin Bowei 秦伯未 and other prominent physicians entitled *Shisi gangyao bianzheng* 十四纲要辨证 ("The Fourteen Principal Rubrics of Pattern Differentiation"), published in January 1961 in the *Journal of Chinese Medicine*.[3]

4. A model proposed by Fang Yaozhong 方药中 in his book *Bianzheng lunzhi yanjiu qi jiang* 辨证论治研究七讲 (*Seven Lectures on Pattern Differentiation and Treatment Differentiation Research*), published in 1979.[4]

The four models are presented in order to further substantiate the argument made in chapter 7. They document the diversity (but also the similarities) between different attempts at systematizing pattern differentiation. For each model I present an overview in graphic form (as a diagram or table) to make its inner structure apparent. Explanatory notes have been added to further explicate this structure.

Model 1: *Outline of Chinese Medicine*

The *Outline* was the first textbook of Chinese medicine compiled on behalf and under the supervision of the Ministry of Health. It was designed to serve as a textbook for the Nationwide Classes for Physicians of Western Medicine Studying Chinese Medicine (Quanguo juban xiyi xuexi zhongyi ban 全国举办西医学习中医班) instituted in the 1950s. The need for such a textbook had become obvious in the course of teaching the first and most prominent of these classes in Beijing between 1955 and 1958. The first edition of the *Outline* was published in 1958. A second revised edition followed shortly afterward in 1959. Thereafter, the *Outline* became a standard textbook for courses in Chinese medicine at universities and colleges of Western medicine, as well as for revision and self-study classes in Chinese medicine until the outbreak of the Cultural Revolution. The *Outline* has, furthermore, significantly shaped the global transmission of Chinese medicine. The entire text has been translated into Japanese, while its core model of pattern differentiation has been employed virtually unchanged in English-language publications such as the *Essentials of Chinese Acupuncture.*[5]

The initial project for the writing of the *Outline* was developed by the MOH in 1956 under the working title *Zhongyixue gangyao* 中医学纲要 (*Essentials of Chinese Medicine*) under the personal supervision of the deputy health minister, Guo Zihua 郭子化. The Jiangsu Province Chinese Medicine Teacher Improvement School (Jiangsusheng zhongyi shizi jinxiu xuexiao 江苏省中医师资进修学校) was initially commissioned to compile the work.[6] Writing commenced in 1957 and initially involved a group of mainly young scholars that included Wu Yigu 吴贻谷, Ding Guangdi 丁光迪, Yin Huihe 印会河, Xu Jiqun 许济群, Wang Mianzhi 王绵之, Wang Yuchuan 王玉川, Fa Xilin 法锡麟, Yan Zhenghua 颜正华, Chen Shennong 程莘农, Cao Zhongling 曹种苓, Xu Junzhi 许浚之, and Wang Youren 汪幼人. The finished text was tried out as teaching tool at the Nanjing school, whose students were mainly practitioners of Chinese medicine. It was commented on by older staff at the college and then further tested in Chinese medicine classes for physicians of Western medicine at the Jiangsu Province Ministry of Health Cadre School (Jiangsusheng weisheng ganxiao 江苏省卫生干效) and the Nanjing College of Medicine (Nanjing yixueyuan 南京医学院).

In the spring of 1958 the MOH formally decided to publish the *Essentials* and a final editorial committee was established at Nanjing that included Wu Yigu 吴贻谷, Ding Guangdi 丁光迪, Fa Xilin 法锡麟, Song Liren 宋立人, Li Hongkui 李鸿逵, Ni Hexian 倪和宪, and Zang Zaiyang 臧载阳. Further input from the teaching and research group at the school and from renowned Jiangsu clinicians resulted in significant changes to the text, which now comprised two volumes and was called *Zhongyixue jiben lilun gangyao* 中医学基本理论纲要 (*Essential Basic Theory of Chinese Medicine*). Additional changes were made after the manuscript was presented to the MOH and following consultation with staff at the Beijing College of Chinese Medicine (Beijing zhongyi xueyuan 北京中医学院) including Ren Yingqiu 任应秋, Yu Daoji 于道济, Yuan Hongshou 袁鸿寿, Xiao Xi 肖熙, Yin Huihe 印会河, and Wang Yuchuan 王玉川. This version was accepted by the MOH and finally published in September 1958 after yet another title change to its final version, the *Outline of Chinese Medicine*. Authorship was conferred onto what had by then become the Nanjing College of Chinese Medicine reflecting both the origin of the text and also the fact that the revisions in Beijing involved physicians, like Yin Huihe, who had originally come from the south.

The systematization of Chinese medicine worked out in the *Outline* became the paradigm for teaching the subject at colleges and universities throughout China. Western descriptions of Chinese medical practice — whether written for a clinical audience or an academic one, such as Farquhar 1994a, Kaptchuk 1983, Maciocia 1989, or Sivin 1987 — reflect the hegemonic status of this paradigm. It is thus merely summarized here. For more detailed descriptions in English, any of the above texts may be consulted.

THE MODEL

As described in chapter 7, the *Outline* constructs patterns (*zheng*) as the pivot of Chinese medical practice and then designates the eight rubrics (*ba gang*) as the basic matrix of Chinese medical diagnostics. This was intended to mean that the principles they embody can be found in various manifestations in all the specific methods of pattern differentiation and treatment determination. According to Hu Xin 胡欣 and Ge Xiumei 葛秀梅 (1994: 86–88), the eight rubrics are the "epitomization of the diverse principles of pattern differentiation" (*ge zhong bianzheng gangling de gaikuo* 各种辨证纲领的概括) "with regard to which the other principles of pattern differentiation assume a subordinate relationship" (*qita bianzheng gangling zhi jian shi yi zhong lishu guanxi* 其它辨证纲领之间是一种隶属关系). In clinical practice, however, all the methods of pattern differentiation described in the *Outline* and taught in contemporary undergraduate courses can be used individually or in combination with one another without needing to reduce them to the eight rubrics.

COMMENT

Of the four models presented here, the *Outline* is the only one produced by a committee under MOH supervision. Although, according to my informants, books edited by committees can be heavily influenced by the views of their chairpersons, the diversity of methods of pattern differentiation described in the text and their presentation without an ultimate unity reflect, in this instance, the text's institutional production and the diverse opinions of the

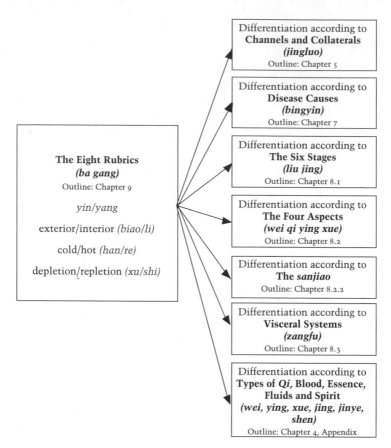

FIGURE A.1. Pattern differentiation according to the *Outline of Chinese Medicine*

writers who contributed to it. The many changes made to the text during its production corroborate this hypothesis.

Furthermore, the *Outline* was intended as a teaching text for Western physicians studying Chinese medicine, and its composition must be understood as a specific response to the needs of that audience. As we shall see below, physicians of Western medicine made known their preference for a systematic presentation of Chinese medical theory and practice that matched basic premises of the biomedical model regarding coherence and systematization. The political imperatives directing the study of Chinese medicine by physicians of Western medicine at the time—the unification of both medicines to form one new medical system—implicitly required that Chinese medicine be set up in such a way as to allow for maximum compatibility with Western medicine.

Finally, while the intended audience of the *Outline* consisted of Western medicine physicians, the actual producers of the text were Chinese medicine scholar-physicians, each with their own views and opinions. Thus, although later simplifications of pattern differentiation clearly originate here, these were not necessarily intended by the authors of the *Outline*.[7] Subsequently, many of the original authors contributed to the writing of the textbooks used in contemporary Chinese medicine colleges and universities.[8] Some, like Yin Huihe 印会河, also went on to produce personal syntheses of pattern differentiation that, in their own words, "are different from standard presentations of Chinese internal medicine" (*yiban zhongyi neikexue you bie* 一般中医内科学有别).[9]

Model 2: Chongqing Western Medicine Physicians

The Chongqing Research Class of Physicians of Western Medicine Seconded from Work to Study Chinese Medicine was convened in February 1956. Following the establishment of the Chengdu College of Chinese Medicine it was directed from there and renamed the Chongqing Branch of the Chengdu College of Chinese Medicine Research Class of Physicians of Western Medicine Seconded from Work to Study Chinese Medicine. The class compiled *Zhongyi bianzheng shuyu de shentao* as a contribution to the systematization of Chinese medicine under way at the time. In the foreword they describe their reasons for doing so:

> Regarding pattern terminology in Chinese medicine, particularly with respect to its meaning, previous generations undoubtedly have carried out much work. However, because the perspectives of different schools were not the same, discrepancies exist, particularly in terms of their designation. Therefore, in terms of meaning the terminology of patterns at present still lacks systematization and formalization. The use of pattern terminology in clinical contexts remains complicated and we Western medicine physicians studying Chinese medicine feel it is difficult to employ and not easy to come to terms with. We feel that the Chinese medicine reference materials in this area are equally unhandy. Hence, we have attempted the task of an initial systematization in this respect.[10]

I have therefore included the Chongqing model as a representation of the direct contribution of Western medicine physicians to the development of *bianzheng lunzhi*.

TABLE A.I. Pattern Differentiation according to the Chongqing Research Class of Physicians of Western Medicine Studying Chinese Medicine

Liver *yang* trespasses upward (*ganyang fan shang* 肝阳犯上)

Disease location (*bingwei*)	The liver (*gan*) visceral system
Disease character (*bingqing*)	Headache, dizziness, red complexion, and wiry pulse representing persistently flourishing liver *yang* (*ganyang pian wang* 肝阳偏旺)
Disease cause (*bingyin*)	Kidney *yin* depletion (*shenyinxu* 肾阴虚) resulting in water failing to moisten wood (*shui bu han mu* 水不涵木) so that liver *yang* trespasses upward

THE MODEL

The Chongqing students define patterns to be distinct from diseases and symptoms following the manner of the *Outline*. They furthermore define patterns as being characterized by three factors (*tiaojian* 条件): disease cause (*bingyin* 病因), disease character (*bingqing* 病情), and disease location (*bingwei* 病位). Disease causes are specified by means of the three causes (*san yin* 三因) of disease taken over from classical medical theory.[11] Disease location specifies the place where a pathology is present, again defined via classical concepts such as visceral systems of function, channels and collaterals, *qi*, and blood. Disease character refers both to the key symptoms and signs (*bingzhuang* 病状) that define a given pattern and to the nature (*xingzhi* 性质) of the pathology they represent. Discussion of the pattern "liver *yang* trespasses upward" (*ganyang fanshang* 肝阳犯上) serves as an example.

The number of patterns described and the terminology employed for their labeling vary from those used by the *Outline* and later textbooks. Like the *Outline*, the overall number of patterns is quite small. Unlike the *Outline*, which sticks closely to the eight rubrics in differentiating between patterns, the Chongqing physicians employ a much more idiosyncratic labeling of patterns. The pathology of the liver and gall bladder visceral systems, for instance, is condensed into just five patterns: (1) liver *yang* upward counterflow (*ganyang shang ni* 肝阳上逆), (2) liver wind moving internally (*ganfeng nei dong* 肝风内动), (3) liver *qi* not spreading (*ganqi bu shu* 肝气不舒), (4) liver kidney *yin* depletion (*gan shen yinxu* 肝肾阴虚), and (5) liver gall bladder not quiet (*gan dan bu ning* 肝胆不宁). We can compare this with the four patterns listed in the *Outline* and with modern textbooks, which generally list eight patterns (see case 6.3).

The model of the Chongqing Western Medicine Physicians represents the input of Western medicine physicians into the formation of *bianzheng lunzhi*. The reasons for the compilation of the text stated in the foreword succinctly summarize the contingencies driving the emergence of *bianzheng lunzhi* during the late 1950s that are analyzed in chapter 7.

While the intentions of the authors broadly match those of the Chinese medicine scholar-physicians who wrote the *Outline*, this work uses a different method of systematization in its presentation of patterns. The terminology for many patterns, too, is significantly different from that of the *Outline* and that of contemporary textbooks. This demonstrates that the modern orthodoxy of pattern differentiation does not represent any kind of natural essence of Chinese medicine.

In spite of the sincerely good intentions of its authors, the Chongqing model was not adopted as a basis of later systematization. The reasons for this are not clear to me. Most likely, however, is the hypothesis that its authors were not part of the networks that determined the direction of later systematizations.

Model 3: Qin Bowei's Fourteen Rubrics

During the Nationalist era, Qin Bowei emerged as one of the most eminent scholar-physicians among the graduates of Ding Ganren's 丁甘仁 Chinese Medicine Technical College in Shanghai. He was called to Beijing in 1955 as an adviser to the MOH and a teacher at the first research class of Western medicine physicians studying Chinese medicine. He later taught and practiced at the Dongzhimen Hospital of Chinese Medicine, the first affiliated teaching hospital of the College of Chinese Medicine established in 1956. Qin Bowei was a prominent spokesperson for the development of an independent Chinese medical tradition, and his contributions to the *bianzheng lunzhi* debates are significant because of his eminent standing as a scholar-physician.

In January 1961 Qin Bowei together with Li Yinglin 李英麟, Yin Fengli 殷凤礼, Jiao Shude 焦树德, Kang Tingpei 康廷培, Wu Zemin 武泽民, Geng Fusi 耿富思, and Liao Jiamo 廖家模, many of whom have since become well-known scholar-physicians in their own right, published a draft program for the systematization of *bianzheng lunzhi* that consisted of fourteen rather than eight principal rubrics. In the introduction to this proposal its authors acknowledge that *bianzheng lunzhi* is characterized by a combination of rule-bound and flexible elements. They lament, however, the unsystematic state of affairs in

The Fourteen Principal Rubrics of Pattern Differentiation *Shisi gangyao bianzheng* 十四纲要辨证		
Rubric 纲	Principal Patterns 主证	Combined Patterns 兼证
Wind *feng* 风	wind damage [*shangfeng* 伤风] wind stroke [*zhongfeng* 中风] internal wind [*neifeng* 内风]	wind cold (see *Cold*), wind warmth (see *Fire*), wind fire [*fenghuo* 风火], wind dampness [*fengshi* 风湿], pestilential wind (see *Epidemics*)
Cold *han* 寒	cold damage [*shanghan* 伤寒] cold stroke [*zhonghan* 中寒] depletion cold [*xuhan* 虚寒]	wind cold [*fenghan* 风寒], cold damp (see *Damp*), cold enveloping fire [*han bao huo* 寒包火]
(Summer)heat *shu* 暑	(summer)heat damage [*shangshu* 伤暑] (summer)heat stroke [*zhongshu* 中暑] hidden (summer)heat [*fushu* 伏暑]	(summer)heat damp [*shushi* 暑湿] (summer)heat wind [*shu feng* 暑风]
Damp *shi* 湿	damp damage [*shangshi* 伤湿] collecting damp [*tingshi* 停湿] accumulated water [*jishui* 积水]	wind damp (see *Wind*), cold damp [*hanshi* 寒湿] (summer)heat damp (see [*summer*]*heat*), damp heat (see *Fire*), phlegm damp (see *Phlegm*)
Dryness *zao* 燥	autumn dryness [*qiuzao* 秋燥] liquid and blood dessication dryness [*jin xue kuzao* 津血枯燥]	
Fire *huo* 火	full fire [*shihuo* 实火] depletion fire [*xuhuo* 虚火] warm pathogen [*wenxie* 温邪] damp heat [*shire* 湿热]	wind fire (see *Wind*), cold enveloping fire (see *Cold*), damp fire [*shihuo* 湿火], wind warmth [*fengwen* 风温], damp warmth [*shiwen* 湿温], warm poison [*wendu* 温毒], warm epidemic (see *Epidemics*)
Epidemics *yi* 疫	warm epidemic [*wenyi* 温疫] pestilential wind/leprosy [*lifeng* 疠风] miasmic toxin [*zhangdu* 瘴毒]	

The Fourteen Principal Rubrics of Pattern Differentiation
Shisi gangyao bianzheng 十四纲要辨证

Rubric 纲	Principal Patterns 主证	Combined Patterns 兼证
Phlegm *tan* 痰	phlegm turbidity [*tanzhuo* 痰浊] phlegm nodes [*tanhe* 痰核] phlegm-rheum [*tanyin* 痰饮]	wind phlegm [*fengtan* 风痰], cold phlegm [*hantan* 寒痰] damp phlegm [*shitan* 湿痰], hot phlegm [*retan* 热痰]
Food *shi* 食	food damage [*shangshi* 伤食] inability to eat [*bu shi* 不食] food wasting [*xiaoshi* 消食]	
Worms *chong* 虫	worm pain [*chongtong* 虫痛] worm consumption [*laochong* 劳虫]	
Essence *jing* 精	insufficient essence [*jing bu zu* 精不足] insecurity of the essence gate [*jingguan bu gu* 精关不固]	
Spirit *shen* 神	spirit depletion [*shenxu* 神虚] deranged spirit [*shen luan* 神乱]	
Qi *qi* 气	*qi* depletion [*qixu* 气虚] *qi* depression [*qiyu* 气郁] *qi* counterflow [*qini* 气逆]	*qi* and blood both depleted [*qi xue liang xu* 气血两虚]
Blood *xue* 血	blood depletion [*xuexu* 血虚] blood heat [*xuere* 血热] blood stagnation [*xuexhi* 血滞] blood loss [*shixue* 失血]	*qi* and blood both depleted (see *Qi*)

this most important aspect of Chinese medicine, which requires each individual physician to learn by trial and error. To rectify this shortcoming they propose to order *bianzheng lunzhi* according to fourteen rubrics, summarized here by means of a direct transcription of the table that precedes the detailed exposition of these rubrics in the main body of the text.

THE MODEL

In the main body of the article the authors discuss each rubric, or pattern, under two headings. The first, "Principle Symptoms and Signs" (*Zhuzheng*

主症), lists the main symptoms and signs for the pattern, explains their pathogenesis, and indicates from which other patterns it needs to be differentiated. The second, "Treatment Methods" (*zhifa* 治法), considers appropriate treatment strategies for each pattern and suggests formulas that represent these strategies. Thus, for the pattern wind damage (*shangfeng*), which needs to be differentiated from cold damage (*shanghan*) and the initial stages of warm [pathogen] disorders (*wenbing* 温病), three treatment strategies are discussed: (1) "Method for Diffusing the Lung with Acrid and Dissipating [Medicinals]" (*xuanfei xinsan fa* 宣肺辛散法); (2) "Method for Securing the Exterior and Dispelling Evil [*Qi*]" (*gubiao quxie fa* 固表祛邪法); and (3) "Method for Regulating and Harmonizing Constructive and Defensive [*Qi*]" (*tiaohe ying wei fa* 调和营卫法). In addition, Qin lists for each rubric a selection of essential formulas (*fangji xuanyao* 方剂选要) and presents a classification of drugs according to the treatment methods reviewed (*yaowu fenlei* 药物分类).

COMMENT

Qin Bowei's project differs from that of the *Outline* in attempting to use just one model to approach all possible illnesses. It does this by drawing into the model aspects of the various traditions that have been kept separate in the *Outline* such as the *shanghan* and *wenbing* streams. Inasmuch as the *wenbing* stream drew on preexisting *shanghan* models, the authors can be said to have every right (in terms of precedents within the Chinese medicine tradition) to do so.

The basic structure of this model is based on disease causes (*bingyin* 病因),[12] expanded here from a smaller number of such causes in the *Outline*. To achieve internal consistency the model requires the formulation of a number of novel terminological concepts that, while allowing for a systematic presentation of the material, are at odds with the terminology of many important classical texts. One example is the authors' use of "wind damage" (*shangfeng*), which in the *Shanghan lun* tradition is referred to as "wind stroke" (*zhongfeng*)—though the polysemy of that concept caused considerable discussions in later times, as noted in chapter 8. Another is their separation of "wind stroke" (*zhongfeng*) and "internal wind" (*neifeng*). Qin et al., following classical theory, subdivide "wind stroke" into "true wind stroke" (*zhenzhongfeng* 真中风)—caused by the invasion of external evils—and "windlike stroke" (*leizhongfeng* 类中风)—caused by internal pathomechanisms—and keep "internal wind" for wind due to blood and *yin* depletion. The problem here is that for many classical authors and modern physicians "windlike stroke" would be a subcategory of "internal wind." Furthermore, according to the contemporary Chinese critic Zhang Weiyao 张维耀 (1994: 355), Qin et al. also mix up disease classification (*bingming* 病名) and pattern differentiation. Zhang is entitled to this criticism inasmuch as in the *Shanghan lun* (which, as we have seen, is widely taken to be the classical model for contemporary pattern differentiation) terms such as "wind stroke" and "cold damage" designate types of illness caused by common pathogens which are then subdivided into different patterns according to the location and mechanism of the pathology.

Thus, what the model gains in terms of coherence and consistency it loses in terms of being able to hold together various aspects of the Chinese medical tradition. Having studied with one of Qin Bowei's students, I am convinced that his model is highly practicable. Furthermore, it has allowed me personally to tie together (both theoretically and practically) diverse aspects of Chinese medical practice without homogenizing them. Why, then, has the model been forgotten?

Modern Chinese authors such as Zhang Weiyao attribute this to the model's logical errors. Identifying a problem of representation (and thus of truth) as the cause, they hold open the possibility of a future correct solution to an apparently desired model of pattern differentiation that overcomes the heterogeneity still implicit in the *Outline*.[13] Two other interrelated factors already mentioned in chapter 7 seem more important to me: the institutional support accorded to the *Outline* and the inability of Qin's model (lacking institutional authority and power) to reflect the plurality of different theoretical and practical approaches of the Chinese medical tradition with respect to which contemporary practitioners, after all, still define themselves. The *Outline* model, on the other hand, acknowledges heterogeneity—at least on the surface. Yet, by prioritizing some practices over others (namely, those that most easily converge with or express the eight rubrics, especially the differentiation of visceral system patterns), it was from the beginning prone to later homogenization and simplification that is now criticized by eminent *laozhongyi*.

Model 4: Fang Yaozhong's *Seven Lectures*

Fang Yaozhong, whose contributions to the emergence of *bianzheng lunzhi* were pointed out in chapter 7, summed up his theoretical reflections on the topic in the *Seven Lectures on Pattern Differentiation and Treatment Determination Research*. The foreword explicitly acknowledges the importance of integrating disease and pattern differentiation as an achievement of the integration of Chinese and Western medicine but admonishes that the systematization of pattern differentiation is an unfinished aspect of the larger project.

Fang's approach advances from the assumption that visceral manifestation (*zangxiang* 脏象) theory, in spite of heterogeneous and discordant opinions on many of its specific aspects, constitutes the core of Chinese medical theory and therapeutics. In this he follows the lead of the *Outline* and differs from Qin Bowei's emphasis of disease causes as main rubrics for pattern differentiation.[14] In lecture 5, entitled "My Humble Proposal for a Seven Step [Methodology] of Pattern Differentiation and Treatment Determination" (*Bianzheng lunzhi qi bu chuyi* 辨证论治七步刍议) Fang develops an innovative seven-step method for applying pattern differentiation to clinical practice which is graphically summarized and described below.

THE MODEL

TABLE A.3. Pattern Differentiation according to Fang Yaozhong

Step 1	Determining the Location [of the Illness] in the Visceral Systems and/or Channels and Network Vessels (*zangfu jingluo dingwei* 脏腑经络定位)

• On the basis of presenting symptoms and signs
(Hereby is meant the projection of symptoms and signs onto the trajectory of channels and network vessels or the location of visceral systems in the body, e.g., of the relation of lower abdominal or genital pain to the liver.)
• On the basis of visceral functions
(Hereby is meant an awareness of the interrelation of pathology and visceral system physiology, e.g., of blood stasis or *qi* stagnation pain to the liver's function of coursing and expansion of *qi* or of insomnia to the liver's function of storing the human soul and the blood.)
• On the basis of evidence from characteristic reflections of visceral functioning
(Hereby are meant reflections of visceral system function onto particular phenomena governed by their five-phases associations, e.g., of the liver to the sour taste, the green color, the shouting voice, the rancid odor, etc.)
• On the basis of the interrelation of visceral systems, seasons, climates, etc.
(E.g., of the liver to the spring and to wind.)
• On the basis of the interrelation of visceral systems and particular disease causes
(E.g., of the liver with anger and depression.)
• On the basis of taking into account constitutional factors, body types, age, sex, etc.
(Hereby is meant an awareness of the liver as the root of the female and therefore its importance in gynecological problems, or of the liver's association with growth and development and therefore with pediatric problems.)

• On the basis of illness development and treatment response
(Hereby is meant, for instance, an awareness of the liver's location in the lower *jiao* and therefore its involvement in the later stages of warm diseases, i.e., those that have penetrated to the lower *jiao*.)

Step 2	Determining the Nature [of the Illness Process] in terms of yin/yang, *qi*/blood, interior/exterior, depletion/repletion, wind, fire, damp, dryness, cold, and toxicity (*yin yang qi xue biao li xu shi, feng, huo, shi, zao, han, du dingxing* 阴阳气血表里虚实风火湿燥寒毒定性)

• On the basis of the characteristics of clinical symptoms and signs
(Hereby is meant the fact that illness processes exhibit characteristic features that can be characterized by the above qualifiers, e.g., of red eyes or burning urination as being related to fire.)
• On the basis of the onset and development of an illness
(Hereby is meant, for instance, an awareness that *yang* type problems are relatively acute, reflect a short illness process, occur relatively more often in children or before middle age, etc.)

Step 3	Determining both Location and Character [of the Illness Process] (*dingwei dingxing hecan* 定位定性合参)

• Referring to a more precise differentiation of the illness process by jointly considering visceral system function and physiology/pathology and of the illness process as described by the categories wind, fire, damp, dryness, and cold
(Hereby is meant a process whereby the physician arrives at a designation of an illness process as being one of, for instance, liver wind, liver fire, liver damp, liver dryness, or liver cold.)

Step 4	Giving Priority to Earlier [Phases of the Illness Process] in Terms of the Five Types of Overcoming (*bi xian wu sheng* 必先五胜)

• Referring to reflecting on the illness process in terms of five-phases visceral system relationships
(Hereby is meant the interpretation of changes of symptoms and signs that have occurred in the course of the unfolding of an illness in terms of their five-phases relationships, e.g., of a lung illness being located solely within its own domain of structural or functional unfolding or of it having been caused by an illness in any of the other visceral systems via the producing [*sheng* 生] or controlling [*ke* 克] cycles.)

Step 5   "To Sort Each into Its Category" (*ge si qi shu* 各司其属)

• While referring in a wider sense to all the above processes, the proverb is used here to the alignment of therapeutic strategies with previously diagnosed illness processes

(Hereby is meant the selection of formulas and drugs according to specific treatment strategies that correct the previously diagnosed problematics: e.g., the selection of drugs and formulas to course the liver [*shu gan* 疏肝] for an illness process located in the liver which is relatively acute and characterized by depression [*yu* 郁] and anger [*nu* 怒]).

Step 6   "To Treat the Illness, Seek the Root" (*zhi bing qiu ben* 治病求本)

• Treating not only the illness as determined in steps 1–3, but also its cause as determined in step 4

(Hereby is meant the selection of a treatment strategy according to the same criteria discussed in step 5 to treat the root).

Step 7   "Develop [Treatment] ahead of the Dynamic [of the Disorder]" (*fa yu ji xian* 发于机先)

• Considering physiological visceral system interrelations even where they are not actively implicated in the presenting illness

(This means taking into account visceral system interrelations according to the producing and conquering sequences of five-phases theory even where these visceral systems are not yet involved in the pathology: e.g., as in cases of liver exuberance there is a danger of either the spleen or the lungs being adversely affected, the relationship between these visceral systems and the liver may be taken into account in the formulation of treatment strategies).

COMMENT

I have chosen to present Fang Yaozhong's contribution to the systematization of *bianzheng lunzhi* for a variety of reasons. First, because in the arrangements of its seven steps it is more clearly than Qin Bowei's model concerned with clinical rather than representational ends (though the differences here are those of relative weightings rather than of categorically different objectives). I find Fang's clear commitment to treating what is not yet ill (*weibing* 未病) as an important aspect of routine medical practice particularly interesting. It is an important difference from Qin Bowei's model, which focuses (at least in the way it is presented) solely on the root of present conditions.

Second, Fang's model shows how the same elements included in the other models can be recombined in yet another way. Fang also uses the eight rubrics, but he merges them with disease causes into a category of tools that then are used as secondary classifiers of visceral function. Each model thus can be said to use the same set of tools, to synthesize a different type of clinical practice.

Third, Fang's model emphasizes yet another core aspect of traditional Chinese medicine: five phases (*wu xing* 五行) theory. Although both Fang's model and the contemporary textbooks that derive from the *Outline* use visceral functions as central rubrics,[15] only the former brings them to life by emphasizing their five-phases interrelations while the latter highlight biomedically influenced physiological transformations of substances.

My aim is not to discuss these differences in detail at this point. My presentation suffices to demonstrate the heterogeneity of pattern differentiation in contemporary Chinese medicine even as it underlines the commitment of its practitioners to develop systematic practices.

NOTES

Introduction

1 These reach from academic works such as Farquhar 1994a; Lu and Needham 1980; Porkert 1978; Sivin 1987; and Unschuld 1985, 1986a, 1986b to texts for practicing clinicians such as Bensky and Barolet 1990; Bensky and Gamble 1993; Maciocia 1989; Nanjing College of TCM 1990; Porkert 1983; Porkert and Hempen 1986 to introductory texts for the general reader such as Hoizey and Hoizey 1993; and Kaptchuk 1983. For an accessible introduction to Chinese medicine that provides readers with all the background necessary to follow the argument in this book, readers may wish to consult Bray 1993.

2 See the discussions by Needham and Lu (1975), Sivin (1997), and Wiseman (1995: 1–80) and the essays collected in Unschuld 1989.

3 Besides Wiseman's dictionary (1995), these included Bensky 1998; Porkert 1978; and Sivin 1987.

4 I have long struggled with this issue. Methodologically, my ethnography is based almost entirely on the observations of friends, teachers, and acquaintances. At the same time, I entirely share the doubts regarding the use of other people for our private purposes at the basis of such research. Such doubts are expressed most emphatically by Farquhar (forthcoming: chapter 1). Use of pseudonyms is a bad compromise. While it would not take too many investigative skills to uncover the real identity of the persons I describe, it nevertheless adds a layer of nontransparency over what should ideally be open.

1. Orientations

1 Dunn's (1976: 147) early analysis of the adaptive capacities of Chinese medicine has since been supported by the more detailed scholarship of historians such as Sivin (1987) and Unschuld (1985, 1986a). Francesca Bray (1993) provides the most easily accessible overview of the historical development of Chinese medicine for nonexperts.

2   While these statements are based on my own fieldwork experience, additional evidence can easily be found in the voluminous writings that detail the case histories of famous physicians in the history of Chinese medicine. Representative collections from premodern China are Qin Bowei 亲伯未 1928; Shi Qi 施杞 and Xiao Mincai 萧敏材 1993; and Wang Xinhua 王新华 1998. For contemporary examples, see Chen Youbang 陈佑邦 and Deng Liangming 邓良明 1987; Dong Jianhua 董建华 1990; and Shi Yuguang 史字广 and Shan Shujian 单书健 1992. Translations into Western languages of various quality include Chen 1988; Hammes and Ots 1994; and Zhang 1994.

3   The literature documenting plurality and syncretism within medicine and science is too large to list in detail. Exemplary ethnographies of non-Western therapeutic practices include Brodwin 1996; Fardon 1995a; Greenwood 1992; Last 1992; Leslie 1992; and Obeyesekere 1992. Plurality and syncretism in biomedicine are documented by an increasing number of studies, for example, Berg and Mol 1998; Hahn 1983; Lock and Gordon 1988; and Rhodes 1990. For examinations of plurality in science at large, see Galison 1996; and Gieryn 1999.

4   I use the terms "first" and "second-order inquiries" because I find that more conventional distinctions, such as descriptive/analytic, emic/etic, and analytic/metaanalytic, do not capture the intended difference. Both first- and second-order inquiries are analytic and metaanalytic, while certain second-order inquiries are not only carried out by scientists but are part of the Chinese medical tradition itself. And is an examination of Chinese medicine by a Chinese scholar versed equally in Chinese medicine and Western aesthetics (Wang Xudong 王旭东 1989) emic or etic?

5   Sivin 1987: 25–26.

6   The dissociation of what I call second-order inquiries from first-order inquiries is a product of the separation between scholarship and practice that occurred as a result of the formation of the modern academy. In medical history, for instance, this separation occurred in the course of the nineteenth century. Before that time physicians in the West continued to utilize the texts of earlier physicians to guide their own practice, something Chinese medical physicians but also Western homeopaths and herbalists continue to do to this day. See Rosenberg 1992: 1.

7   These subjects are taught as academic subdisciplines at universities and colleges of Chinese medicine; see, for example, Qiu Peiran 裘沛然 and Ding Guangdi 丁光迪 1992; and Zhen Zhiya 甄志亚 and Fu Weikang 傅维康 1991. Both disciplines are sometimes referred to as "academic disciplines devoted to sorting out the Chinese medical literature" (zhongyi wenxian zhengli zhuanye 中医文献整理专业); for example, Wang Songbao 汪松葆 1987: 63. The field of history of Chinese medicine emerged in China during the early part of this century when Chinese medicine was under threat by modernizers, as shown by Hinrichs (1998).

8   Baer et al. 1997: 9. Medical pluralism emerged as a topic of anthropological research during the 1970s among ethnographers particularly of Asian societies,

where health care experts struggled to explain the continued vitality of traditional medical practices long after the introduction of biomedicine. The dominant perspective at the time was modernization theory, which held that medical practices were reflections of theoretical models about the world and that obsolete models would eventually yield to better ones. Anthropologists, instead, suggested that viewing medical traditions as cultural systems provided better explanations of actual behavior. The anthropological literature on medical pluralism and the different theoretical positions elaborated within it is too large to review here. Researchers working in Asian settings who made important contributions to the establishment of the discipline include Dunn (1976), Kleinman (1980), Kunstadter (1976a, 1976b), Leslie (1976b, 1980), Lock (1980), and Unschuld (1973, 1975).

9 Kleinman's (1980) study of health care in Taiwan is an influential example of this approach. The study first sets out the structure of the Taiwanese health care system, differentiating between three distinct health care sectors (popular, folk, and professional) and various medical traditions and beliefs. Kleinman then analyzes health-seeking behavior in terms of individual movements through these sectors. During a given illness episode a patient might originally rely on personal knowledge and advice from family and friends. When such treatment does not work, the patient will cross from the popular to the professional health care sector and choose a practitioner on the basis of culturally specific explanatory models. Treatment within the folk medical sector, at a local shrine or with a shamanic healer, frequently is the last choice for patients who are not helped by professional treatment. At each point of interaction between patients and healers negotiations between different explanatory models regarding the illness episode take place, and the outcome shapes the form treatment takes.

10 Brodwin (1996: 14–16, 190–201) supplies a cogent critique of the standard model of medical pluralism based on his own fieldwork in Haiti.

11 Hsu (1991) and White (1999) show that in both urban and rural Yunnan Province Western medical treatment techniques and pharmaceuticals are appropriated by both Western and Chinese medical practitioners and inserted into explanatory frameworks informed by indigenous discursive categories. The term "traditional Chinese medicine," on the other hand, is the official Ministry of Health translation of the Chinese term *zhongyi* (Chinese medicine) and was coined as such only in the 1950s (Taylor, 2000: chapter 3). The influence of Maoist and post-Maoist policy shifts in the constitution of this medicine is analyzed from different perspectives by Croizier (1976), Farquhar (1987, 1994a), Hsu (1999), Sivin (1987), Taylor (2000), and Unschuld (1985, 1992). Biomedicine is a powerful influence in the shaping of such modern "traditional" medicines, not merely in China but also in other contexts such as Japan (Lock 1980, 1990a), Korea (Son 1999), Tibet (Janes 1995, 1999), Hong Kong (Gauld 1998), and Taiwan (Chi et al. 1996). For a more general discussion, see particularly Worsely 1982.

12 These issues were raised for the first time in exemplary fashion by Charles Leslie

(1976a) in the introduction to *Asian Medical Systems: A Comparative Study*, a collection of essays that marked a breakthrough in challenging previous analyses of Asian medicines carried out in terms of positivist or modernist discourse. See also the follow-up volume edited by Leslie and Young (1992).

13 There are two types of proponents of this argument. The first is positivist and accords value to Chinese medicine merely as a repository of empirical knowledge (Chen 1961). This line is taken frequently by biomedical practitioners (including proponents of Western medicine in China) in their struggles with Chinese medicine. The second school opposes such positivism and grounds medical practice in a mixture of specific effects, myths, ritual, and so on, but arrives in this way at a view of Chinese medicine as being constituted by "unrelated and irreconcilable" systems (Cooper 1973: 270).

14 Sivin 1987; Farquhar 1994a.

15 This implication underlies Porkert's (1978) effort to reconstitute through philology an originally systematic Chinese medicine that according to him has been lost in the process of its transmission. Sivin (1990) makes a similar suggestion but attributes the loss of authenticity to the effects of modern (i.e., post-1949) transformations, an observation shared by Porkert (1998) in later essays. Both authors are quite explicit about the negative effects of this perceived loss of authenticity on clinical practice.

16 Unschuld 1992.

17 Farquhar 1994a: 223.

18 "Traditional Chinese Medicine" is the official English translation used by the state to designate the state-authorized practice of Chinese medicine in contemporary China. Its origin dates to 1955 (Taylor 2000: chapter 3).

19 Seltzer 1992: 6.

20 In contemporary postcolonial writings the term "Orientalism" is most commonly employed to denote the manner in which the non-Western is represented to the West so as to facilitate its exploitation and suppression within imperialist and neo-imperialist practices. This reading of the term originates with Said's (1985) path-breaking work on the Middle East. A less critical use of the term sees in Orientalism the various ways in which the West employs Asian thought to solve its own intellectual or practical problems (Clarke 1997).

21 STS is an interdisciplinary field with disciplinary links to anthropology, cultural studies, feminist studies, history, philosophy, political science, rhetoric, social psychology, and sociology of science and technology. Useful reviews and overviews of the field are provided by Golinski (1988), Franklin (1995), Hess (1997a, 1997b), Traweek (1993), and Woolgar (1988).

22 I say "quasi apprenticeship" to distinguish it from the formal apprenticeships described in chapter 6. However, inasmuch as my teacher frequently refers to me as "his disciple" when introducing me to colleagues and friends, it would be more correct to say that our relationship attests to the plurality of discipleship in contemporary Chinese medicine.

23 The main reason for this is undoubtedly Beijing's role as the state capital and its dominance in the control and allocation of state funds, but also the fact that, as in the United Kingdom, experimental policies are often tried out first in faraway regions.

24 Such informal tests consisted in assessing my diagnostic skills, acupuncture needle technique, memorization of classical prescriptions, and familiarity with the teachings of famous physicians. They were used to define my status as a student as much as to provide entertainment to my interlocutors and their patients—or, if I should be able to come up with the right answer, to increase their face vis-à-vis their patients by showing just what sort of foreigner came to study with them.

25 One aspect of this is my deliberate focus on prominent physicians who lived and worked in Beijing throughout the various case studies presented in this book. Because I am attempting to examine transformations of Chinese medicine, it seemed appropriate to focus on physicians whose influence on these transformations is documented. Thus, when I speak of "famous" or "influential" physicians, I mean that they were known to all my informants, or that their case histories or biographies have been published, or that their influence on the shaping of Chinese medicine is acknowledged by contemporary Chinese historians. Besides the specific sources cited, bibliographic information on these physicians can be found in Li Jingwei 李经纬 1988; Li Yun 李云 1988; and Shi Yuguang 史宇广 1991.

26 One might read, for instance, Ong 1995; and Yang 1988, 1995 in the context of the debates narrated by Wang (1996).

27 The relation between official and folk practices in contemporary China is constantly evolving. While, on the one hand, official efforts at scientizing practices such as qigong 气功 continue unabated (Kubny 1995: 10.1), mainland research into spirit-medium practices has recently "developed a cachet" (Hinrichs 1998: n. 26).

28 Taylor (1999) shows that the negative connotations associated with the term jiu 旧 (which I have translated as "old and backward") emerged in the course of the communist revolution, a period marked by a great pressure for all things to become "new" (xin 新)—a new China, a new economy, a new culture, a new medicine. The term "old" (jiu 旧) thus came to stand for all things backward that had to be got rid of in order to establish the new. One of the terms used for Chinese medicine at the time was "old medicine" (jiu yi 旧医). From the mid 1950s onward, when more value was again placed on the merits of indigenous Chinese culture, this term was phased out and the term "ancient medicine" (gudai yixue 古代医学) was employed instead to refer to the Chinese medicine of the past that could be adapted to the needs of the present "Chinese medicine" (zhongyi). The designation "traditional Chinese medicine" (known in the West under its acronym, TCM) was reserved exclusively for foreign-language publications. Taylor argues that this was due to the different effects intended by the use of these various terms. Whereas within China it was important to emphasize that the past could be transformed to suit the present, in the West the continuity of tradition provided a more favorable image.

29 Biographies of Hua Tuo are contained in both the *Sanguo zhi* 三国志 (*Record of the Three Kingdoms*) and the *Hou han shu* 后汉书 (*History of the Later Han*). See De-Woskin 1983: 140–53 for translations. Regarding the apotheosis and iconography of Sun Simiao, see Unschuld 1994. For biographical details, see also Sivin 1968: 81–144. For an exemplary biography of a physician within the Chinese medicine establishment who consciously draws on Buddhist, Daoist, and empirical medical traditions, see Ilg 2001.

30 Farquhar 1996a, 1996b; Hsu 1992; Ots 1994. The encounter between the state and the popular *Falungong* 法论功 movement that was ongoing while I was complet-ing the manuscript for this book will provide valuable insights into articulations between the religious, medical, and scientific domains in contemporary China.

31 *Journal of Chinese Medicine News* 1997; Wang Zhipu 王致谱 and Cai Jingfeng 蔡景峰 1999, 67–70.

32 Ma Boying 马伯英 et al. 1994; Unschuld 1986.

33 Various aspects of the modernization of Chinese medicine throughout the last cen-tury are discussed in Andrews 1996, 1997; Ågren 1974; Croizier 1968, 1976; Deng Tietao 邓铁涛 1999; Hsu 1999; Jia 1997; Lei 1998; Sivin 1987; Taylor 2000; and Zhao Hongjun 赵洪钧 1989.

34 The assimilation of Chinese medicine into therapeutic practice in the West is ana-lyzed by Baer et al. (1998), Barnes (1998), and Hare (1993). Hsu (1995, 1996) docu-ments the transformation of therapeutic practices in the commerce between China and the West.

35 By "contemporary" I mean the 1980s and 1990s, though I have tried to contextual-ize it at least to the period from 1949 to the present. By "China" I mean the People's Republic of China, though see my notes regarding Beijing above. I make no claims to have thereby defined the boundaries of "contemporary China."

36 Appadurai 1990, 1995; Featherstone 1990; Hannerz 1992; and Robertson 1992 pro-vide different influential perspectives on the issue of globalization, a topic that has become too large to summarize or reference.

37 Markus and Fischer 1986; and Clifford 1988 are seminal works in this respect. See also the essays collected in Ahmed and Shore 1995.

38 Sahlins 1993: 15–16.

39 Asad 1973; Said 1985.

40 Latour 1993.

41 Strathern 1995a, 1995b.

42 I could, of course, also have used etic categories derived from anthropological dis-course such as "cosmopolitan medicine." This would have presented me with the even greater problem, however, of having to justify my choice vis-à-vis both Chi-nese medicine and medical anthropology.

43 He Yumin 何裕民 1987: 1–17.

44 For examples, see Chen Li 陈离 1991; Jia Dedao 贾得道 1993; Shi Lanhua 史兰化 1992; and Zhen Zhiya 甄志亚 and Fu Weikang 傅维康 1991.

45 One of the most prominent and influential of these theoreticians was the scholar-physician Ren Yingqiu 任应秋 (1914–1984), whose collected writings (1984a) are representative of this effort. Ren, in turn, draws on earlier efforts by scholars such as Xie Guan 谢观 1935. See also the work of Qin Bowei 秦伯未, whose concerns for standardization begin in the 1920s (1929) and extend to the 1960s (1983e).

46 While this particular historical vision is firmly rooted in Marxian dialectic materialism and associates medical practices and ideas with specific social formations, it never surrenders to an entirely Western modernism in which the older is consecutively replaced by the newer. The old can still possess value within the new, and modern physicians, therefore, must continue to study the work of ancient masters. See the discussion on the difference between "old" and "ancient" in note 28 above.

47 Much more could be said on this. I find the analysis of the French philosopher François Jullien (1999) regarding essential differences between Chinese and Western conceptions of agency and efficacy most instructive. If Jullien is correct, then the difficulties described here are a direct result not only of problems in translation but also of our concern for and manner of creating theoretical models.

48 Good 1994; Spivak and Harasym 1990. The same may be said of scientists at large, of course, though this is rarely admitted as yet by natural scientists. Hence, the ongoing efforts by writers within STS to demystify science and the backlash against critical intellectuals by the scientific establishment particularly in the United States—the so-called science wars.

49 Archer 1996: 3. Archer's critical analysis concerns the use of early ethnographic work in the theory of culture. It does not take account of decisive transformations in anthropology since. For a review of distributionist thinking in earlier anthropology, see Pelto and Pelto 1975.

50 This is the view of Sir Edmund Leach (1964: 7).

51 Hannerz 1992 is an attempt to rethink cultural complexity within the boundaries of classical culture theory as a problem of the flow of meaning. The book includes a brief review of distributionist anthropology since the 1970s (10–15 and 271–72, n. 10).

52 The term "holism" carries many meanings. I do not use it here as reflecting the connection, in anthropological explanation, of elements from heterogeneous social domains (which I endorse), but rather as the search for explanations that see culture as one interconnected whole.

53 Schwartz 1993.

54 Appadurai 1986: 357. In my opinion this is not a "reverse Orientalism" but simply Orientalism, for Orientalism is the very practice by which the other can be so constructed as to always occupy an inferior or subaltern position. I have left the quote, however, as it appears in the original.

55 Latour (1987) notes that Western colonial discourse tends to imagine that culture is something that distinguishes others but does not apply to itself. The very foundation of STS is the disallowance of such asymmetrical explanation (Bloor 1976).

56 Farquhar and Hevia 1993: 486. A similar point is made by Latour (1987), who shows that the aggregation of anthropological knowledge in Western metropolitan centers reflects imbalances of trade and capital accumulation.

57 Turner (1994: chapter 1) identifies Ihering and Burkhardt as the authors most influential in bringing the role of *Sitten*, or culturally variant suppositions, to the attention of mainstream philosophy and social theory in Germany. Among British political theorists he refers to Hobbes, Berkeley, and Hume. See Kuper 1999 for a detailed investigation of the anthropological idea of culture from early twentieth-century accounts to the theories of Geertz, Schneider, Sahlins, and their successors.

58 Luhmann 1995: 28.

59 The Kantian influence on anthropology is discussed by Bloch (1985). On Montesquieu as the first comparative sociologist, see Baum 1979. Montesquieu's essay *De l'esprit des lois* argued that each social system has its own law of development, a "holistic" view clearly akin to British structuralist-functionalist anthropology and the concepts of culture, tradition, and so on, discussed above.

60 See McLennan 1995 for a succinct overview of contemporary interpretations of pluralism and their problems.

61 Rosaldo 1995: xv. The terms "hybrid" and "hybridity" are much used in postcolonial theory and also in STS. See Shaw and Stewart 1994 for a discussion regarding the use of terms such as "syncretism," "hybridity," "creolization," and "bricolage."

62 George Marcus (1995) perceptively links this monist bias of anthropology and the framework of accommodation and resistance that it generates (see n. 59 above) to the focus on single fieldwork sites in conventional anthropology. He suggests that this is being overcome by the current movement within the discipline toward "multisited ethnography." It is interesting that Marcus, too, identifies STS as an important inspiration for this shift. See chapter 2 in this volume for further discussion.

63 This implies not a rejection of anthropology but rather the assertion that even though researchers in SSK had borrowed from anthropology, they did not have to refer back to that tradition for approval. Three main uses of the ethnographic method in the SSK literature can be distinguished. The first involves extensive fieldwork at a laboratory site in order to familiarize oneself with how science works. For Collins and Pinch (1982) the goal was an interpretive understanding of scientific practice, for Latour and Woolgar (1986) a demystification of science by recording the mundane nature of its functioning. A second perception of ethnography characteristic of STS is its intent to distance itself from science (something about which educated sociologists of science as well as their readers will have certain ideas) by perceiving and portraying it as something "strange" (Latour and Woolgar 1986; Woolgar 1988). The third use borrows from anthropology the idea of reflexive ethnography to problematize one's own writings (Woolgar and Ashmore 1988).

64 Hess 1997.

65 Rouse 1992; Hess 1997a; Haraway 1991; and Traweek 1992 all make different suggestions in this direction. See also the essays collected in Downey and Dumit 1997, which demonstrate the seminal influence of Haraway's cyborg model for this kind of intervention. Neither of the lables used (STS, SSK-STS, critical STS) implies that we are dealing with homogeneous traditions. For a review of its diversity but also the many existing interconnections between these traditions and between STS and other academic disciplines such as anthropology, history, and cultural studies, see Hess 1997b.

66 This distinguishes my ethnography from that of anthropologists of science such as Traweek (1988) and Gusterson (1996), who examine science through established anthropological frameworks. There are several excellent explorations of medicine situated at the borderland of medical anthropology, STS, feminist scholarship, and cultural studies—which, however, all examine biomedicine; for example, Cussins 1988; Haraway 1993; Martin 1987; Rapp 1997; and Young 1995. By thus excluding other medical traditions from its purview, even critical STS strengthens the very borders it apparently questions: "Science for the West, Myth for the Rest?" (Scott 1996). More recently, though, Lei (1999) has examined the modernization of Chinese medicine from an STS perspective.

67 MacIntyre 1984.

2. Plurality and Synthesis

1 The translations are taken from Ames 1984. In Chinese each term carries additional connotative meanings from its uses in particular types of discourse. In neo-Confucianism, for instance, ti 体, the essence of something, is opposed to yong 用, its manifestations or uses.

2 Some examples are debates about the relation of the spirit (shen 神) to the heart (xin 心) and brain (nao 脑) (e.g., Deadman and Al-Khafaji 1995: 32–33; and Ma et al. 1994: 480–85); the emergence, recently, of the new subdiscipline of Chinese medical psychology (zhongyi xinlixue 中医心理学) (e.g., Wang Miqu 土米渠 et al. 1986); and the existence of different perceptions about the relation between body and mind even within one textual tradition (e.g., Chiu 1986). Both Sivin (1987: 81) and Farquhar (1994b) see this openness as resulting from a focus in Chinese medicine on body process rather than structure.

3 Suwen 8; Lingshu 18.

4 Nanjing 25 and 38; see also Nanjing 31.

5 Bensky (1996: 64 n. 58, 105), Porkert (1978: 158–62), Sivin (1987: 120, 125 n. 13), and Unschuld (1986b: 356) provide various summaries of these debates from the first mentioning of the sanjiao occurrence in the Shiji (Historical Records) of the first century B.C. to the late 1970s.

6 Zhang Xichun 张锡纯 (Yixue zhongzhong canxi lu, 2:194–96), for instance, asso-

ciates the *sanjiao* with the great omentum, in which he follows Tang Zonghai 唐宗海. Cf. *Zhongxi huitong yijing jingyi* 中西汇通医经经义 (*The Essential Meaning of the Medical Classics from the Perspective of the Convergence of Chinese and Western Medicine*): *Zangfu zhi guan* 脏腑之官 (*Offices of the Internal Visceral Systems*), 1: 22. Porkert (1978: 161) cites the two German acupuncturists Bachmann and Schmitt as establishing links between the *sanjiao* and the endocrine system instead.

7   *Suwen* 8 states that the *sanjiao* "holds the office of clearing drains; the water pathways emerge from it" (*juedu zhi guan, shuidao chu yan* 决渎之官, 水道出焉). *Nanjing* 46 states that the *sanjiao* "is a special envoy that transmits the original influences" (*yuanqi zhi bie shi ye* 原气之别使也). For a summary of the ensuing debates in the history of Chinese medicine, see Zhang Weiyao 张维耀 1994: 294–96.

8   *Lingshu* 10 and 12 pair the *sanjiao* with the pericardium. *Lingshu* 47 pairs it instead with the bladder.

9   Several authors have examined the historical diversity of thinking about disease in Chinese medicine. Epler (1977) illustrates a wide range of ideas concerning disease and its nature, pathology, and etiology current in the scholar-officialdom of third-century China. Chiu (1986) finds at least three different models for perceiving health and illness in the *Neijing* tradition. Furth (1988, 1999) examines in detail the development of *fuke* 妇科 (gynecology) in Chinese medicine from its origins in the Song. She argues that women's medicine was informed by quite specific concerns regarding a "female gestational body" (vis-à-vis the "androgynous body of generation" of classical medicine). Any internal unity of thought and practice had to be enforced from above, as Hinrichs's (1995) examination of the "transformations of southern customs" in the Northern Song shows. For general overviews, see Ma Boying 马伯英 1993 and Unschuld 1985; as well as Hinrichs's 1998 bibliographic review of recent Chinese and Western scholarly research.

10 "Die chinesische Medizin passt sich der modernen Welt an," Xinhua News Agency, 2–11 November 1992, cited in *ChinaMed* 1 (1), 1993.

11 These are differentiations of patterns (*bianzheng* 辨证) according to pathologies of the *zangfu*; the channels and collaterals (*jingluo* 经络); the four aspects *wei, qi, ying, xue* (卫气营血); the six stages (*liu jing* 六经); the *sanjiao*; according to disease causes (*bingyin* 病因); and according to pathologies of spirit (*shen* 神) *qi*, blood (*xue* 血), and body fluids (*jingye* 津液). For more detailed discussions, see Farquhar 1994a: chapter 4; and Deng Tietao 邓铁涛 1987. See also chapter 7 on the emergence of pattern differentiation as the "pivot" of contemporary Chinese medicine.

12 I have in mind here such methods as differentiation of disharmony between "ascending" (*sheng* 升) and "directing down" (*jiang* 降), differentiation on the basis of presumed constitutional types, "disease differentiation" (*bianbing* 辨病) in contradistinction to the more often described pattern differentiation, and the "moving *qi* doctrine" (*yunqi xueshuo* 运气学说). For a detailed discussion of currently employed diagnostic methods, see Ma Zhongxue 麻仲学 1991.

13 The Chinese state is trying, though, to establish these by enforcing standards of diagnosis and treatment. See chapter 7 and Wang Zhipu 王致谱 and Cai Jingfeng 蔡景峰 1999, 60.

14 Unschuld 1987.

15 Kuriyama 1986: 75–86 includes a concise summary of historical debates regarding pulse diagnosis. See also Zhao Enjian 赵恩俭 1990 for a more complete discussion.

16 Since the mid-1950s an entire subdiscipline of academic Chinese medicine has been devoted to researching medical streams (*yixue liupai* 医学流派) and scholarly disputes (*xueshu zhengming* 学术争鸣). See the introduction to Qiu Peiran 裘沛然 and Ding Guangdi 丁光迪 1992 for a historical overview of such traditions and contemporary Chinese research. The emergence of this tradition can be dated to the early Republican period, when the first books on the history of Chinese medicine were produced from within the field of Chinese medicine itself. Xie Guan's 谢观 *Zhongguo yixue yuanliu lun* 中国医学源流论 (*On the Origins and Development of Chinese Medicine*), published in Shanghai in 1935, is frequently referred to as the seminal text in the tradition.

17 The commentaries on the *Nanjing* collected by Unschuld (1986b) provide a telling example. Contemporary Chinese scholars provide us with similar collections of divergent commentaries on other classics, such as Cheng Shide 程士德 1987 for the *Huangdi Neijing*; Li Peisheng 李培生 and Liu Duzhou 刘渡舟 1987 for the *Shanghan lun* 伤寒论 (*Discussions of Cold Damage*); Li Keguang 李克光 1989 for the *Jingui yaolue* 金匮要略 (*Essentials of the Golden Casket*); and Xu Jiqun 许济群 and Wang Mianzhi 王绵之 1995 for the study of formulas. Published case records are a genre used by many physicians, past and present, to demonstrate their superior skills and knowledge. Numerous examples can be found in Shi Qi 施杞 and Xiao Mincai 萧敏材 1993.

18 One example is the acumoxa method known as "draining the south and supplementing the north" (*bu beifang xie nanfang* 补北方泻南方), first mentioned in *Nanjing* 75. I personally have encountered three different interpretations in practice. For a discussion of the medical literature on the topic, see Wang Ziqiang 王自强 1994: 336–41.

19 This point is emphasized in Sivin 1987: 21.

20 Unschuld 1979: 118. See also Bodenschatz in preparation; Hsu 1999; Hymes 1987; and Wu 1993 for ethnographic and historical examinations of changing conceptions of what it means to be a physician of Chinese medicine.

21 Throughout this book I use the term "stream" to translate the Chinese *pai* 派, which has the original meaning "to branch off, like a river." I will discuss this important term in a forthcoming study. I am grateful to Marta Hanson for discussing its meaning with me. Wu (1993, 4: 37 n. 5) shows how diverse modes of transmission can all be found within one medical stream. What precisely constitutes a medical stream and how such streams should be defined and analyzed is not at all clear to contemporary scholar-physicians within the Chinese medical tradition. See, for

example, Ren Yingqiu 任应秋 1981, Gu Zhishan 顾植山 1982, and Qiu Peiran 裘沛然 and Ding Guangdi 丁光迪 1992: Introduction.

22　The development of Chinese medicine in contemporary China is discussed in chapter 3.

23　Guo Mingxin 郭铭信 1980.

24　Andrews 1996; Deng Tietao 邓铁涛 1999: 31–100; Ma Boying 马伯英 et al. 1994; and Unschuld 1985: chapter 9.2 provide historical accounts of the influence of Western medicine on and its assimilation into Chinese medicine up to the Republican period.

25　Kwok (1965) discusses the rise of scientism in China in the first half of this century, while Hua (1995) surveys its influence in post-Mao China. According to Hua (ibid.: 145), "the Chinese obsession with science was disrupted only twice in the last century"—during the Great Leap Forward and the Cultural Revolution. See, however, Hui 1997, which shows that the connotations of what science stood and stands for in China were channeled through historically particular exegetical paradigms.

26　Lei (1998) provides the most detailed analysis of this process in English. He argues that during the Republican period Western medicine doctors succeeded in establishing dominance over Chinese medicine doctors by controlling the state's medical machinery. After Western medicine doctors turned the construction of a national medical-administrative system into a state project in 1929, Chinese medicine doctors, in order to survive, were forced to compete within this system and to accept its perception of science and modernity. For other analyses of this struggle, see Croizier 1968; Xu 1997; and Zhao Hongjun 赵洪钧 1989.

27　The transformation of Chinese medicine after 1949 is the subject of Kim Taylor's doctoral dissertation at the University of Cambridge (Taylor 2000).

28　Various aspects of this process are analyzed in Andrews 1996, 1997; Deng Tietao 邓铁涛 1999: 74–93, 228–68; Hsu 1996; Scheid 1995a, 1999; Taylor 2000 and White 1993, 1999.

29　The introduction to Zhang Weiyao 张维耀 1994: 1 contains a discussion of these terms from a contemporary Chinese perspective. See also Taylor 1999.

30　This, at least, is the conclusion reached by various Western commentators such as Sivin (1987) and Unschuld (1992). It is confirmed by my own fieldwork.

31　For an illustrative case study, see Liscomb 1993. This influence is attested in the life and work of many other classical and contemporary physicians such as Xue Shengbai 薛生百 (1681–1770), Fei Boxiong 费伯雄 (1800–1879), Cheng Menxue 程门雪 (1902–1972), Qin Bowei 秦伯未 (1901–1970) and Qiu Peiran 裘沛然 (1916–) and was emphasized by many of my own teachers. The connection between art and Chinese medicine is discussed in Qiu Peiran 裘沛然 1995. The small volume includes poems and calligraphies by the author, an eminent scholar-physician in Shanghai (see Zhongguo kexue jishu xiehui 中国科学技术协会 1999: 263–80). See also Hay 1984. The topic clearly deserves to be studied in much greater detail.

32　See Barnes 1998; MacPherson and Kaptchuk 1996; Scheid 1995b; and Unschuld 1997: 106–33 for examples.

33 See Hsu 1995 for a fascinating case study. In the following I will place "traditional" and "modern" in quotation marks to indicate that I think of them as constructed and not as given categories of analysis.

34 See, for instance, Kubny 1995.

35 Some examples are the transformation of madness from a medical into a legal problem in late imperial China discussed by Ng (1990); the integration of neurasthenia into Chinese medical practice in the early part of the twentieth century and its translation into the indigenous illness category *shenjing shuairuo* 神经衰弱, which was facilitated by its affinity to established Chinese medical illness categories; the current transformation of *shenjing shuairuo* into the popular "Western" disease category of depression (*yiyuzheng* 抑郁症) discussed by Lee (1999); and the emergence of women's medicine (*fuke* 妇科) as a specialist discipline of Chinese medicine from the Song onward (Furth 1999).

36 I have in mind here the debate regarding the relation of Chinese medical practice to the literary canon or that between advocates of culture and practice theories in anthropology. Plurality of practice is thus variously interpreted as a loss of the systematicity inherent in canonical texts (Porkert 1978) or of its as yet insufficient systematization (Lu and Needham 1980), as a reflection of a timeless cultural aesthetic (Unschuld 1990) or the constellation of practice (Farquhar 1994a).

37 The quote is from Hua 1995: 145. Regarding scientism in China, see note 25 above. For a general overview of the history of modernization in China since the Qing, see the *Cambridge History of China* (Twitchett et al. 1978: vols. 10–15).

38 That "modern" and premodern Chinese medicine are different is today an orthodoxy in China expressed in the terms "ancient medicine" (*gudai yixue* 古代医学) used to refer to the old Chinese medicine and "Chinese medicine" (*zhongyi* 中医, officially translated as "traditional Chinese medicine") used to refer to contemporary Chinese medicine (Taylor 1999). Western authors who appear to hold this view include Andrews 1996; Hsu 1999; Lei 1998; Sivin 1987; Taylor 2000 and Unschuld 1992.

39 There are innumerable ways to define modernity, and my list is by no means meant to be complete. Weber (1968) provides the most commonly cited reference, pointing to such factors as rationalization, mechanization, bureaucratization, secularization, and the disenchantment of social and religious life. More recent attempts to define the uniqueness of modernity include Berman 1982; Foucault 1979; Giddens 1990, 1991; and Habermas 1987.

40 Two exemplary studies relevant to the Chinese context are on policing (Wakeman 1995) and education (Bailey 1990).

41 Interestingly, Andrews (1996) discusses modernization and specifically defers an examination of the influence of nationalism to a later date while Croizier (1968) emphasizes the latter.

42 Hsu (1999), for instance, separates three distinct types of knowledge transmission associated with what she perceives of as modern and traditional types of reasoning, while Lei (1998) teases out a distinct point of transition.

43 In the literature a distinction is often made between "needling" (*cifa* 刺法), referring to needle selection and insertion, and "manipulation" (*shoufa*), referring to the manipulation of the needle after insertion in order to achieve a supplementing (*bu* 补) or draining (*xie* 泻) effect. In conversation *shoufa* seems to encompass both aspects.

44 Chen Kezheng 陈克正 1992; He Puren 贺普仁 1989; Zhang Ji 张吉 1994.

45 Hsu 1995 documents and analyzes the rapid assimilation of auricular acupuncture developed in France in the 1950s into "traditional" Chinese medicine.

46 The different modernity offered by noncapitalist and non-Western societies has been the stimulus in homogenizing perceptions of modernity as derived from the Enlightenment and the Industrial Revolution in the West. Examples of such critiques with special relevance to the Chinese case are Ong 1995, 1997; Rofel 1992, 1999; and Yang 1988.

47 The process of this construction is discussed in detail in chapter 7. For a detailed description and analysis of pattern differentiation, see Farquhar 1994. The difference between Farquhar's position and my own is that what she identifies as a stable form of cultural agency underlying the plurality of actual practice is for me a process tending to the standardization of such practice.

48 Personal information provided by Professor Li Ding 李鼎, Shanghai. See also Zehentmayer and Scorzon 2000. Professor Li has been instrumental in the development of acumoxa since the 1950s, developing, for instance, the charts of channels on which teaching in contemporary schools and universities is based.

49 There are several theoretical frameworks through which these issues are discussed in the anthropological literature. Two particular influential perspectives are Foucault's (1980, 1990) conceptualization of power/knowledge and the postcolonial examination of the "subaltern" (people's voices that came into existence as effects of colonial power relations but are written out of official histories) originating from the work of a group of mainly Indian scholars known as the Subaltern Studies Group (see Prakash 1990). For exemplary ethnographies relating to China, see Dutton 1998; Ong 1987; and Yang 1994. A critical examination of what has been called "the romance of resistance" is carried out by Lila Abu-Lughod 1990.

50 Porkert (1998), Sivin (1990), and Unschuld (1992) are prominent examples. Many Western practitioners of Chinese medicine, too, perceive a loss of tradition in contemporary China that needs to be recovered in the West, as Barnes (1998) demonstrates. The resonance between these academic and professional positions points to shared but unacknowledged background assumptions regarding the relation of tradition and modernity in their production.

51 Latour 1990, 1993, 1997; Pickering 1995. For some critical perspectives, see Amsterdamska 1990; Bloor 1999; Gingras 1995, 1997; and Shaffer 1991.

52 The model of the mangle is elaborated in Pickering 1995. For commentaries and criticisms, see Gingras 1997; Hacking 1996; Lynch 1996; Pinch 1999; Rheinberger 1999; Schatzki 1999; and Turner 1999.

53 Pickering 1995: 225.

54 Ibid.: 22. Pickering is very specific about the fact that his notion of resistance is quite different from the language of constraint that marks classical social theory.

55 Similar models, which eschew notions of an ultimate reality or truth that causes the world to be as it is, can be found in philosophy, ethnography, and other contributors to the STS literature, most influentially in Latour's (1987, 1988) actor-network model and Haraway's (1991) concept of the cyborg. What characterizes Pickering's model is its concern for temporal processes of transformation rather than their structural articulations.

56 Hess 1997: 108–9.

57 Rouse 1997: 148–51.

58 Some readers may object to my attempt to find resonances between Pickering's mangle and Chinese conceptions of *qi* transformation, arguing that the purpose of cultural studies is the examination of native categories by means of social theory, not the translation of social theory into native discourse. The distance between categories in native and social scientific culture, in this view, provides the space necessary for meaningful explanation. Given that Pickering's model of the mangle was developed without any reference to Chinese medicine, this space is not eroded, while, at the same time, the resonances I point out do no undue violence to Chinese medicine.

59 He Yumin 何裕民 1987: 2. I make no claim that my interpretation of agency is that of official textbooks or of particular individuals in contemporary China. In fact, given the widespread scientism among members of the Chinese medical community, there is much evidence for attempts to move Chinese medicine closer to the model of agency espoused by the natural sciences. Yet, as the above quote and other material presented throughout this book show, this is never pushed to the limits, and the other possibilities of perceiving agency that I discuss here are never far from the surface of even introductory teaching materials.

60 Sivin 1987: 47.

61 Porkert 1978: 167; Unschuld 1985: 67–73. The most extensive study of the concept of *qi* in the history of Chinese thought including its translation into Western thought and language is Kubny 1995.

62 Brief overviews of the visceral systems of function in Chinese medicine can be found in Farquhar 1994a; Porkert 1978: 107–96; and Sivin 1987: 124–33. Farquhar (1994b) discusses particularly the multiplicity inherent in Chinese views of the body.

63 *Suwen* 8, 1992: 126–27.

64 Hay 1983.

65 Farquhar 1994a: 96 n. 39; Zito 1994: 121. I gratefully acknowledge the help of Nathan Sivin in guiding me toward this understanding.

66 The statements in this and preceding paragraphs have been collated from a wide variety of verbal and written sources. Most can be found in introductory textbooks

or teaching aids such as Beijing zhongyi xueyuan 北京中医学院 1986. See Wiseman and Boss 1990 for a convenient listing.

67 *Lingshu* 8, 1989: 83–84. My translation follows Bensky 1996: 23.

68 Examples can be found in the vast case history literature of Chinese medicine. See, for instance, the cases discussed in the chapter on depression (*yu* 郁) in the influential *Linzheng zhinan yi'an* 临证指南医案 (*A Compass of Clinical Patterns Based on Case Histories*), by the Qing dynasty physician Ye Tianshi 叶天士 (1959 [1766], 6: 300–306).

69 Fung 1953: 533.

70 *Bei xi zi yi* 北溪字义 (*Philosophical Glossary of Neo-Confucian Technical Terms*) chapter 2: 5b, cited in Needham 1956: 563–64.

71 Needham 1956: 565–70.

72 Ibid.: 567.

73 Rouse 1997: 152.

74 This makes us aware of the inevitability of why things are "just so" without reducing the process of emergence to anything outside itself. In addition, this perspective effectively defends an emergent model of culture against charges of relativism or subjectivism to which it would otherwise be subject. In this sense, "just so–ness" constructs culture or practice without reifying it.

75 I am inspired in this analysis by the work of de Certeau (1988) and Serres (1995). See Sivin 1987 for a detailed study of how the past of Chinese medicine is reworked in the present.

76 A similar critique is at the basis of the emergence of the cultural studies of science or critical STS (Hess 1997a, 1997b). This emergence is motivated, on the one hand, by a political desire to actively manipulate how science configures life in the postmodern world. On the other, it stems from epistemological considerations that view early constructivist models of scientific practice as unnecessarily limited. Haraway, for instance, criticizing both Kuhn's model of paradigm shifts and Latour's actor-network model, argues that change in science depends on more encompassing transformations: "Even to imagine destabilization, one must be formed at a social moment when change is possible, when people are producing different meanings in many other areas of life" (1989: 303).

77 Thus, the history of "modern" science is not merely a process of knowledge creation but one of continued self-definition through boundary work. For a review of boundary work in STS and examples from the history of science, see Gieryn 1995, 1999. Anthropology and sociology, of course, have always attached great importance to how cultural boundaries are constructed and maintained (Douglas 1966; Berger and Luckman 1967).

78 That "synthesis" (from the Greek verb *syn-tithēmi*, to put or place together) is a process at the very heart of anthropological inquiry has been stated by other writers, of whom Lincoln (1989) is a pertinent example, if one who remains tied to a discourse- (rather than performance-) based analysis.

79 Marcus 1995: 102. The article provides a useful summary of the emergence of multisited ethnography, including its conjunction with and borrowings from the social studies of science and technology.

80 It can be argued that Pickering's emphasis on the distinction between practice and practices is a reflection of his own boundary work as he seeks to distinguish his personal concern with *practice* from the analyses of *practices* developed by competing research traditions within STS.

81 As in my portrayal of Chinese medicine as consisting of multiple partially related networks in chapter 6, my description of how patients shape medical practice in chapter 4, and my analysis of the global development of Chinese medicine as a result of multiple individual but nevertheless interconnected choices in chapters 5 and 7. For detailed studies of decentered agency and partial connectedness, see, for instance, Haraway 1991; and Strathern 1991.

82 The term "infrastructures" is borrowed from Gasché's (1986: 148–53) discussion of the preontological and prelogical nature of text in relation to Derridean philosophy, where it is used in an entirely different context of inquiry and with entirely different connotations. This definition of synthesis is opposed to the classical definition of synthesis as proceeding via thesis and antithesis and thus, incidentally, also rejects the teleology that underpins the discourse of modernity.

83 Wang Ji 王琦 1993; Zhang Weiyao 张维耀 1994: 14.

84 The notion of "field" has a long history in anthropological and sociological theory and "fieldwork" is, of course, the very paradigm of ethnographic activity. Implicit in early anthropological conceptualizations of "political fields" was a clear desire to move away from institutions and rules as a basis for understanding political action and toward process, conflict, and change (Swartz et al. 1966: 7–11). More recently, the concept has been applied in an influential manner by Bourdieu (1993), though in a more structuralist reading than used in this book. Bourdieu does, however, make the important observation that a field is a dynamic entity defined through the positions of agents within it.

85 See, for instance, Fang Yaozhong 方药中 1993a.

86 Pickering (1995) discusses these issues in detail in the concluding chapter of his book.

87 On the importance of gift giving in China, see Xu Ping 许平 1990; partially translated in Dutton 1998: 40–41, 204–7; and also Kipnis 1997; Yan 1996; and Yang 1994.

88 As I discuss in greater detail in chapter 4, this leads to decentering of the resistance and accommodation framework that informs much valuable anthropological work in a direction more immediately related to Pickering's use of these terms.

89 Fields of practice have two characteristics. The first is the alignment of infrastructures with each other. I use the term *topography* to refer to the description of such alignment. The *Oxford English Dictionary* defines topography as mapping the surface of a body with reference to the parts beneath it, making it a particularly fitting term for my examination of syntheses built from infrastructures. However, the

mapping of a body or field is not an objective process. Whether we (as agents/observers) visualize social relations as networks, as expanding waves of agency radiating outward from diverse centers, or as fluid spaces that are forever expanding and contracting is as critical to the results of our analysis as the organization of space itself. My awareness of this effect is indexed by reference to the notion of topology. See Mol and Law 1994 and Serres and Latour 1995: 60 for critical discussions.

90   Marcus 1995. While Marcus identifies a shift in methodology as indicating or even leading to a changed epistemology, it is implicit in my entire argument that the influence is always moving in both directions at the same time.

3. Hegemonic Pluralism

1   The material presented in this chapter is drawn predominantly from secondary sources to which further reference will be made only in case of quotation or reference to a specific person or event: Cai Jingfeng 蔡景峰 et al. 2000; Croizier 1968; Lampton 1977; Ma Boying 马伯英 1993; Meng Qingyun 孟庆云 2000; Wang Zhipu 王致谱 and Cai Jingfeng 蔡景峰 1999; Wang Songbao 汪松葆 1987; Zhang Weiyao 张维耀 1994; and Zhen Zhiya 甄志亚 1987. A doctoral dissertation examining the transformation of Chinese medicine in early Maoist China was in preparation at the time of this writing at the University of Cambridge (Taylor 2000). I am obliged to Kim Taylor for pointing me in the right direction on many occasions. There also exist some impressionistic personal assessments of this period, such as Chen 1989; and Sidel and Sidel 1974. The Chinese government (Zhonghua renmin gongheguo weishengbu zhongyisi 中华人民共和国卫生部中医司 1985) has published official documents relating to Chinese medicine for the period 1950–80. Material drawn from these sources has been supplemented by information gathered from interviews and conversations collected and conducted during my fieldwork with physicians who participated in the transformations described.

2   It is beyond the scope of this book to examine these ruptures and continuities in detail. I am currently working on an examination of this transition by following several medical streams from the late Qing to the present. In general, Western historians of medicine tend to emphasize ruptures, focus on the distinctiveness of a specific historical period, and see Chinese medicine after 1949 as different from Chinese medicine prior to that time (e.g., Andrews 1996; Sivin 1987; Unschuld 1992; Taylor 2000), whereas Chinese histories emphasize continuity within a framework of historical materialism (e.g., Deng Tietao 邓铁涛 1999).

3   See Zhang Weiyao 张维耀 1994: 14–18; and Cui Yueli 崔月梨 1980.

4   Lampton (1977), for instance, traces at least seven periods for the years 1949–77.

5   Regarding Guo Murou, see Croizier 1968: 155; and Louie 1986. Guo, like many other prominent modernizers and revolutionaries of the time, had studied Western medicine in Japan for a while. Mao Zedong (no date: 54) wrote in the 1940s that

"old doctors, circus entertainers, snake oil salesmen, and street hawkers are all of the same sort."

6   It is no coincidence that many influential reformers and politicians of the Nationalist era (e.g., Sun Yat-sen and Lu Xun) had studied Western medicine. Efforts to outlaw Chinese medicine culminated in a proposition passed by the first legislative session of the Central Ministry of Public Health on 26 February 1929 that was later reversed owing to organized protest by Chinese medical physicians, who could draw on widespread public support. Regarding the history of Chinese medicine during the Nationalist period, see Andrews 1996; Croizier 1968; Deng Tietao 邓铁涛 1999; Lei 1988; Ma Boying 马伯英 et al. 1993: chapter 12; Xu 1997; Zhao Hongjun 赵洪钧 1989; and Zhen Zhiya 甄志亚 1987.

7   Taylor 2000: 251.

8   During the Communists' stay in the Yan'an area, for instance, efforts to establish model health villages included attempts to root out all shamanistic beliefs and superstitions (Ma Boying 马伯英 et al. 1993; Zhen Zhiya 甄志亚 1987: 288).

9   Tang et al. 1994. The first conference, in July 1950, advanced only the first three principles; the fourth, the integration of mass campaigns and health work, was added at the second conference, in April 1952 (Wang Zhipu 王致谱 and Cai Jingfeng 蔡景峰 1999: 6).

10 Both Ma Boying 马伯英 et al. (1993: 577) and Taylor (2000) argue that the Communist Party's aim at this point was to create a single new medicine by a total unification of Western and Chinese medicines. Lampton (1977) and especially Taylor (2000) provide detailed examinations of these struggles.

11 Croizier 1968: 158. This view is shared by Lampton (1977: 36) and Taylor (2000: 54–79).

12 Taylor 2000: 63–64. A biographical sketch of Yu Yunxiu is provided by Zhongguo yixuehui Shanghai fenzhi yixueshi xuehui 中国医学会上海分支医学史学会 1954. For evaluations of Yu's role on the struggles between Chinese and Western medicine in Nationalist China, see Andrews 1996: 166–71; Lei 1999; and Ma Boying 马伯英 et al. 1993: 547–55. It should not go without notice that as late as 1954 Yu was able to publish through the MOH publishing organ, the People's Health Publishing House (Renmin weisheng chubanshe 人民卫生出版社). Cf. Yu 1954.

13 Guo Taomei 郭桃美 1988, cited in Guojia zhongyiyao guanliju 国家中医药管理局 1997: 218. See also Yu Yunxiu's article "Unification" (*Tuanjie* 团结), originally published in October 1950 in the journal *Yiyao shijie* 医药世界 (*Medical World*), reprinted in Zhao Hongjun 赵洪钧 1989: 281–87.

14 Other restrictions that handicapped the Chinese medical profession were the fact that the newly instituted health insurance system did not include treatment by Chinese medical doctors, great problems concerning the production and distribution of the medical herbs, and decline in the training of competent Chinese medical practitioners during the period of the Sino-Japanese War and the Civil War (Taylor 2000: chapter 3).

15 I am aware of at least one such course run at Beijing Medical Hospital (Beijing yixueyuan 北京医学院). See the biographies of Fang and Tang in Zhongguo kexue jishu xiehui 中国科学技术协会 1999: 361 and 396.

16 Mao Zedong, cited in Li Zhizhong 李致重 1997b: 155. The context of this quote brings out its meaning even more clearly. Mao said, "China has great contributions to make to the world. I think of Chinese medicine as being one. . . . Chinese and Western medicine definitely must be united, Western medicine definitely must smash sectarianism" (Zhongguo dui shijie you da gongxiande, wo kan zhongyi shi yi xiang . . . zhongxi yi yiding yao tuanjie, xiyi yiding yao dapo zongpaizhuyi 中国对世界有大贡献的, 我看中医是一项 . . . 中西医团结, 西医一定要打破宗派主义). It is significant, too, that the improvement schools did not train new physicians but reeducated already practicing physicians, increasing their knowledge of Western medicine and awareness of politics (Taylor 2000: 111).

17 Representation of Chinese medicine among the people was very strong because every village used to have a Chinese medicine physician. Forcing these physicians out of their jobs (as the early policies of the MOH did) led to widespread unemployment with resulting social consequences (Taylor 2000). Lampton (1977), like almost all the Chinese physicians I know, thinks that Mao Zedong's idiosyncratic interest in Chinese medicine was a major factor in its institutionalization. I think, however, that this estimation needs to be revised in two directions. First, Mao's interest in Chinese medicine never appears to have been guided by a desire to establish it as an independent medical tradition, but rather as a contribution to a specifically Chinese medicine; second, although Mao's support of Chinese medicine appears to be the most obvious, it was shared by other high-ranking leaders. Evidence can be found in many anecdotes dispersed through the literature and the personal recollections of senior physicians. Furthermore, as China's new political leaders began to age, many would naturally turn to Chinese medicine with its ideas of health preservation in an effort to shore up their physical powers. He Shi-Xi 何时希 (1997: 232), who worked at the Academy of Chinese Medicine in Beijing from 1955 to 1966, thus links the academy where many of the experts brought to Beijing worked and practiced to the Imperial Medical Academy at the Qing court. Just as an aside, one may note that Yue Meizhong 岳美中, the first physician at the academy to enter the CCP and therefore a physician with much cachet among the leadership, became an expert in geriatric medicine.

18 Liu Shaoqi on 9 July 1954, cited in Wang Zhipu 王致谱 and Cai Jingfeng 蔡景峰 1999: 9.

19 See Li Zhizhong 李致重 1997b: 155.

20 Taylor 2000: 112. It should be noted that promoting the spread of "Chinese" medicine throughout the world was not something invented by Mao or the Communists. As early as 1929, Qin Bowei 秦伯未, a Chinese medicine physician and educator who served as an adviser to the MOH in Beijing from 1955 onward, began

publishing the *Zhongyi shijie zazhi* 中医世界杂志 (*Chinese Medicine World Journal*). For more than a decade the title page of the journal showed a map of the world with the slogan "Transform Chinese medicine into a world medicine" (*hua zhongyi wei shijie yi* 化中医为世界医) written across it.

21 Personal communication from two students of the first class assembled in Beijing in 1955. See also Ma Boying 马伯英 et al. 1993: 583–84 for personal accounts of some students.

22 The intellectual hub of Chinese medicine for at least the preceding four centuries had been located in Jiangnan 江南, south of the Yangtze River, especially in Jiangsu and Zhejiang. For biographies of the physicians mentioned in this paragraph, see Zhongguo kexue jizhu xiehui 中国科学技术协会 1999.

23 Wang Zhipu 王致谱 and Cai Jingfeng 蔡景峰 1999: 14.

24 Ma Boying 马伯英 et al. 1993: 575.

25 Taylor 2000: 168. See also Lou Shaolai 楼绍来 and Ren Tianluo 任天洛 1998. There are other reasons why Chinese medicine was able to gradually assert its autonomy. The concentration of eminent scholar-physicians in Beijing and their newly secured status certainly allowed them to work toward the independence of their tradition rather than its integration with Western medicine. Also, Western medicine physicians had little to gain from the policy of integration. Mao's influence waned decisively after the disaster of the Great Leap Forward.

26 Wang Songhao 汪松葆 1987: 20–26. Although it is sometimes claimed that education in Chinese medicine prior to 1949 was entirely apprenticeship based, this is not actually the case. He Shixi 何时希 (1997: 68–91) lists a total of 162 schools, colleges, societies, and other institutions providing education in Chinese medicine established in China between 1885 and 1945.

27 For biographies of Ding Ganren and Shi Jinmo, see Zhongguo kexue jizhu xiehui 中国科学技术协会 1999: 23–29 and 47–56.

28 Nanjing zhongyi xueyuan 南京中医学院 1958. The compilation of this important textbook is described in the foreword to the third revised edition (Meng Jingchun 孟景春 and Zhou Zhongying 周仲瑛 1994). For a more personal memory, see "Lü Bingkui cong yi 60 nian wenji" weiyuanhui 吕炳奎从医６０年文集编辑委员会 1993: 7. According to personal information from participants, the first class of Western doctors as well as the first two classes at the Beijing College of Chinese Medicine were taught from original texts rather than textbooks. For this and other reasons they generally consider themselves more authentic practitioners of Chinese medicine than later graduates. See also Taylor 2000: chapter 3.

29 For a complete listing of teaching materials and the teaching and research groups that produced them, see Taylor 2000: 224–31.

30 Taylor 2000: chapter 3; "Lü Bingkui cong yi 60 nian wenji" weiyuanhui 吕炳奎从医６０年文集编辑委员会 1993: 6. Altogether Lü brought more than forty teachers to Beijing from the south, including Dong Jianhua 董建华 and Yang Jiasan 杨甲三

at the Dongzhimen Hospital, Wang Mianzhi 王绵之 and Yan Zhenghua 颜正华 at the Beijing Chinese Medicine University, and Yin Huihe 印会河 at the China-Japan Friendship Hospital.

31 The letter is reprinted in Ren Yingqiu 任应秋 1984: 3–6.

32 Taylor 2000: 226–27. See chapter 6 and also Hsu 1999 for an analysis of the effects of this shift in knowledge transmission.

33 While Mao Zedong himself officially declared the "Great Proletarian Cultural Revolution" to be over in 1969, Chinese today refer to the entire decade from 1966 to 1976 as the Cultural Revolution or the "ten lost years" (Ogden 1992: 48).

34 There are as yet no detailed analyses of Chinese medicine during the Cultural Revolution. White (1993, 1998, 1999) presents some data from provincial Yunnan, but her ethnography is situated in the late 1980s. Hillier and Jewell (1983) is an impressionistic account.

35 These figures are from Meng Qingyun 孟庆云 2000: 744. From 1970 onward, education at Chinese medicine schools and colleges was resumed following a "leftist" line with much-reduced duration of courses and simplified contents. Graduates of this period are not well respected now because of their perceived low levels of academic achievement. The views expressed by Wang Zhipu 王致谱 and Cai Jingfeng 蔡景峰 (1999: 87) are those shared by the majority of my informants.

36 The encyclopedia provides monographs for 5,767 different drugs. Many of these drugs were assimilated from folk knowledge and some have since become standard ingredients in contemporary medical practice.

37 Wujinxian weishengju bianshi xiuzhi lingdao xiaozu 武进县卫生局编史修志领导小组 1985: 196–97.

38 The information in this and the preceding paragraph is from my own notes. It should be borne in mind, of course, that if my informants remembered—whether for me or to themselves—a "trusting" time before 1966, such memories tell us as much about now as they do about then.

39 Baum 1982; Ong 1995: 65.

40 Henderson 1989. I use the term "plural health care system" to denote that in this phase the state acknowledged the coexistence of different medicines without implying any longer that these would eventually be merged into a single medicine. Although a de facto plural health care system has, of course, always existed in China (not just since the importation of Western medicine), it was established de jure only in the 1980s. It might also be argued that the integration of Chinese medicine into the National Insurance Scheme in the 1950s marked the official recognition of Chinese medicine. Again, I would argue that it marked a factual rather than a legal acceptance of actual plurality. Ultimately, though, these distinctions are academic and all I am after is a convenient designation.

41 "Lü Bingkui cong yi 60 nian wenji" weiyuanhui 吕炳奎从医６０年文集编辑委员会 1993: 12–13; Zhang Weiyao 张维耀 1994: 16–17; Zhonghua renmin gongheguo weishengbu zhongyisi 中华民共和国卫生部中医司 1985.

42 "Lü Bingkui cong yi 60 nian wenji" weiyuanhui 吕炳奎从医６０年文集编辑委员会 1993: 11; Yu Shenchu 俞慎初 1983: 510.

43 *Guomin jingji he shehui fazhan shi nian guihua he di bage wu nian jihua gangyao* 国民经济和社会发展十年规划和第八个五年计划纲要 (*Ten-Year National Economic and Social Development Plan and Principles for the Eighth Five-Year Plan*) published April 1991. Cited in Guojia zhongyiyao guanliju 国家中医药管理局 1997: 219.

44 White 1999.

45 Cui Yueli 崔月梨 1980. See also the recent essays by Li Zhizhong 李致重 (1997a, 1997b), a high-ranking member of the Association of Chinese Medicine.

46 The official translation is "State Administration of TCM." For reasons previously noted, I eschew use of the term TCM. I have replaced it with my translation in order to avoid unnecessary confusion.

47 Previously Chinese medicine had been administered by a subsection of the general office of the MOH (Chen 1984: 63–66).

48 The letter, signed by Dong Jianhua 董建华, Wang Mianzhi 王绵之, Ren Jixue 任继学, Shi Dianbang 施奠邦, Liu Duzhou 刘渡舟, Lu Zhizheng 路志正, Cheng Xinnong 程莘农, Fang Yaozhong 方药中, Deng Tietao 邓铁涛, and Zhang Qi 张琪, is reprinted in Cui Yueli 崔月梨 1997: 30–32.

49 Chen 1984: 69–71; Shi Yuguang 史宇广 1989: 1, 30, 34

50 Shi Yuguang 史宇广 1989: appendixes 1 and 2; Wang Songbao 汪松葆 1987: 20–26.

51 This was a new observation I made in Shanghai in 1999. During my first period of fieldwork in Beijing, when tuition fees had just been introduced, I did not encounter this problem.

52 At the time of this writing the MOH was about to introduce a new examination to be taken by all practicing physicians that would group them into one of three categories: physician of Western medicine, physician of Chinese medicine, and physician of Western and Chinese medicine. Only those in the third group would in future be able to prescribe and carry out both Chinese and Western medicine treatments.

53 Chen Minzhang 陈敏章 1997: 296–97.

54 Shi Yuguang 史宇广 1989.

55 Zhang Weiyao 张维耀 1994: 17.

56 For a full listing of these institutes, see Shi Yuguang 史宇广 1989: appendix 4.

57 Chen Minzhang 陈敏章 1995.

58 Wang Qiaochu 王翘楚 1998: 68; Zhang Mingdao 张明岛 and Shao Jieqi 邵洁奇 1998: 136. In 1997 Beijing had twenty-two Chinese medicine hospitals, more than any other municipality (Meng Qing-Yun 孟庆云 2000: 927). In 1989 45.3 percent of Beijing clinics (including those providing Western medicine) were privately operated. This compares with 2.3 percent in Shanghai and 85.5 percent in Anhui according to figures provided by Henderson (1993: 109 n. 14). Huang's (1988) study of the transformation of health care in rural China in the 1980s elucidates and confirms

my informants' views. Farquhar (1996), Jia (1997), and White (1998) provide detailed ethnographic descriptions of private Chinese medical practices in rural China. Examples of private practice on different ends of a continuum that I encountered in Beijing were a Manchu acupuncturist celebrated for his treatment of strokes and famous older physicians practicing in big hotels for a foreign clientele. Many physicians in the state sector treat private patients in the evenings (and sometimes also during work) to supplement their incomes.

59 Meng Qingyun 孟庆云 2000: 923–33; Chen Minzhang 陈敏章 1997: 294–95.

60 Xu and Fan 1980: 137.

61 At the end of the Eighth Five-Year Plan in 1995 the gross value of Chinese medicine products produced had reached RMB 17.570 billion, an increase of 212.6 percent over the 1990 figure, while the revenue generated from sales had increased by 122.6 percent to RMB 1.573 billion (Wang Zhipu 王致谱 and Cai Jingfeng 蔡景峰 1999: 22).

62 Wang Zhipu 王致谱 and Cai Jingfeng 蔡景峰 1999: 25–28.

63 Baer et al. 1986; Banerji 1985; Elling 1980; Foster 1986; Gruenbaum 1981; Zimmerman 1978.

64 Lock 1990: 45.

65 For additional relevant overviews of health care reform in China during the 1980s and 1990s consulted but not cited so far, see Henderson et al. 1994; Liu et al. 1994; World Bank 1996; and Zheng and Hillier 1995.

66 See Cui Yueli 崔月梨 1997: 30–32.

67 I am following here an argument made by James Scott (1998) that is taken up in more detail in chapter 9. Detailed evidence for state centralization in various domains will be provided in subsequent chapters: with respect to education (chapter 6), with respect to medical practice (chapter 7), and with respect to research (chapter 8). Evidence for state centralization can also be found in the work of other authors, such as Hsu (1999) on education and Shao (1999) on hospital practice.

68 For relevant policies, see Zhonghua renmin gongheguo weishengbu zhongyisi 中华民共和国卫生部中医司 1985.

69 Chen 1984: 304–6; Wang Songbao 汪松葆 1987.

70 Quoted in the publisher's preface to the Self-Study Material for Chinese Medicine Correspondence Courses of National Further Education Colleges and Schools 全国高等中医院校函授教材, Hunan kexue jishu chubanshe (1985: 358).

71 Chen 1984.

72 Ibid.: 1–33.

73 Ibid.: 1–46. Compare Guangzhou, with eleven of twenty-three work-units under MOH control; Shanghai, with three of forty; and Tianjin, where all thirty-one work-units are locally administered.

74 Quoted in Shi Yuguang 史宇广 1989: 14.

75 Cui Yueli 崔月犁 1990: 1.

76 Wang Zhipu 王致谱 and Cai Jingfeng 蔡景峰 1999: 14. In 1996 the MOH affirmed

its policy to promote Chinese medicine abroad on the basis of the maxim "correct guidance, exerting advantages, maximizing favorable factors and minimizing unfavorable ones, and promoting development" (Chen Minzhang 陈敏章 1997: 123).

77 A very useful example was the mobilization of the health care sector in the government-directed campaign against the *Falungong* movement that occurred in the summer of 1999 while I was revising this chapter. This mobilization was deemed necessary for two reasons. First, because the movement had many devotees in the health care sector. According to my informants there was at least one active practitioner in each department. Second, because health maintenance through "scientific" means was one of the major strategies chosen by the government in its ideological campaign against *Falungong*. Government policy was communicated downward through meetings. All hospital staff had to attend meetings in which heads of departments conveyed government directives that they themselves had learned of during special meetings directed by MOH personnel, who were in turn directed by CCP cadres.

78 Guojia zhongyiyao guanliju yizhengsi 国家中医药管理局医政司 1991; Guojia zhong-yiyao guanliju zhengce fagui si 国家中医药局管理局政策发规司 1992: 146–47.

79 Guojia jishu jianduju 国家技术鉴督局 1994, 1995, 1997a, 1997b, 1997c. See also Latour 1987 regarding the importance of standardized systems of recording in the operation of power.

80 Chen Minzhang 陈敏章 1997: 122.

81 Du Ruzhu 杜如竹 1994.

82 WHO Regional Committee for the Western Pacific 1994.

83 Moore 1992, cited in Tang et al. 1994.

84 No statistical data are available for Chinese medicine. Studies of general health care changes do, however, paint a picture of the rapid adoption of "high-tech" medicine, even if patients have to share part of the costs. See Henderson 1989; Liu and Hsiao 1995; and Tang et al. 1994.

85 Dan Bensky (August 1996, personal communication) attended such discussions in Chongqing in 1985. See also Huang Xingyuan 黄星垣 1985.

86 Manfred Porkert (1998) reduces the entire problem to one striking observation. He argues that in the last one hundred years not a single physician has been taken to court for incompetency as evaluated according to Chinese medical standards. At the same time, charges of incompetency as evaluated by Western medical standards are a constant threat to physicians of Chinese medicine.

87 In general, I found morale among graduate students of Chinese medicine to be not very high. Young graduates in Beijing expected to earn about RMB 1000, while their friends in private enterprises or the media expected starting salaries of RMB 5000–6000 and above. Even the promise of a secure job no longer exists due to cutback of public subsidies. Many students, furthermore, felt that securing a job and career advancement depended more on their personal connections than on their

grades. Not surprisingly, seeking a career in the pharmaceutical industry or out-side the Chinese medical sector altogether is becoming a preferred option for many graduates.

88 The quote is taken from a report of the First Plenary Meeting of the Chinese Medi-cine Expert Consultative Committee, chaired by the State Administration of Chi-nese Medicine, in September 1996. This summarized the official understanding of Chinese Medicine since the establishment of the State Administration (Chen Min-zhang 陈敏章 1997: 119).

89 Guojia zhongyiyao guanliju yizhengsi 国家中医药管理局医政司 1991; Guojia jishu jianduju 国家技术鉴督局 1994, 1995, 1997a, 1997b, 1997c.

90 *Guojia zhongyiyao guanliju yizhengsi* 国家中医药管理局医政司 1991, 11–12. The latest regulations for all hospitals of Chinese medicine concerning the writing of medical histories (Zhongyi bing'an shuxie guifan 中医病案书写规范) and the case history cover sheet (Zhongyi bing'an shouye 中医病案首页) came into force on 1 February 1992. As is made clear by Wang Zhipu 王致谱 and Cai Jingfeng 蔡景峰 (1999: 60), these rules can only be understood in the wider context of state-controlled regularization and standardization, extending from the nomenclature of acupuncture point names and locations to hospital administration and nursing.

91 Besides my Chinese informants I wish to thank Brenda Hood and Eric Karchmer for talking to me about the composition and function of case records in contem-porary Chinese medicine hospitals.

92 Regarding the historical development of the genre of medical case statements in Chinese medicine, see the contributions by Andrews and Cullen in Hsu 2001.

93 Shao 1998.

94 In driving home this without doubt important and correct analysis Shao Jing would appear to reduce the multiple functions and layers of inpatient notes (their plu-rality) to a single scheme of explanations. In their totality, case notes are also medi-cal tools, legal documents, and billing records. My thanks to Eric Karchmer for pointing out to me these additional functions.

95 Shao 1998. While it is true that many students and interns find writing case notes bothersome, especially because it does not impinge on actual treatment decisions, they also appreciate its function in developing their skills in analyzing disease mechanisms (*bingji* 病机), which is of old the main purpose of a Chinese medical diagnosis.

96 Undoubtedly, it will have occurred to many readers that the current phase in the history of Chinese medicine is only partially captured by examining its political integration into an officially plural health care system. Increasingly important is the assimilation of Chinese medicine to global technoscience. Carrying out an analysis of this process will be an important task of future ethnographies but ex-ceeds what is possible in the present book. Such an analysis will show that this assimilation is a process mediated but certainly not controlled by the Chinese state. In that sense, it will support the conclusion presented here of the state as a

powerful disciplining agent that is itself disciplined in its encounter with Chinese medicine.

4. Dilemmas and Tactical Agency

1 The Beijing Chinese Medicine Hospital Study is cited from *ChinaMed* 3 (1994: 5). Similar claims have been made by Ots (1990a: 140–44) based on fieldwork in Beijing, by Lee (1980: 359) for Hong Kong, and by Unschuld (1976: 311–15) for Taiwan. See also Kleinman 1980: 184–85, 266, 273.

2 Ots 1990a: 140–41; Hsu 1992: appendix 6.

3 Jia 1997: 84–86; White 1999. Views of patients interviewed by social scientists differ dramatically from the actual decisions patients make when embarking on a course of treatment. This was brought home to me most directly one night when I interviewed a young doctor of Chinese medicine. In the course of our conversation she repeated all the above stereotypes and said that she would never use Western medicine for chronic problems. "What about your hyperthyroidism, then?" asked her husband, producing a packet of pills his wife was apparently taking regularly. "Well, that is entirely different," countered his wife, explaining that this was not what she meant by a chronic problem.

4 The belief/action model underpins the work of all researchers working with a conception of culture as an ideational system. The most influential theorist of this tradition for social theory and anthropology is Talcott Parsons (1968). In a systematic overview of anthropological theories of human phenomena Hahn and Kleinman 1983b: 310–11, however, list under the categories of "epiphenomenal idealism" and "idealism" not only the theories of Parsons, but also those of the symbolic interactionists; Wittgensteinian culturalists such as Winch, Geertz, Sahlins, and Lévi-Strauss; and phenomenologists such as Berger and Luckman. The most influential representatives of the cultural systems approach in medical anthropology are cognitivists (reviewed in detail in Good 1994: 48–52) and Kleinman's (1980: 104–18) explanatory model framework. The convergence between cognitive health belief models and Kleinman's explanatory model framework has been criticized by Young (1981). The criticism is rejected by Good (1994: 53 n. 31). However, many anthropologists, as Rubel (1990: 123) and Pelto and Pelto (1990) show, persist in thinking of explanatory models as cognitive constructs; that is, as "sets of beliefs or understandings." For a critique of the culture theory approach with specific relevance to Chinese studies, see Farquhar and Hevia 1993.

5 *Qi ju dihuang wan* is a commonly used prescription for such conditions first mentioned in the *Yiji baojian* 医级宝鉴 (*Precious Mirror for the Advancement of Medicine*) of 1777. See Xu Jiqun 许济群 and Wang Mianzhi 王绵之 1995: 269.

6 This formula is a commonly used gynecological formula first mentioned in *Jingui yaolue*, chapter 20. Dr Sun has extended the use of the formula to treat all kinds of conditions in which blood and fluid stasis concur.

7   The relevance of such *guanxi* 关系 relations for Chinese medicine is discussed in chapter 6.

8   Many physicians who work on a ward do, in fact, continue to see patients they have treated on a private fee-for-service basis after the patients have been discharged. However, as such consultations have to be carried out after hours or during work, they are much more difficult to arrange for both patients and physicians.

9   In the course of the economic reforms implemented since the 1980s, health facilities throughout China are increasingly forced to generate most of their own revenue and managers are allowed to pay bonuses to employees and invest in equipment out of surpluses they earn. This means that the desire to earn bonuses is becoming an important influence on diagnostic and therapeutic decision making. See Bloom and Gu 1997 for a summary of health care reforms and their impact on medical practice.

10 The other types are public insurance for government workers (*gongfei yiliao* 公费医疗) and collective welfare for village residents (*hezuo yiliao* 合作医疗). Many rural insurance schemes based on prepayment have collapsed since the early 1980s, and peasants in rural China therefore meet most health expenses out of their own pockets. The situation is different for formal-sector workers in both rural and urban China, who are still financed largely by insurance schemes. The increasing number of people employed in private or joint venture companies, however, also rely on private funds or privately financed health insurance (Liu and Hsiao 1995). Ongoing economic and political reforms cause this sector to be in a continuous state of transformation. A new system of health insurance, intended to reduce the burden placed on the state by the current system, was under consideration by the Department of Labor and Social Security at the time of this writing and planned to come into effect at the end of 1999. This system is based on the idea of co-payment, whereby urban employees would pay 2 percent of their wages into an insurance fund and employers would contribute an amount equal to 6 percent of the entire payroll. Of this money, 30 percent would be used to create individual accounts to cover outpatient services and less expensive inpatient services, and all other treatment would be funded from the other 70 percent. See EIU 1998: chapter 5.

11 Epidemiological data indicate that patients are becoming older and suffer more from chronic diseases (Henderson 1993: 117). Costs and wages in the health care sector rose considerably during the 1980s and 1990s, reflecting both a general rise in living standards and a consumer-led shift to high-tech hospital medicine. In response, health care providers have increased fees for drugs and services and shifted from preventive care to high-income-generating diagnostic and therapeutic services. This, in turn, is why insurers find it increasingly difficult to meet the burden of expenditure placed on them (Liu and Hsiao 1995; Bloom and Gu 1997). Negotiating preferential rates with specific institutions and limiting treatment to care at those institutions is one way insurers have responded to this constellation of forces.

12 *Yin qiao wan* is probably the most popular classical formula for the treatment of colds and flu available in many different over-the-counter preparations. It was first mentioned in the *Wenbing tiaobian* 温病条辨 (*Systematic Differentiation of Warm [Pathogen] Disorders*) of 1798. See Xu Jiqun 许济群 and Wang Mianzhi 王绵之 1995: 70–72.

13 *Huoxiang zhengqi pian*, commonly used for the treatment of summer flu, are derived from a classical formula first mentioned in the *Taiping huimin hejiju fang* 太平惠民和剂局方 (*Prescriptions of the Public Pharmacy of the Era of Great Peace and of the Bureau of Medicines*) published after 1078. See Xu Jiqun 许济群 and Wang Mianzhi 王绵之 1995: 478–81.

14 Self-prescribing with both Chinese and Western medicines is common practice among Chinese patients. Significant differences exist, however, between different regions and, presumably, between urban and rural areas. In Guangdong, for instance, the use of Chinese medicines as an ingredient in ordinary cooking is far more widespread than in Beijing or Shanghai. Hence, in my limited experience, patients from Guangdong are also much more open to the use of Chinese medicine in case of illness.

15 And even where it does matter, as in Zhengnan's case, beliefs may need to be given up, or at least suspended, if more important considerations require it.

16 This sentence, which can also be translated "Do not take the drugs of a physician who is not acquainted with the texts of three traditions," is first mentioned in the *Zhouli* 周礼 (*Book of Rites*), dating presumedly from the Zhou but actually from the Han dynasty. The three texts are usually taken to be the *Huangdi zhenjiu* 黄帝针灸 (*The Yellow Lord's Acumoxa [Classic]*), an acupuncture text that is no longer extant; the *Sunu maijue* 素女脉诀 (*The Simple Woman's [Classic] on Pulse Diagnosis*), a manual of pulse diagnosis that is also no longer extant; and the *Shennong bencao* 神农本草 (*The Divine Husbandman's Materia Medica*). See Qiu Peiran 裘沛然 and Ding Guangdi 丁光迪 1992: 3.

17 Another indication of the renewed economic viability of Chinese medicine is the increase in pharmacies specializing in Chinese medicine products. When I returned to Beijing in 1996 I noted that several new businesses had opened in prominent trading positions within the space of only one year.

18 Such registration fees (*guahaofei* 挂号费) can amount to RMB 500 for half a day's work. For comparison, a junior physician in 1994 earned about RMB 300 per month, and a senior consultant RMB 1000 plus benefits.

19 It should be clear that I do not claim that patients' agency is not influenced by stereotypical efficacy attributions, shared symbols, institutional arrangements, etc. What I do claim is that such factors do not determine behavior and are themselves open to transformation.

20 The stereotype is rooted in perceptions of Chinese medicine, being primarily concerned with illness prevention. The story that Chinese patients used to pay their physicians as long as they stayed healthy and expected free medical treatment

when ill is a typical example. There is, of course, an interesting overlap between older concerns for the extension of life and techniques for health preservation (*yangsheng* 养生) and the Maoist emphasis on preventive medicine. Also, while Chinese medicine practiced in the state sector like its biomedical other focuses on the treatment of disease, the older focus on health preservation continues to influence people's behavior through a literature that draws on the medical classics but is aimed specifically at a modern clientele. See Farquhar (forthcoming) for an exemplary discussion of these issues.

21 This is particularly so in the case of Western medicine due to the high prestige accorded to Western medicine physicians and their apparently miraculous powers when biomedicine was first introduced to China. Patients often feel more comfortable with physicians of Chinese medicine, who, up to now, at least, depend on patient cooperation in making a diagnosis. The increasing utilization of biomedical technology by Chinese medicine is rapidly changing this picture. While I have not carried out any meaningful investigation of patients' views, I have met a number of younger physicians of Chinese medicine who have little interest in their patients as people but instead consider them entities to be processed by a system.

22 See Zhonguo zhongyi yanjiuyuan 中国中医研究 1984, 1987; Zhongyi bingming zhenduan guifan keti zu 中医病名诊断规范课题组 1987; Zhang Baiyu 张伯臾 et al. 1988.

23 Ots 1990b.

24 Farquhar 1994a: 45.

25 Ots 1990a: 147–48.

26 Farquhar 1994a: 41–44 provides a good description of the typical clinical encounter in Chinese medicine.

27 My observations confirm those of Ots (1990a: 144), who notes that the acquisition and use of ultrasound scanners in Chinese medical hospitals during the 1980s is a direct result of patient pressure. See also Jia 1997, which documents the influence of patients shopping for health care on the delivery of that health care.

28 Some authors such as Kleinman (1986) and Ots (1990a: 159–64, 1990b) suggest that many of the terms used by Chinese patients to refer to their discomforts express culture-specific cognitive ordering of "uncognized universal psychobiological experience" or "primary affects." What precisely is meant by "uncognized universal psychobiological experience" and how we are to gain access to it is more problematic. Farquhar (1994a: 62–70), more simply, argues for the importance of bodily awareness in Chinese patients as being related to the fact that this awareness is prized in Chinese medical practice. Historically, knowledge acquisition in Chinese culture has been associated with memorization (Liu 1986). In cognitive tests, for instance, the memory ability of Chinese subjects is usually higher than that reported for Americans, so the fact that they remember more about their bodies may be a consequence of better memorization in general.

29 Zhang Xichun 张锡纯, *Yixue zhongzhong canxi lu*, 1: 167.

30 I make no claims that these data are representative. According to my colleague Dan Bensky (1996), who studied Chinese medicine in Taiwan and Macao during the mid-1970s, this percentage was much higher among the patient population he encountered there. I certainly did meet some laypeople who possessed considerable knowledge of Chinese medical theories.

31 Product information for *Yaotong kang* 腰痛康 (Health [from] Back Pain) produced by Huangdonghua tianbao yaodian 黄东华天宝药店.

32 Qian Zifen 钱自奋 et al. 1993: 17; Qin Bowei 秦伯未 1983d.

33 Opposition to such innovation appears to have come from literary-oriented scholar-physicians such as Ren Yingqiu 任应秋, e.g., 1984b.

34 See also the listing of all Chinese medical practitioners in Anonymous 1992.

35 An exhaustive listing of relevant ethnographies is beyond the scope of this study. Studies that have influenced my thinking and are not cited elsewhere include Comaroff 1985; Fabrega 1973; Frankel and Lewis 1989; Lewis 1975; and Zimmerman 1978.

36 Explorations of health-seeking behavior as concerned with the search for meaning, derived from phenomenological and interactionist models in sociology, have also deepened our understanding of individual behavior and its embeddedness in cultural networks of signification. The narrow focus of this research tradition with individual life-worlds, however, frequently hides the shaping of these worlds by globally situated systems of power. The opposite problem applies to structural analyses of health care systems. These succeed in delineating the determination of individual behavior through the global characteristics of a health care system at the price of exploring in detail the local constitution of agency. The label "critical medical anthropology," like all such labels, is given different meanings by different authors. It would be of little value to discuss these definitions and their politics within the present context. Exemplary ethnographies in the sense that I have applied to the category have been produced by writers such as Good 1977, Martin 1987, Lock 1993, Scheper-Hughes 1992, and Young 1980, 1995.

37 Although Foucault is often invoked by theorists of resistance, his use of that notion is, as Talal Asad 2000: n. 15 remarks, rather distinctive in that it represents a "limit" of power. "There is indeed always something in the social body, in classes, groups and individuals themselves which in some sense escapes relation of power, something which is by no means a docile or reactive primal matter, but rather a centrifugal movement, an inverse energy, a discharge." Cited from Foucault 1980: 138.

38 I am thinking here about the Greenpeace-led activism that forced Shell not to sink the Brent-Spar oil platform; popular resistance against genetically modified food; and the generation of more plural health care systems in the West over recent years, a process in which consumers have had a considerable input. Chinese medicine in the West, for instance, has become respectable not because biomedical physicians have advocated it but because patients have elected to see Chinese medicine

practitioners for their health care problems. On the dangers of romanticizing the discourse of resistance, see Abu-Lughod 1990.

39 A possible exception would be the influence of economically or politically powerful individuals (such as Mao Zedong) or of synthesized individual power, such as in the formation of political movements.

40 For a discussion of these issues, see Hanson 1997.

41 *Fei Shengfu yihua yi'an* 费绳甫医话医案 (*Fei Shengfu's Medical Essays and Case Histories*), section on *shanghan* 伤寒 illness, reprinted in Zhang Yuankai 张元凯 et al. 1985: 273.

42 *Lenglu yihua* 冷庐医话 (*Medical Stories from Cold Cottage*), 63.

43 *Ding Ganren yi'an* 丁甘仁医案 (*Ding Ganren's Case Records*), foreword by Cao Yingfu 曹颖甫.

44 On the use of tactics and their differentiation from strategies, see de Certeau 1988: 29–44. The essays collected in Laderman 1996 show what can be gained by moving performance to the forefront of inquiry in medical anthropology. On the notion of "ideological dilemmas," see Billig et al. 1988, particularly chapter 6, "Health and Illness." For a concise overview of various models of patient behavior in the anthropological literature, see Good 1994: 25–65.

45 Note that the notions of resistance and accommodation still inform this model, but each is now perceived from various angles simultaneously. Such perspectival pluralism enables the perception of plurality in opposition to the monism of a world systems perspective. See, however, McLennan 1995 on the conceptual problems of distinguishing descriptive and prescriptive (methodological, epistemological) pluralism. Pickering's (1995) "mangle of practice" discusses explicitly the concepts of accommodation and resistance, while Marcus (1995) shows how surrendering the anthropological focus on local life-worlds placed in opposition to a global system encompasses a surrendering of widely held attachments to subaltern points of view.

46 See the volume edited by Bermingham and Brewer 1995 for a series of investigations into cultural consumption that mirror recent theories in literary criticism focusing on the consumption of texts by their readers.

5. Shaping Chinese Medicine

1 Farquhar 1994a: 228. I would like to acknowledge the support of Elisabeth Hsu, whose careful editing of a previous version of case 5.4 and of the introduction and conclusion has greatly benefited the writing of this chapter. Cf. Hsu 2000: 370–404.

2 Scheper-Hughes and Lock 1987; Lock and Scheper-Hughes 1990.

3 On the distinction between "practices" as being concerned with "atemporal cultural mappings" and "practice" as designating an interest in the "temporality of cultural extensions," see Pickering 1995: 4.

4 Ots 1990a: 176–77, for instance, claims that state-run Chinese medicine offers little help to patients with psychosomatic illness.

5 This term is an example of the ambiguous use of terms in contemporary Chinese medicine. *Xinshen* refers here to cardiology and urology as much as to the heart and kidneys of Chinese medical discourse.

6 Throughout my period of observation in 1994, the demand for Professor Zhu's services was considerably greater, but he had specifically instructed the reception desk to limit the number of patients to a maximum of ten (a number that was always exceeded in the end) because he wished to have ample time for each consultation.

7 Ma Boying 马伯英 et al. 1994: 580.

8 Professor Zhu is aware that Chinese medical drugs can have side effects, of course. But in contradistinction to biomedical treatment, in which such side effects are accepted as a routine aspect of therapy, they are considered by him signs of the inappropriate use of drugs in Chinese medicine.

9 See Hay 1994; Liscomb 1993; and Qiu Peiran 裘沛然 1995 for investigations into the relationship between art and medicine in the Chinese tradition.

10 Farquhar 1994a: 190.

11 The total number of formulas available to Chinese physicians is unknown. The *Zhongyi fangji dacidian* 中医方剂大辞典 (*Great Encyclopaedia of Chinese Medicine Formulas*) compiled by the Nanjing College of Chinese Medicine (Nanjing zhongyi xueyuan 南京中医学院 1997), which runs to eleven volumes, lists 96,572 formulas. Clinical dictionaries like the *Jianming fangji cidian* 简明方剂辞典 (*Concise Dictionary of Formulas*) by Jiang Keming 江克明 and Bao Mingzhong 包明蕙 (1989) still contain more than 7,500 formulas. Students and doctors I asked claimed to know on average 200 formulas by heart, though some knew considerably more and many far fewer. In practice, some doctors are famous (and others infamous) for basing their entire practice on the use of only a handful of formulas. Others draw from a large base of memorized formulas.

12 The two extremes here are those who would tend to use the classical formulas (*jing-fang* 经方) of the Han, and those who would use modern formulas (*shifang* 时方), often their own.

13 According to some of my informants their use is derived from Shi Jinmo 施今墨. See Lü Jingshan 吕景山 1982 for a detailed study. It is discussed independently, however, by Qin Bowei 秦伯未 1983b and probably dates back much further. Shi Jinmo was thus an important popularizer rather than an inventor.

14 Professor Zhu used the older pronunciation *bo* rather than the modern colloquial *bai*. Although a thoroughly modern physician, Professor Zhu frequently also uses unsimplified characters in his writing. His patients and students pointed out to me his beautiful handwriting on many occasions.

15 *Shanghan lun* 34. See Li Peisheng 李培生 and Liu Duzhou 刘渡舟 1987.

16 Beijing's *si da mingyi* were Xiao Longyou 肖龙友 (1870–1960), famous for successfully treating Sun Yat-sen in 1924; Shi Jinmo 施今墨 (1881–1969) an important figure, both intellectually and politically, in preparing the way for the integration of Chinese and Western medicine; and Kong Bohua 孔伯华 (1885–1955), who established the Association of Chinese Medicine and Pharmacology in Beijing in 1929 together with Wang Fengchun 汪逢春 (1882–1948). Brief biographies and case studies that confirm Professor Zhu's assertion are in Dong Jianhua 董建华 1990: vol. 3. See also Jia Dedao 贾得道 1993: 359–60.

17 *Jingui yaolue* 12.5. See Li Keguang 李克光 1989: 328.

18 *Buzhong yiqi tang* is the flagship formula of Li Gao's *Piwei lun* 脾胃论 and thus of the important *yishui* 易水 school of medical thought. See Qiu Peiran 裘沛然 and Ding Guangdi 丁光迪 1992: 145, 154–65; Xu Jiqun 许济群 and Wang Mianzhi 王绵之 1995: 235–43.

19 Ibid.

20 *Shanghan lun* 141. See Li Peisheng 李培生 and Liu Duzhou 刘渡舟 1987; Xu Jiqun 许济群 and Wang Mianzhi 王绵之 1995: 538–40.

21 Zhang Xichun 张锡纯, *Yixue zhongzhong canxi lu*, particularly 1: 5–11, 181–83, and 3: 122–24, 132–34. Regulating uplifting and directing downward was an important concern to Zhang. He was clearly influenced in this by the *Yishui* 易水 school, which therefore also has influenced Professor Zhu. Cf. Qiu Peiran 裘沛然 and Ding Guangdi 丁光迪 1992: 708–22 and Scheid 1995a.

22 Jiang Keming 江克明 and Bao Mingzhong 包明蕙 1989: 23.

23 *Lizhong wan*, another formula from the *Shanghan lun*, had been memorized by this student to treat the stomach vacuity cold patterns with which it is linked in internal medicine textbooks; for example, Zhang Baiyu 张伯臾 et al. 1988: 271.

24 Edwards and Bouchier 1991: 770.

25 Xu Jiqun 许济群 and Wang Mianzhi 王绵之 1995: 522–25; Zhang Baiyu 张伯臾 et al. 1988: 334–35.

26 This combination is used by Zhang to treat painful obstruction, such as in his famous formula *Huoluo xiaoling dan* 活络效灵丹 (Miraculously Effective Elixir to Quicken the Collaterals). Cf. Zhang Xichun 张锡纯, *Yixue zhongzhong canxi lu*, 1: 185–87.

27 Gao Luwen 高渌纹 1993: 75–81; Yan Zhenghua 颜正华 1991: 304–5.

28 Xu Jiqun 许济群 and Wang Mianzhi 王绵之 1995: 227–31.

29 Zhang Xichun 张锡纯, *Yixue zhongzhong canxi lu*, 1: 383–85.

30 On the life and work of Sun Simiao, see Qiu Peiran 裘沛然 and Ding Guangdi 丁光迪 1992: 497–512; Sivin 1968: 81–144; and Unschuld 1994. A translation of Sun's treatise on "great physicians" (*dayi* 大医) is in Unschuld 1979: 29–33.

31 The original text of the *Xin tang shu* 新唐书 and a later reference to it by Zhang Jiebin 张介宾 are in Duan Yishan 段逸山 1986: 62, 196–97.

32 *Chengqi tang* formulas are a class of purgative decoctions first mentioned in the *Shanghan lun*. *Yizong bidu* 医宗必读: "Xingfang zhiyuan xinxiao danda lun" 行方智

圆心小胆大论 (Discussion regarding moral comportment, comprehensive knowledge, carefulness, and courage [of physicians]) 1.14: 87.

33 In passing he also, of course, reaffirms Chinese medicine's view of the body/person by means of the association between carefulness and a "little heart" (*xin xiao*), and courage and a "large gall bladder" (*dan da*).

34 Edwards and Bouchier 1991: 843.

35 Li Anmin 李安民 and Long Yurong 尤玉荣 1993; Zhang Baiyu 张伯臾 et al. 1988: 439–50.

36 Different textbooks arrive at different patterns for dizziness. The *Zhongyi dacidian* (1987: 286), for instance, states that there are at least eight principal patterns that can be further subdivided: *fengyun* 风晕 (wind dizziness), *shiyun* 湿晕 (dampness dizziness), *tanyun* 痰晕 (phlegm dizziness), *zhongshu xuanyun* 中暑眩晕 (summerheat dizziness), *zaohuo xuanyun* 燥火眩晕 (dry fire dizziness), *qiyu xuanyun* 气郁眩晕 (*qi* depression dizziness), *ganhuo xuanyun* 肝火眩晕 (liver fire dizziness), and *xu yun* 虚晕 (depletion dizziness).

37 The use of the term *xing* (type) rather than the more classical *zheng* (pattern) is common in clinical papers that take biomedical disease categories as their starting point. In practice, patterns are often designated as types, though types are stable whereas patterns are ephemeral. Clinical research is thus often carried out on the basis of types. See also chapter 7.

38 Deng Tietao 邓铁涛 1987: 426–39. Contemporary understandings of liver disorders are derived, in the main, from the three rubrics (*san gang bianzheng* 三纲辨证) of liver *qi*, liver fire, and liver wind as proposed by the Qing physician Ye Tianshi 叶天士 (1667–1746). See Li Xiaohai 李晓海 1988 for an overview of Ye Tianshi's theories regarding liver disorders and their influence on other Qing physicians.

39 For *shengjiang* theory, see Kou Huaxing 寇华胜 1990.

40 In both verbal and written discourse Chinese physicians sometimes use terms that would, strictly speaking, refer to a particular channel and/or to one of the six stages in the *shanghan* model of disease when they mean the visceral system (*zangfu*) and its associated channel, as in the present case. They can, of course, make the necessary distinction between the two if they so choose.

41 *Shanzhi tan zhe, bu zhi tan er zhi qi, qi shun ze yishen zhi jinye yi sui qi er shun* 善治痰者, 不治痰而治气, 气顺则一身之津液亦随气而顺. This quotation, widely cited today, is attributed to Pang Anshi in the *Zhengzhi zhunsheng* 证治准绳 (*Indispensable Tools for Pattern Treatment*), vol. 1, section 1, p. 203.

42 Deng Tietao 邓铁涛 1987: 377.

43 The opposition between the tangible, or formed (*xing*), and the intangible, or formless (*wu xing*), is a recurrent topos of Chinese medicine, but is applied to phlegm for the first time in Chinese medical textbooks of the late 1950s. Steve Clavey, 1996: personal communication.

44 Feng Zhaozhang, 冯兆张 *Miannang milu* 绵囊秘录 (*Secret Records of the Cotton Bag*), 12.9: 383.

45 It is common practice not to specify amounts but to leave these to the discretion of individual practitioners.

46 An important antecedent formula frequently employed by Professor Zhu in which *Haematitum* is used for this purpose is *Zhengan xifeng tang* 镇肝熄风汤 (Settle the Liver and Extinguish Wind Decoction), which was composed by Zhang Xichun 张锡纯 (*Yixue zhongzhong canxi lu*, 1: 312–18, and 2: 42–55). For the different roles drugs can assume in Chinese medical formulas, see Xu Jiqun 许济群 and Wang Mianzhi 王绵之 1995: 14–15; and Farquhar 1994a: 181–84.

47 The chief antecedent formulas here are *Erchen tang* 二陈汤 (Two-Cured Decoction) and its variation *Daotan tang* 导痰汤 (Guide [Out] Phlegm Decoction). The former was first mentioned in the *Taiping huimin hejiju fang* 太平惠民和剂局方 (*Formulas of the Public Pharmacy of the Era of Great Peace and of the Bureau of Medicines*), 4.19: 141, published after 1078, and has since become the representative formula for drying dampness and transforming phlegm (*zaoshi huatan* 燥湿化痰). The latter is a variation first mentioned in the *Jisheng fang* 济生方 (*Formulas to Benefit the Living*) of 1253, cited in Xu Jiqun 许济群 and Wang Mianzhi 王绵之 1995: 529–32.

48 There is a certain degree of overlap between these categories. *Trichosanthis fructus*, for instance, is a drug for treating phlegm, and *Pinelliae rhizoma* also directs *qi* downward. My presentation simplifies even more complex relations.

49 Cheng Shao'en 程绍恩 et al. 1990: 154–55; Yan Zhenghua 颜正华 1991: 334–36; Zang Kuntang 臧坤堂 and Wu Keqiang 吴克强 1990: 59–61.

50 Deng Tietao 邓铁涛 (1987: 37), for instance, quotes the first chapter of the Qing dynasty *Cuncunzhai yihua gao* 存存斋医话稿 (*Medical Notes from the Hall of Actuality*) as saying "phlegm belongs to damp, it is a transformation of the fluids" (*tan shu shi, wei jinye suo hua* 痰属湿, 为津液所化).

51 Zhang Baiyu 张伯臾 et al. 1988: 146. This is the most common view today, though there are quite different interpretations, of which the work of Cheng Menxue 程门雪 (1902–1972), former principal of the Shanghai College of Chinese Medicine, is a prominent example (1986: 76–83).

52 Zhongshan yiyuan "zhongyi fangji xuan jiang" bianxiezu 中山医院 "中医方剂选讲" 编写组 1983: 232.

53 Edwards and Bouchier 1991: 843.

54 Yan Zhenghua 颜正华 1991: 327.

55 Xu Jiqun 许济群 and Wang Mianzhi 王绵之 1995: 531.

56 Ibid., 445–46.

57 On biomedical drugs, see Zhang Xichun 张锡纯, *Yixue zhongzhong canxi lu*, 2: 141–65. Zhang employed biomedical theories in his understanding of the *sanjiao* 三焦 (ibid.: 194–96) and in the formulation of novel formulas for wasting thirst (*xiaoke* 消渴), which he equated with diabetes. See 1: 76–78.

58 Last 1992; Sivin 1987, 1990; Unschuld 1992.

59 For related ethnographies of syncretism in the development of Chinese and Ayurvedic medical practice, see Obeyesekere 1992; and Hsu 1995, 1996.

60 What I label "Western medicine" here is likewise (although I have not examined it)

not a universalized abstract practice but Professor Zhu's idiosyncratic use of biomedical theories, drugs, tools, and so on, within specific institutional and historical contexts.

61 A detailed discussion of this transformation by Christine Bodenschatz forms part of a forthcoming doctoral dissertation in progress at the Department for the History of Medicine, Ludwig-Maximillian-University, Munich. Ding Guangdi 丁光迪 1999 is an analysis of the same transformation from a contemporary Chinese perspective. See also Miyashita 1986.

62 For reasons of economy I have not described here in detail the unfolding of individual case histories over successive treatment episodes. Several such descriptions are available, however, in Farquhar's (1992a, 1992b, 1994a: 46–55) ethnographic studies of Chinese medicine. We can observe there Chinese medical practice as an unfolding interaction, where interpretations of a disease stated in the present lead to treatment formulations, the effects of which lead to new interpretations, and so on.

63 Qiu Peiran 裘沛然 and Ding Guangdi 丁光迪 1992: 19–112; Yan 1993: 34–55; Bodenschatz forthcoming.

64 The social history of the emergence of the *wenbing* stream during the Qing is discussed by Hanson (1997). For examples of modern attempts at reconciliation known as *hanwen tongyi* 寒温统一 (the unification of cold and warm [pathogen disorders]), whose political imperatives are briefly discussed in chapter 7. Also see the brief overview in Meng Shujiang 孟澍江 1985: 14–15.

65 On the composition, action, and origin of these formulas, see Xu Jiqun 许济群 and Wang Mianzhi 王绵之 1995: 509–12, 532–34, 546–47; and Li Keguang 李克光 1989: 328–31, 340–41.

66 My discussion is based on the overview in Li Anmin 李安民 and Long Yurong 尤玉荣 1993: 329–33.

6. Students, Disciples, and the Art of Social Networking

1 Farquhar (1994a) created the term "knowing practice" to describe the clinical encounter in Chinese medicine.

2 Henriques et al. 1984: 204. The notion of a universal Enlightenment self is challenged by studies from within a variety of research traditions that expose the social construction of body (e.g., Dissanayake 1993 and Lock 1993b; cognition (e.g., Schleifer et al. 1992; and Varela et al. 1995); emotion (e.g., Harré 1986; and Lutz 1988); and person and self (e.g., Shweder and Bourne 1982, 1985; and Taylor 1989). It is further challenged by both historical and anthropological studies which show that the individual never has been a stable focus of inquiry and is increasingly difficult to define as such at the end of the twentieth century (e.g., Dodds 1973; Geertz 1977; Haraway 1993; Rabinow 1996; Shore 1982; Strathern 1992a, 1992b; White and Kirkpatrick 1985; and Young 1990).

3 Lock 1993b: 138. The historical process by which the Enlightenment subject was

established is described by Toulmin 1990. On the definition of subjectivity as an object of study, see Henriques et al. 1984. For definitions with particular relevance to Chinese studies, see Farquhar and Hevia 1993; and Zito and Barlow 1994b.

4   The seminal study here is Mol and Law 1994. See also Serres and Latour 1995: 60.

5   Other routes existed, too. These reached from the use of folk remedies and ready-made formulas at one end of the spectrum to self-study and training at the Imperial Academy (Taiyiyuan 太医院) at the other.

6   A good example is the Shanghai Technical College of Chinese Medicine (Shanghai zhongyi zhuanmen xuexiao 上海中医专门学校) founded by Ding Ganren 丁甘仁 in 1916, which later changed its name to Shanghai College of Chinese Medicine (Shanghai zhongyi xueyuan 上海中医学院). Students at the college completed two years of classroom teaching before being apprenticed to a physician with whom they would complete another year of internship ("Mingyi yaolan" bianshen wei-yuanhui 《名医摇篮》编审委员会 1998).

7   The reason for this was the desire to increase the number of Chinese medicine physicians more rapidly than could be achieved merely by means of the newly opened colleges. In Shanghai, for instance, 1,447 physicians were trained through various apprenticeship courses between 1957 and 1960 (Wang Qiaochu 王翘楚 1998: 83).

8   Wang Zhipu 王致谱 and Cai Jingfeng 蔡景峰 (1999: 32) provide the entire list of physicians and students. See also Croizier 1968: 181–82; and Taylor 2000: chapter 3). This scheme has been continued since then in various ways.

9   The biography of the physician Chunyu Yi 淳于意 (fl. 180 B.C.) contained in the *Shiji* 史记 (*Memoirs of the Grand Astrologer*; c. 100 B.C.) 105: 45, documents his training with his master, Gongcheng Yangqing 公乘阳庆. See Sivin 1995: 177–82 for a translation. Cf. also Keegan 1988: 222–36.

10   Sivin 1995: 200.

11   See Chao 1995; and Wu 1998 for a discussion of these issues. My own research into late imperial and Republican medical traditions in Jiangsu and Shanghai suggests that personal transmission was of the utmost importance even for the most paradigmatic literati physicians.

12   These relationships are enumerated in their standard sequence for the first time by Mencius (3a.4, 3b.9, 4a.2), who also joins them with their appropriate emotive tenor. Although formulated within the context of family kinship, their content applied equally to relations outside the family. See Eastman 1988: 35.

13   Cf. Eberhardt's (1971: 6) dictum (cited in Eastman 1988: 35) that Chinese society is based on the assumption that "no two persons are ever equal; always one is higher than the other."

14   Smith 1983: 115.

15   Watson 1982; Yang 1961.

16   On the notion of "face" (*mianzi* 面子, *lian* 脸), see Ho 1975; Hu 1944; and Hwang 1987. Power distance "is the extent to which the members of a society accept that

power in institutions and organizations is distributed unequally" (Hofstede 1980: 83, 1983). On value change in modernizing Chinese cultures, see the contributions to the special spring 1991 issue of *Daedalus*.

17 It was not easy to speak with disciples about their teacher, because commenting on him in any judgmental way or revealing intimate knowledge could have amounted to a betrayal of the ethos of that relationship. It was not, for instance, possible for me to speak much with Professor Rong's disciples. I had very good relations, though, with his students and with the personal disciples of three other famous Beijing physicians. I have also spoken to many Chinese physicians about their views on discipleship, to disciples of less famous physicians and physicians studying within family traditions, and to Westerners who have been accepted as disciples of Chinese physicians. See also the biographies of contemporary physicians such as Fang Yaozhong 方药中 1983; and Liu Duzhou 刘渡舟 1983, which include descriptions of old-style apprenticeship.

18 My knowledge of discipleship is based on accounts in the literature as well as conversations with older physicians who were disciples during the 1930s and 1940s. The biographies collected in Zhou Fengwu 周风梧 et al. 1981–85 present autobiographical accounts by many of China's most famous contemporary physicians that contain details of their apprenticeships.

19 Sivin 1995.

20 Wang Zhipu 王致谱 and Cai Jingfeng 蔡景峰 1999: 41. I spent considerable time attempting to establish how exactly one becomes a *ming laozhongyi* but was unable to arrive at one clear set of criteria. In 1978 MOH statistics accounted for eighty-five *laozhongyi*, of whom twenty-eight were *ming laozhongyi* (Zhonghua renmin gongheguo weishengbu zhongyisi 中华人民共和国卫生部中医司 1985: 294), though the number was later increased more than five hundred. While the subject clearly warrants further investigation, it seems that besides descent, clinical efficacy (rendered visible by a large clientele), and contributions to the textual archive of Chinese medicine as the author of articles and books, political connections and evaluations also play a role.

21 The five factors that worked in Dr. Chao's favor were pointed out to me by Dr. Chao herself on explicit questioning.

22 *Renqing, ganqing,* and their relation to "subjectification" and "subjectivity" in contemporary China are discussed in detail by Kipnis (1997) and Yang (1994).

23 They share it, however, with some other faculty members at the university.

24 I know of children of other Beijing *ming laozhongyi* who carry on the family line abroad. Many children of famous physicians of the Republican period studied Western medicine rather than Chinese medicine. According to my informants, at least sometimes the reason was that families perceived Western medicine to be a better bet for the future.

25 This seems to be a general phenomenon of change in the contemporary period. During my fieldwork I met three female doctors (from Liaoning, Shanxi, and Bei-

jing) who were heirs to a family medical tradition. I also met female students from Taiwan, Japan, and Malaysia who were the heirs to their families' medical lines and had been sent by their families to study Chinese medicine on the mainland.

26 This should not be read to imply that all teachers demand ties only to themselves. Many teachers actively encourage their disciples to study elsewhere, and there are many examples of well-known physicians (such as Ye Tianshi 叶天士) who studied under many different teachers. Many more examinations of these relations and in particular the conjunction of professional, familial, emotive, and economic ties they imply are required before any generalizations can be made.

27 In Professor Rong's line, for instance, is a famous prescription formulated by Professor Rong's father whose ingredients remain secret.

28 *Houhan shu* 侯汉书 (*History of the Later Han*), quoted in Ma Boying 马伯英 1993: 778. A biography of Guo Yu can be found in DeWoskin 1983: 74–76, whose translation I follow.

29 For a summary of these debates, see Ma 1993: 778–85, He Yumin 何裕民 1987: 15–16, and Liao Yujun 廖育群 1999. In these discussions the notion of *yi* is used not only to signal the difficulty of teaching the craftlike aspects of medical knowledge but as a constitutive aspect of the medical *habitus* that is the foundation of clinical success and medical innovation. Polanyi's (1958) assimilation of scientific inquiry to implicit and therefore personal knowledge is derived from a quite different context of debate, as shown by Fuller 2000: 139–53.

30 On the context of situated learning as legitimate peripheral participation, a perspective of learning developed from within a framework of Vygotskian activity theory, see Lave and Wenger 1991 and Lave 1993. This perspective situates itself against notions of knowledge as something that simply can be transmitted from one person to another but leaves knowledge itself unchanged. It also deserves to be pointed out that literati physicians such as Xu Dachun 徐大椿 (1693–1771) depicted learning medicine through peripheral participation, that is, within discipleships, as absolutely essential only for hands-on subdisciplines like external medicine (*waike* 外科). See his *Yixue yuanliu lun* 医学源流论 1757, 6.12: 216–17.

31 See Hsu 1999: 102–4. Hsu has devoted an entire book to examining the transmission of knowledge in contemporary Chinese medicine, differentiating between three distinct contexts and forms of transmission: the transmission of secret knowledge within personal master-disciple relationships; learning as an aspect of classical scholarship; and undergraduate courses within modern Chinese colleges. Her descriptions and analysis are considerably more detailed than those presented here and constitute an essential background to my own work. In a sense, it is the separation of these forms and contexts of learning by Hsu that allows me to focus on their intricate interconnectedness in the person of Professor Rong.

32 He Yumin 何裕民 1987; Wang Songbao 汪松葆 1987.

33 Competition seems to be getting increasingly fiercer. According to my informants, in the 1999 academic year only six undergraduates managed to be admitted to study

for master's degrees at the Beijing University of Chinese Medicine and Pharmacology.

34 For the kind of examinations typical of Chinese medicine state education, see Quanguo gaodeng jiaoyu zixue kaoshi zhidao weiyuanhui 全国高等教育自学考试指导委员会 1986.

35 Medical examinations in the Song dynasty were equally stereotyped, pointing to an important historical continuity which also may have a bearing on the composition of modern exams (Lu and Needham 2000: 95–113). I am indebted to Nathan Sivin for pointing out this connection. Zhu Chenyu 祝谌予, the first dean of the Beijing Chinese Medicine College, emphasizes in his biography that memorization (beigong 背功) constitutes a traditional yet essential method of learning in Chinese medicine (Qian Zifen 钱自奋 et al. 1993: 21). This view is shared by all senior physicians I have asked about this issue.

36 In a detailed examination of textual and ethnographic sources Hsu (1992) identifies five important changes in the way Chinese medicine is taught to Chinese medicine undergraduate students as a result of this process: (1) an increasing separation of theory from clinical practice, (2) a visible emphasis on the systematic presentation of material and a change in the presentation of concepts from mnemonic devices to descriptions and propositions so that truth and contradiction became visibly problematic, (3) a reversal of the emphasis on matter over function in the explication of key concepts such as blood (xue) and body fluids (jinye), (4) the importation and integration of concepts derived from various European traditions (Marxism, biomedicine, natural science) with classical knowledge, and (5) changes to the manner in which students gained access to classical knowledge (excerpts from classical texts replaced the careful reading of source texts, dialogue was replaced with monologue).

37 Li Jingwei 李经纬 and Deng Tietao 邓铁涛 1995: 1282.

38 I was told by my informants (students at the Beijing College of Chinese Medicine in the 1950s and 1960s) that the various networks that formed around these key teachers had very cordial relations but were nevertheless clearly bounded.

39 See Sivin 1987 for details.

40 These textbooks, published by Shanghai Science and Technology Press, are compiled by special commissions under the guidance of the MOH. The most recent series of textbooks, compiled during the Eighth Five-Year Plan (1990–95) encompasses thirty-eight specialized subjects from basic theory to pharmacology.

41 Formulas are Professor Rong's proclaimed area of theoretical expertise. Clinically Professor Rong professes to specialize in the "treatment of difficult conditions within the fields of internal medicine, pediatrics, and gynecology" as well as in "externally contracted heat diseases" (from the biography in his clinic).

42 Medical efficaciousness as embodied practice discussed in terms of linghuo is discussed in detail by Farquhar (1994a, 1996: 246). Feuchtwang (1992) discusses similar uses of ling by temple-goers in Taiwan, referring to the magical powers of gods and

the efficaciousness of embodied actions by gods, humans, and other agents. The verb *biantong* 变通 expresses the same ability to adapt oneself to circumstance. Regarding essential differences in Chinese and Western perceptions of efficacy, see also Jullien 1997, 1999.

43 The distinct pattern of symptoms and signs associated with a formula that is memorized by students can, if found in a patient, provide a diagnosis. This kind of practice is commonly referred to today as *bianfang* 辨方 (differentiation by prescription). It allows physicians to agree on the use of a formula without necessarily agreeing on the underlying disease mechanism or the action of the formula. As both Farquhar (1994a), Qin Bowei 秦伯未 (1983a) and Qin Bowei 秦伯未 et al. (1961) make clear, such practice cannot, however, be equated with simple empiricism but must be seen in the wider context of pattern differentiation in which diagnosing a disease mechanism and deciding on a treatment strategy mutually enable one another.

44 See Schoenhals 1993 for a discussion of how education in China is concerned with helping students to embody socially sanctioned models of virtue.

45 In Beijing I observed student groups ranging in size from one to twelve during clinical training. Students rarely followed the same physician for longer than two to three months.

46 In 1994 it was impossible, for instance, to study for a doctoral degree in pediatrics (*erke* 儿科) in Beijing because no professor there was entitled to supervise such a degree.

47 Examining the role and meaning of secret formulas in contemporary and classical Chinese medicine goes far beyond the scope of my present investigation. They are mentioned here for two reasons only: as an example of another crossover point between differently situated contexts of learning, and as an example for how old tools are adapted to new contexts. For a more complex and detailed study of the transmission of secret knowledge and secret formulas in Chinese medicine, see Li 1997; and also Hsu 1999.

48 I follow here the argument made by Yan (1996: 74) and King (1994: 114) that none of the English translations available for *guanxi* can grasp its rich connotational meanings in Chinese and that it should therefore be left untranslated.

49 Fei Xiaotong's *Xiangtu zhongguo* (1992) is the most interesting and influential of these. It is particularly important inasmuch as it represents a genuine attempt to furnish a sociology of China based on native rather than Western sociological categories. See also Wang Songxing, "The Lineage of the Han People," unpublished manuscript cited in King 1994: 115. Jacobs (1979) gives as the most common attributes for building networks: locality, kinship, co-worker, classmate, sworn brotherhood, surname, and teacher-student. King (1994: 115) compares Chinese family ethics based on individual relationships with Japanese ones based on group membership and thereby follows Fei Xiaotong's lead.

50 Oi 1989: 131, 228; Walder 1986: 6–7.

51 Kipnis 1997; Yan 1996; Yang 1994. See also the more general discussion in Nathan 1993.

52 Yan 1996: 75, 88; Yang 1994: chapter 3.

53 Kipnis 1997: 7.

54 This list was established on the basis of biographical entries in Shi Yuguang 史宇广 1981; and Li Yun 李云 1988.

55 Chen 1989: 182; Ma Boying 马伯英 et al. 1994: 574–76. Evidence for personal contact and informal connections between political leaders and leading Chinese medicine scholar-physicians can be found in the biographies of many of these physicians. In 1953, for instance, Yue Meizhong 乐美中 presented a memorial regarding the development of Chinese medicine to the state council that he had composed together with Li Dingming's son Li Zhensan 李振三. Yue is also said to have treated many members of the political elite, including Mao Zedong and Zhou Enlai (Zhongguo kexue jizhu xiehui 1999: 132). Shi Jinmo had several audiences with leading politicians, including Mao Zedong and Zhou Enlai (ibid.: 54). Zhou seems to have known many of the leading physicians of Chinese medicine. Another physician, Zhang Cigong 章次公, who was an adviser to the MOH from 1955 to 1959, treated Mao Zedong, Zhou Enlai, Zhu De 朱德, Deng Xiaoping, He Long 贺龙, and other leading members of the politburo at the time, according to a biography by his daughter (Zhu Liangchun 朱良春 2000: 420). He Shixi 何时希 (1997) compared the Academy of Chinese Medicine, where he worked from 1956 to 1966, to the Imperial Medical Academy (Taiyiyuan 太医院), which provided medical services to the imperial family.

56 The subjective nature of such decisions regularly leads to discussions in journals of Chinese medicine debating the content of textbooks. See, for example, Gu Zhishan 顾植山 1982; and Lu Zhongyue 陆中岳 and Hong Shenglin 洪胜林 1988. According to my informants such debates take place between participants who are not connected to each other within guanxi networks so that the exchange of views is not subject to obligations or effects of power.

57 Nanjing zhongyi xueyuan 南京中医学院 1958: 146–47.

58 Deng Tietao 邓铁涛 1987: 426–38.

59 My case study is based on the examination of articles published in Chinese medical journals between 1984 and 1995 and on conversations with physicians and students. For overviews of relevant debates in Chinese medical history, see Hu Yulun 胡玉伦 1986; and Chen Baoming 陈宝明 and Zhao Jinxi 赵进喜 1994.

60 Yizong bidu 医宗必读 (Essential Readings from the Medical Ancestors), 1: 1.11, 1999: 85. Authors subscribing to this view argue that supplementation of the liver must proceed indirectly via the supplementation of the kidneys.

61 Hu Yulun 胡玉伦 (1986) cites passages from Suwen 1, 2, 9, 58, and 80, and from Lingshu 8, 10, and 54 as well as from other canonical works from the Han onward.

62 Zhang Jiebin 张介宾 (Collected Treatises of [Zhang] Jingyue), cited in Chen Baoming 陈宝明 and Zhao Jinxi 赵进喜 1994: 6.

63 Wang Qinlin's thirty methods are contained in *Xixi shuceng yehua* 西溪书层夜话 (*Nighttime Essays from the West Stream Library*). They are reprinted in Huang Zili 黄自立 1988: 43–45.

64 See Li Xiaohai 李晓海 1988 for an overview of Ye Tianshi's theories and their influence on other Qing physicians.

65 Sivin 1987: 113.

66 Zhongyi bingming zhenduan guifan ketizu 中医病名诊断规范课题 1987; Guojia jishu jianduju 国家技术鉴督局 1995: 38–40.

67 Tang discusses the role of liver *qi* in an influential passage in the *Xuezheng lun* 血证论 (*Discussion of Blood Patterns*) 1.3 and 7: 76–77. Zhang Xichun 张锡纯 (*Yixue zhongzhong canxi lu*) discussed the role of liver *qi* and its depletion in many different contexts. These are analyzed by Han Zhirong 韩智荣 and Liu Jinsheng 刘金声 (1990) and Zhang Yingcai 张英才 (1993).

68 Hu Yulun 胡玉伦 1986: 52.

69 Guojia jishu jianduju 国家技术鉴督局 1997b.

70 This holds true for both the fifth (Deng Tietao 邓铁涛 1984) and the sixth editions (Zhu Wenfeng 朱文锋 1995).

71 Exemplary here is the work of Chen Jiaxu 陈家旭 (1992, 1993, 1994a, 1994b), a former graduate student of Professor Yang, with whom I discussed this issue and who confirmed my analysis.

72 Yang Weiyi 杨维益 1988: 105. Although I have attempted to contact Professor Zhu Wenfeng personally and via two of his students, I have not succeeded in obtaining information regarding the reasons for the exclusion of these patterns from the official textbooks or the process of discussion and deliberation within the committee.

73 It is not discussed, for instance, in Deng Tietao 邓铁涛 1987; and Zhang Baiyu 张伯臾 et al. 1988.

74 Guojia jishu jianduju 国家技术鉴督局 1995.

75 Qiu Peiran 裴沛然 and Ding Guangdi 丁光迪 1992: 607.

76 *Buzhong yiqi tang* is one of the most important supplementing formulas in Chinese medicine. It was composed by the Jin dynasty physician Li Gao 李杲 in the *Piwei lun* 脾胃论. *Shengxian tang* is discussed in Xu Jiqun 许济群 and Wang Mianzhi 王绵之 1995; but not, for instance, in Yang Yiya 杨医亚 1994. I discuss this topic at length in Scheid 1995.

77 Compare Zhao Shaoqin 赵绍琴 et al. 1982 with Meng Shujiang 孟澍江 1985. According to information by other informants, the process of textbook composition is more complex and more varied than made out by my teacher. It may also have changed over time. I was told that today the role of committee chairpersons is often a purely ceremonial one (reflecting status and position within Chinese medicine as a state institution) without real power or influence. The chief editor(s) of many textbooks may therefore have had no role in their composition, the task having been carried out instead by younger physicians and academics under direction of the state administration.

78 Maciocia 1996.

79 For a historical case study of the relation between painting and clinical practice in Chinese medicine, see Liscomb 1993.

80 The new importance of *guanxixue* in Chinese society and its historical transformation is discussed by Kipnis (1997), Yan (1996), and Yang (1994).

81 See chapter 7.

82 I am thinking here, for instance, of Wu's (1993–94) illuminating prosopographical study of Liu Wansu 刘完素 and his disciples from the Jin to the early Ming. Much may also be gained from trawling the (auto)biographies of Chinese physicians such as those collected by Zhou Fengwu 周风梧 et al. (1981–85), a task already begun by Farquhar (1992b).

83 Zito 1994.

84 Hay 1983b, 1983c.

85 Note that the nonsimplified character for *mai* 脈 shares its phonetic element with *pai* 派. On the connection between the phonetic component of Chinese characters and their meaning, see Boltz 1994: 95–99.

86 de Certeau 1988: 117.

87 Farquhar 1994a: 96 n. 39; Hay 1983a; Zito 1994: 121.

88 Ames 1994; Hsu 1971; Tu 1994. For attempts to capture such relational efficacy in social psychological models of social influence, see Latané and Wolf 1981; and Tanford and Penrod 1984.

89 Such observations are confirmed by Schoenhals's (1993) detailed study of education in the People's Republic. Based on participant observations in a Chinese secondary school (*zhongxue* 中学) Schoenhals argues that a paradox of power exists in cultures of face and shame such as China's. This cedes to inferiors a certain power over superiors in spite of the hierarchical character of the system. Superiors have more face but are constantly onstage and must live up to the standards expected of them. This, according to Schoenhals, gives each class session the character of a performance.

90 Ames 1994.

91 Latour 1987.

92 For a critique of the network metaphor in relation to Latour's actor-network model, see Mol and Law 1994; and Pickering 1995: 11, 221.

93 The concept of synthesis (elaborated to a much greater extent) features prominently in the work of Deleuze and Guattari (1983), which has provided much stimulation for my own reflections, and from which the distinction between conjunctive and connective syntheses is borrowed.

94 de Certeau 1988: 201.

95 Serres and Latour 1995: 60.

7. Bianzheng lunzhi

1 My focus on voices from within the Chinese medicine community narrows the scope of my exploration sufficiently to make it practicable and also directly extends

the discussions of chapters 5 and 6. It relates to the other studies of pattern differentiation available in the Western academic literature on Chinese medicine, specifically Farquhar 1994a and Sivin 1987, but also to debates within the Chinese medicine community in the West (Flaws 1992; Hammer 1991). Finally, this approach accords with the specific orientations of this study outlined in chapter 1. I feel vindicated in my choice of representative persons (a choice made in 1995) inasmuch as all are included among the thirty-seven scholar-physicians of Chinese medicine whose biographies were published by the China Science and Technology Association (Zhongguo kexue jishu xiehui 中国科学技术协会) in 1999. Furthermore, they have recently been acknowledged as the main influences on the shaping of pattern differentiation by Meng Qingyun 孟庆云 (2000: 81), who is himself an important contributor to the ongoing development of the practice.

2 Ke Xuefan 柯雪帆 (1987: 31–38), for instance, differentiates ten distinct types of pattern differentiation with even more subtypes.

3 Another term, *zheng* 征, denoting manifestations arising from a certain condition, exists but is less used in medical discourse.

4 For example, Deng Tietao 邓铁涛 1987: 295; Ke Xuefan 柯雪帆 1987: 9–24; Ouyang Qi 欧阳琦 1993: 2–5; Zhonguo zhongyi yanjiuyuan 中国中医研究院 1984: 1–7, 1987: 1–17.

5 For most physicians I observed, the notion of *bing* would include, in Eisenberg's (1977: 11) terms, "experiences of disvalued changes in states of being and in social function" rather than mere "abnormalities in the structure and function of body organs and systems." Furthermore, the semantic range of *bing* covers not only diseases but also such states as broken bones and wounds. Sivin (1987) therefore translates *bing* as "disorder," while Farquhar (1994a) decides on "illness" for *bing* and "disease" for *jibing*. If I nevertheless use "disease" to translate *bing*, this is to make clear the close association the term now has in both professional and public discourse with the biomedical notion of disease.

6 Farquhar (1994a: 58) translates *zheng* 征 as "sign" to distinguish it from *zheng* 症, "symptom." However, *zheng* 症 includes both subjective symptoms and objective signs, and I thus translate it as "symptoms and signs."

7 Pei Xueyi 裴学义 and Kong Xiangqi 孔祥琦 1981: 102. Regarding Beijing's four famous physicians, see chapter 5, note 16.

8 Sivin 1987: 106–15; Farquhar 1987, 1992a, 1992b, 1994a, 1994b.

9 Farquhar 1994a: chapter 5.

10 He Yumin 何裕民 1987: 160. Similar statements are found in many other texts, for example, Hu Xin 胡欣 and Ge Xiumei 葛秀梅 1994: 1; and Ke Xuefan 柯雪帆 1987: 9–24.

11 Zhang Baiyu 张伯臾 et al. 1988: 22.

12 Typical examples are Fang Yaozhong 方药中 1979: chapter 3; and Ke Xuefan 柯雪帆 1987: 9–24.

13 Zhonguo zhongyi yanjiuyuan 中国中医研究院 1987: 1. This view is shared by West-

ern commentators such as Ågren (1986), Farquhar (1994a), Porkert (1983: 1–15), and Sivin (1987: 109–15). Farquhar, Porkert, and Sivin all correlate proficiency in pattern differentiation with clinical efficacy.

14 Chen Li 陈离 1991; Jia Dedao 贾得道 1993: 101; Hu Xin 胡欣 and Ge Xiumei 葛秀梅 1994: 6–31; Ma Boying 马伯英 1993: 285; Shi Lanhua 史兰化 1992: 63; Zhongyi bingming zhenduan guifan ketizu 中医病名诊断规范课题组 1987: 2.

15 Cf. Yang 1995.

16 Wang Xudong 王旭东 1989: 204.

17 The development of Chinese medicine in other countries corroborates this statement. In Taiwan, for instance, national examinations in Chinese medicine are still based on classical texts such as the *Neijing* and *Nanjing* and do not make pattern differentiation a central element. The same is true for Europe prior to the popularization of contemporary Chinese medicine in the 1980s, as evidenced, for instance, by Soulié de Morant 1994.

18 Farquhar 1994a: 171. See also Unschuld 1985: 258.

19 So much is admitted even in contemporary Chinese medical discourse, though from the teleological perspective of historical materialism. Hu Xin 胡欣 and Ge Xiumei 葛秀梅 (1994: 6–31), for instance, divide the development of *bianzheng lunzhi* into three stages: (1) the emergence of basic concepts in the *Neijing*, (2) a gradual development of theories up to the Qing, and (3) its contemporary systematization and reconciliation of previously divergent traditions and practices. Ke Xuefan 柯雪帆 (1987: 3–8) provides a similar historical account.

20 Ke Xuefan 柯雪帆 (1987: 2) takes the origin of *bianzheng lunzhi* two steps further back. Not only does Ke locate the origin of Zhang Zhongjing's six-stage diagnostic system in the *Neijing*, he also detects the distinction between depletion (*xu* 虚) and repletion (*shi* 实) in the manuscripts found in the tomb at Manwangdui, which date back to the Western Han.

21 The book is today separated into two texts: the *Shanghan lun* 伤寒论 (*Discussions of Cold Damage*) and the *Jingui yaolue* 金匮要略 (*Essentials of the Golden Casket*). Li Peisheng 李培生 and Liu Duzhou 刘渡舟 (1987: 4–9) and Li Keguang 李克光 (1989: 4–10) provide contemporary expositions of the therapeutic approach advocated in these texts.

22 *Shanghan lun* 1; *Jingui yaolue* 13 and 20.

23 *Shanghan lun* 149.

24 *Shanghan lun* 2.

25 *Shanghan lun* 18.

26 *Shanghan lun* 14.

27 Compare *Shanghan lun* 96, 103, 104, and 107.

28 *Shanghan lun* 138, for instance, gives *xiao jiexiong bing* 小结胸病 (lesser chestbind disease) as a subpattern of *taiyang* diseases for which *Xiao xianxiong tang* 小陷胸汤 (Minor Sinking into the Chest Decoction) is indicated in the same manner in which otherwise patterns are discussed.

29 *Shanghan lun* 48.

30 *Jingui yaolue* 7.

31 *Jingui yaolue* 9.

32 *Jingui yaolue* 1.

33 These are grouped together under the label "*Shanghan* scholarly stream" (*Shang-han xuepai* 伤寒学派). See Qiu Peiran 裘沛然 and Ding Guangdi 丁光迪 1992: 19–112. For discussions of unresolved issues, see Li Peisheng 李培生 and Liu Duzhou 刘渡舟 1987; and Li Keguang 李克光 1989, which also provide ample evidence of historical debates.

34 See chapter 2, notes 11 and 12. A good historical example of another method is the five-phases-based differentiation of *zangfu* patterns of Chen Shiduo's 陈士铎 *Bian-zheng lu* 辨证录 (*Record of Differentiating Patterns*) (1989 [1687]), a classical text found in almost every medical bookshop.

35 One example is damp jaundice symptom (*shi dan hou* 湿疸候) under the disease category jaundice (*huangbing* 黄病).

36 According to the Zhongyi bingming zhenduan guifan ketizu 中医病名诊断规范课题组 (1987: 2–3), the numbers of diseases listed in each text are 1061, 381, and 714, respectively.

37 Furth (1999: 65–66) refers to pattern diagnosis as an invention of the Northern Song that gradually spread in the twelfth and thirteenth centuries. The reasons for what I prefer to call an emergence rather than an invention cannot be discussed here in detail but must include the following. First, government-sponsored publications of the *Shanghan lun* during the Song helped to establish this text as the foundation of pharmacotherapy. Second, during the Song it became more common for gentlemen to become physicians, gradually generating a new group of scholar-physicians who imported into medicine more complex processes of reasoning and aesthetic sensibilities but also needed to distinguish themselves from the practices of common healers (Chen Yuanpeng 陈元朋 1997; Hymes 1987; Bodenschatz forthcoming). Third, many medical innovators of the Jin-Yuan period focused on the function of visceral systems and assessed their imbalance according to various manifestation patterns (Ding Guangdi 丁光迪 1999). Fourth, focusing on the analysis of symptoms and signs and their grouping into patterns gave physicians another diagnostic system to add to information derived from pulse diagnosis (Xie Guan 谢观 1935: 36a).

38 See the foreword to Wang Ang's (1957 [1682]) *Yifang jijie* 医方集解 (*Medical Formulas Collected and Analyzed*). Other influential authors/texts emphasizing the diagnosis and treatment of clinical patterns as a core aspect of medical practice frequently quoted in contemporary texts and in personal discussions I had with physicians and students are Wang Kentang's 王肯堂 *Zhengzhi zhunsheng* 证治准绳 (*Indispensable Tools for Pattern Treatment*) of 1602, Ye Tianshi's 叶天士 *Linzheng zhinan yi'an* 临证指南医案 (*A Case Record Compass of Clinical Patterns*) of 1766, and the works by Zhang Jingyue and Xu Dachun cited below.

39 *Jingyue quanshu: Chuanzhong lu yinyang pian* 景岳全书: 传忠录阴阳篇 (*Collected Treatises of [Zhang] Jingyue: A Record of Sincere Interpretations—Yin Yang Chapter*) 1991 [1637], 1.2: 4, quoted, for instance, by Yue Meizhong 岳美中 (1978: 3). My thanks to Christine Bodenschatz and Steve Clavey for alerting me to the importance of Zhang Jiebin.

40 Xu Dachun, *Yixue yuanliu lun* 医学源流论 (*Discussions on the Origin and Development of Medicine*) 1988 [1757], 1.19: 173. Translated by Unschuld 1991: 114–16.

41 Ren Yingqiu 任应秋 1984a: 103–4. For a biography and bibliography, see Zhongguo kexue jishu xiehui 中国科学技术协会 1999: 229–43.

42 On the emergence of the *wenbing* scholarly stream in the Qing, see Hanson 1997. Considerable efforts have been made ever since to reconcile differences between the *wenbing* and *shanghan* streams. For some contemporary examples, see Qin Bowei 秦伯未 1983c; and the essays collected in Li Peisheng 李培生 and Liu Duzhou 刘渡舟 1987: 777–81.

43 Cited in Chen Xiaoye 陈小野 1997: 499. The article provides many other examples of the fluid distinction between diseases and patterns in the history of Chinese medicine.

44 Lin Peiqin, *Leizheng zhicai* 类证治裁 (*Tailored Treatments According to Patterns*), author's own foreword (1988 [1839]: 11).

45 Ibid.: "Xintong lunzhi" 心痛论治 (Discussing the treatment of heart pain) (1988 [1839], 6.8: 337–39).

46 Ding Guangdi 丁光迪 1999; Lei 1998; Zhao Hongjun 赵洪钧 1989.

47 Zhang Xichun 张锡纯 (*Yixue zhongzhong canxi lu*, 3: 1–7). I distinguish the formal case histories in volume 3 from the more informal case notes that Zhang Xichun uses throughout his various essays to exemplify the use of particular formulas and treatment principles.

48 On changes in the writing of case histories in Republican China, see Andrews 1996: chapter 7.

49 Zhang was an influential member of the "scholarly stream of convergence and integration" (*huitong xuepai* 汇通学派) who succeeded in assimilating Western medical ideas to classical medicine. See Qiu Peiran 裘沛然 and Ding Guangdi 丁光迪 1992: 708–722 and Zhao Hongjun 赵洪钧 1989: 196–206. Like many so-called streams, this one is as much an invention of later commentators as of the actual physicians who formed it.

50 The meaning of this term has always been vague and in premodern texts often refers to the symptoms rather than to the disease (Sivin 1987).

51 Zhang Xichun 张锡纯 (*Yixue zhongzhong canxi lu*, 3: 103, 121).

52 Zhang Weiyao 张维耀 1994: 352. The constructed nature of pattern differentiation in contemporary Chinese medicine—hidden in most clinical textbooks—is acknowledged by other historical accounts that have been published recently; for example, Cai Jingfeng 蔡景峰 et al. 2000: 287–88; and Meng Qingyun 孟庆云 2000: 81–92.

53 Zhu Chenyu 祝谌予 1982, cited in Zhang Weiyao 张维耀 1994: 352–53. It is unclear to me why Zhang singles out Shi Jinmo in this way, as many other physicians of his time espoused similar views. On the other hand, of the various colleges that existed during the Republican era, Shi Jinmo's Beijing School of Medicine and Pharmacology (Beiping yiyao xuexiao 北平医药学校) appears to have been the only one that taught a course on *bianzheng lunzhi*. See Deng Tietao 邓铁涛 1999: 204, which also lists the curriculum taught by other major Chinese medicine colleges at the time. Shi joined the Communist Party after liberation and became an adviser to the MOH. His enormous personal and intellectual influence in Chinese medical circles (many physicians with whom I studied used his formulas) was reflected in his being invited to several personal audiences with Mao Zedong and Zhou Enlai, as well as his participation in the Second and Third Chinese People's Political Consultative Conferences. For a biography of Shi, see Zhu Chenyu 祝谌予 1985. One of the earliest discussions of symptom and pattern differentiation in Maoist China is Zhu Yan 朱彦 1954.

54 The statement contains references to a famous chapter entitled "Discussion on Using Drugs like Soldiers" (*Yongyao ru yongbing lun* 用药如用兵论 in Xu Dachun's *Yixue yuanliu lun* (1757 [1988], 2.40: 185–86). For a discussion, see Ma Boying 马伯英 1993: 785–91.

55 Andrews 1996: 266. For a brief discussion of Shi Jinmo's role in the reform of Chinese medicine during the Republican era, see Ding Guangdi 丁光迪 1999: 84–86. Shi was inclined to accord Western medicine an important role in the modernization of Chinese medicine. On the history of *jingyan* 经验 (experience) as a term strategically employed by proponents of Western medicine intent on "revolutionizing" (i.e., scientizing) Chinese medicine, see Lei 1998.

56 As a scholar-physician from the south, Qin Bowei complements the northern perspective as embodied in my narrative by Shi Jinmo and Zhu Chenyu. The author of more than fifty books and many articles, Qin Bowei was a scholar, physician, and educator. For brief biographies of Qin Bowei, see Wu Dazhen 吴大真 and Wang Fengqi 王凤岐 1984; and Wu Boping 吴伯平 1985. See also He Shixi 何时希 1997: 197–207 for a very personal account by a former student. Ding Ganren was a leading figure in the modernization of Chinese medicine in the early years of this century. See He Shixi 何时希 1991: 1–4, 1997: 1–17 and Zhang Xiaoping 漳笑平 1991: 32–40.

57 Qin Bowei 秦伯未 (1983a: 36). Note the use of the term *guilu* 规律 already in Zhu Yan 朱彦 1954.

58 Qin Bowei 秦伯未 et al. (1961). By the early 1980s Qin's statement appeared in texts on the subject—for example, Jiao Shude 焦树德 1982: 17—without citation, a clear sign that it had by then become canonical.

59 This point has already been made by Unschuld (1985: 252–60). The Chinese medicine improvement schools set up during the early 1950s and discussed in chapter 3 served not only to raise standards of Western medical knowledge among physicians of Chinese medicine, but also to familiarize them with basic tenets of Maoism.

60 Farquhar 1994a: 171, n. 33. That the basic mode of analysis in Chinese medicine was in fact compatible with the dialectic elaborated by Western philosophy was first proposed by Yang Zemin 扬则民 in the 1930s, as shown by Dong Hanliang 董汉良 and Chen Tianxiang 陈天详 (1981a, 1981b).

61 The tenets hinted at here were developed under the political guidance of the CCP, which ordained dialectical materialism to be one of the guiding principles of the systematization of Chinese medicine including pattern differentiation (Ke Xuefan 柯雪帆 1987: 26). They were gradually developed into substantial theories concerning the dialectical nature of Chinese medicine (e.g., Lu Ganfu 陆干甫 and She Yongxin 谢永新 1986). The teaching of Chinese medical dialectics was facilitated by specially written teaching aids such as Liu Ruchen 刘汝琛 1983.

62 Qin Bowei 秦伯未 1983a: 27.

63 Yue Meizhong 岳美中 1981a: 10. I include Yue Meizhong's views in my narrative because being essentially self-taught, he embodies yet another perspective within Chinese medicine. By all accounts he was an extremely popular teacher and an effective physician. As the first member of the Academy of Chinese Medicine to join the Communist Party he enjoyed considerable influence among the political elite. Yue Meizhong treated many high-standing cadres and foreign dignitaries, including Mao Zedong, Zhou Enlai, and Ye Jianying. In 1962 he helped President Sukharto of Indonesia get rid of kidney stones. He was one of the few well-known physicians who continued to be active during the Cultural Revolution and already in 1972 began to petition MOH leaders to let him organize a class for advanced students that was finally realized in 1976. For a biography and bibliography, see Zhongguo kexue jishu xiehui 中国科学技术协会 1999: 130–46. For a very personal account, see He Shixi 何时希 1997: 176–92.

64 This idiom, used already by Zhang Xichun and other scholar-physicians during the late Qing, was impressed on me more than once by my teachers in Beijing and can be found in the biographies of many modern Chinese scholar-physicians. The biographies of scholar-physicians such as Fang Yaozhong, Qin Bowei, Ren Yinqiu, and many others that I have not included in this account present evidence that the transformation of subjectivity I assert in the text was not limited to a few exceptional physicians.

65 Qian Zifen 钱自奋 et al. 1993: 14–15; Zhu Chenyu 祝谌予 1981. According to my informants, as dean of the newly established Beijing College of Chinese Medicine Zhu Chenyu was an especially integrative figure who labored to unite the different factions and traditions that were brought together there by political fiat. This demonstrates both his modernity and dialectics.

66 Fang Yaozhong 方药中 1993: 3. Fang already was an established Chinese medicine practitioner in Chongqing when he decided to study Western medicine in Beijing from 1952 and 1957 following the political demand for Chinese and Western medicine to unite. From 1957 onward he worked for the Academy of Chinese Medicine. He was a prolific author and contributed to the development of Chinese medicine

through his own innovative ideas as well as by posing difficult questions. Younger than most of the other scholar-physicians I have included in my narrative, he represents the perspective of a generation that came to maturity in Maoist China. For biographies and a useful bibliography, see Zhongguo kexue jishu xiehui 中国科学技术协会 1999: 359–69.

67 A number of young but already established physicians were selected through competitive examinations and enrolled at Beijing Medical College (Beijing yixueyuan 北京医学院). See the biographies of Fang and Tang in Zhongguo kexue jishu xiehu 中国科学技术协会 1999: 361 and 396.

68 Five-phases (*wu xing* 五行) theory had become particularly emblematic of the uselessness of classical Chinese thought in comparison to Western science in the early part of the century. Cf. Andrews 1996; Ding Guangdi 丁光迪 1999: 257–68; and Unschuld 1985: 242–60.

69 Fang Yaozhong 方药中 1953, reprinted 1993: 1–5.

70 The influence of the improvement schools was pointed out by students of the older physicians who had attended them. The influence of Western on Chinese medicine during the Nationalist period is discussed in several of the works previously cited. These transformations were enabled, in turn, by the physicians nowadays classed by Chinese historians as belonging to the "scholarly stream of convergence and integration" (*huitong xuepai* 汇通学派). Based on my observations I venture that the most important of these has undoubtedly been Zhang Xichun. See Andrews 1996; Ding Guangdi 丁光迪 1999; Lei 1998; and Zhao Hongjun 赵洪钧 1989.

71 The use of single drug formulas (*danfang* 单方) in Chinese medicine is very rare. Most prescriptions combine between four and twelve drugs. The idea is that single drugs are too unbalanced in their action, while different drugs used in combination can mutually accentuate and moderate one another, much like using different flavors in cooking to achieve an overall effect.

72 The events described in the paragraph are discussed in Ding Guangdi 丁光迪 1999: 290–322; and Zhao Hongjun 赵洪钧 1989: 213–20.

73 "Bianzheng yu zhibing" 辨证与识病 (Differentiating Patterns and Knowing Diseases), reprinted in Yang Zemin 扬则民 1985: 53–55.

74 Jiang Chunhua 美春华 explains the reason for the deletion of Yang Zemin from the public memory of Chinese medicine in a foreword to the collection of essays by Yang Zemin published in 1985. He does not say, however, who precisely was responsible for branding Yang a reactionary. Yang Zemin's rehabilitation was initiated in the 1980s by means of two short journal articles by Dong Hanliang 董汉良 and Chen Tianxiang 陈天祥 (1981a, 1981b), who also edited the compilation of his essays cited above. Yang's influence on the development of Chinese medicine during the Nationalist period is acknowledged in the two major Chinese-language texts on the subject, namely Deng Tietao 邓铁涛 1999: 398; and Zhao Hongjun 赵洪钧 1989: 188–196. To date, he is not, however, cited in any of the major texts on pattern differentiation. This episode demonstrates in yet another way the powerful

influence exerted by the state on the development of Chinese medicine. An exhaustive account of this influence will be possible only when the penetration of state power into the lives of individual physicians can be accurately traced.

75 Shi Jinmo's proposals were made in a document entitled "Zhongyang guoyiguan xueshu zhengli weiyuanhui tongyi zhongyi bingmin jianyi shu" 中央国医馆学术整理委员会统一中医病名建议书 (Recommendation for the unification of Chinese medicine disease names by the Central Institute of National Medicine's Committee for the Systematization of Knowledge). Yang Zemin was the representative of the Zhejiang Branch of the Institute of National Medicine. His analysis was published as a reply to this paper and originally entitled "Duiyu Zhongyang guoyiguan tongyi zhongyi bingmin jianyi shu" 对于中央国医馆统一中医病名建议书 (Regarding the recommendation for the unification of Chinese medicine disease names by the Central Institute of National Medicine). Shi Jinmo and many others must thus have been aware of Yang's analysis. Dong Hanliang 董汉良 and Chen Tianxiang 陈天祥 1981b; Zhao Hongjun 赵洪钧 1989: 188–196; Zhongyi bingming zhenduan guifan ketizu 中医病名诊断规范课题组 1987: Foreword.

76 Zhu Chenyu 祝谌予 1981: 266–71; see also Qian Zifen 钱自奋 et al. 1993.

77 Fang Yaozhong 方药中 1955, reprinted 1993b: 16–26. It should be emphasized, however, that Zhu, Fang, and others were not advocating here the creation of an entirely new medicine, but rather the development of Chinese medicine they considered necessary by way of assimilating into it specific and narrowly circumscribed aspects of Western medicine. See, for instance, Fang Yaozhong 方药中 1993b: 3–5.

78 For biographies of Pu Fuzhou, see Gao Huiyuan 高辉远 1983; Pu Zhixiao 蒲志孝 1985; and Zhongguo kexue jishu xiehui 中国科学技术协会 1999: 68–79.

79 *Baihu tang* is first mentioned in the *Shanghan lun*, but its use for summerheat warm [pathogen] (*shu wen* 暑温) disorders derives from Wu Jutong's 吴鞠通 *Wenbing tiaobian* 温病条辨 (*Systematic Differentiation of Warm [Pathogen] Disorders*), 1.2: 29.

80 *San ren tang*, too, is first listed in Wu Jutong's 吴鞠通 *Wenbing tiaobian*, 1.4: 34, where it is indicated for damp warm [pathogen] disorders (*shi wen* 湿温). The origin of the formula, like the use of *Baihu tang* for summerheat warm [pathogen] disorders, is derived from Ye Tianshi 叶天士 (1667–1746).

81 Pu Fuzhou, cited in Zhongguo kexue jishu xiehui 中国科学技术协会 1999: 74. I translate *zheng* 症 here as "pattern" because the term "transmuted pattern" has a specific meaning in the context of treating cold damage disorders. See Ke Xuefan 柯雪帆 1987: 5 for an acknowledgment of the importance of this episode in the formation of pattern differentiation theory.

82 I have had the story of Pu Fuzhou's success told to me by many different physicians on many different occasions. Pu Fuzhou's name is often dropped, however, suggesting an affirmation of Chinese medicine rather than that of an individual physician's skills, much in the manner that names are omitted from Western scientific knowledge (Latour 1987).

83 Comparing, for instance, Zhou Weixin 周味辛 1954 with Lin Ganliang 林乾良 1960, one gains a sense of the increasing naturalization of this new status of *bianzheng* developed over a space of only six years. The necessity of creating a theoretically coherent model of pattern differentiation for the purpose of teaching Chinese medicine is explicitly acknowledged by Ke Xuefan 柯雪帆 (1987: 5).

84 A typical example of imputing modern meaning into classical texts is Ke Xuefan 柯雪帆 1987: 9, a text I cite repeatedly because of its authoritative status (the editorial panel is composed of eminent physicians). The authors argue, for instance, that the character 症 was not used in the Han and that physicians employed only the character 证. Hence, it is our task to intuit when a given author is referring to symptoms and signs 症 and when to patterns 证. Nanjing zhongyi xueyuan 南京中医学院 1958: 130. Its now orthodox status is evidenced by three books published by the Academy of Chinese Medicine with explicit support from the MoH: *Zhongyi zhengzhuang jianbie zhenduanxue* 中医症状鉴别诊断学 (1984) (*The Discrimination of Symptoms in Chinese Medical Diagnosis*); *Zhongyi zhenghou jianbie zhenduanxue* 中医证侯鉴别诊断学 (1987) (*The Discrimination of Patterns in Chinese Medical Diagnosis*); and *Zhongyi jibing jianbie zhenduanxue* 中医疾病鉴别诊断学 (forthcoming) (*The Discrimination of Diseases in Chinese Medical Diagnosis*). The introductions to the published texts contain detailed discussions of the topic.

85 Zhu Ziqing 朱子青 1963. One might wish to note here also Farquhar's (1994a: 70 n. 11) comment that the very use of the term *bianzheng lunzhi* in modern medical discourse "seems to insist on a very deep epistemological divide between 'Western' structural, essentialist and representational biases and the practical, collective, and relativistic biases of Chinese medicine."

86 The analysis in this paragraph is based on conversations with participants in the Beijing classes of 1955 and 1956. See also Ke Xuefan 柯雪帆 1987: 5. Chongqingshi xiyi lizhi xuexi zhongyi yanjiuban 重庆市西医离职学习中医研究班 1959, discussed in detail in appendix 1, is an example of the contribution to this process by Western medicine physicians studying Chinese medicine. See also Taylor 2000 for a more detailed discussion.

87 Chongqingshi xiyi xuexi zhongyi yanjiuban 重庆市西医离职学习中医研究班 1959: 1.

88 Cai Jinggao 蔡景高 1962.

89 Sun Shizhong 孙世重 1962; Zhu Liangchun 朱良春 1962.

90 These are differentiation of patterns (*bianzheng* 辨证) according to pathologies of the *zangfu*; the channels and collaterals (*jingluo* 经络); the four aspects *wei, qi, ying,* and *xue* (卫气营血); the six stages (*liu jing* 六经); the *sanjiao*; disease causes (*bingyin* 病因); and pathologies of spirit (*shen* 神) *qi*, blood (*xue* 血), and body fluids (*jingye* 津液). For more detailed discussions, see Farquhar 1994a: chapter 4; and Deng Tietao 邓铁涛 1987.

91 Contemporary textbooks on diagnosis such as Deng Tietao 邓铁涛 1987: 295 describe the *ba gang* as the most important system of pattern differentiation and ex-

trapolate its formation to the *Neijing* and *Shanghan*. In fact, as Wang Huaimei 王怀美 et al. (1998) show, while from the late Ming onward diverse authors such as Zhang Jiebin, Cheng Guopeng 程国彭, and Xu Dachun emphasized the use of the eight principles *yin/yang*, exterior/interior, cold/heat, and depletion/repletion as fundamental to the practice of medicine, the actual term "eight rubrics" was coined as late as 1947 by Zhu Weiju 祝味菊, a physician from Sichuan who studied Western medicine in Japan and later taught and practiced in Shanghai.

92   Nanjing zhongyi xueyuan 南京中医学院 1958: 8–9. Contemporary Chinese commentators affirm this point. Hu Xin 胡欣 and Ge Xiumei 葛秀梅 (1994: 86–88), for instance, state that the *ba gang* have a dual connotation. In one sense, they are the "epitome of the diverse principles of pattern differentiation" relative to which these other methods assume a subordinate relationship. In a second sense, however, the *ba gang* constitute nothing more than a method for differentiating a particular group of diseases, namely *zabing* 杂病 or "miscellaneous diseases." These are perceived to be of internal origin as opposed to *shanghan* or *wenbing* diseases, which are thought to arise from external pathogens penetrating into the organism. Inasmuch as the diseases of this latter group frequently exhibit a seasonal character, or were thought of as being due to unseasonal climatic factors, they are sometimes jointly referred to as *shibing* 时病 or "seasonal diseases." The formulation by Hu and Ge, which seeks to accommodate the perceived root of *ba gang* differentiation in the *Shanghan zabing lun* as well as the modern plurality of differentiation practice, clearly expresses the transformation of the *ba gang* in the course of contemporary developments of *bianzheng lunzhi*.

93   Cited in Zhongguo kexue jishu xiehui 中国科学技术协会 1999: 51. Given his erudition, Shi was probably aware that others before him had already had this idea. The Ming dynasty physician Li Zhongzi 李中梓 (1588–1655), for instance, included blood and *qi* as two of his "seven great methods for differentiating treatment" (*bianzhi dafa* 辨治大法) in his well-known *Yizong bidu* 医宗必读 (*Essential Readings from the Medical Ancestors*) 1.12 (1999 [1637]: 85). Each of these methods equates to one pair of two principles. Besides Shi's ten principles, the other four mentioned by Li are the *yin* and *yang* visceral systems (*zangfu* 脏腑) and root and manifestations (*ben biao* 本标).

94   In addition to the articles already cited, see Cai Jinggao 蔡景高 1962; Li Lianda 李连达 1959; Li Lianda 李连达 and Jing Yuzhen 靖雨珍 1963; and Zhu Ziqing 朱子青 1963. From a different perspective the discussion can be interpreted as a struggle by Chinese medicine physicians to assert control over their practice, responding to demands from above to combine Chinese and Western medicine and from below by Western physicians studying Chinese medicine for a more systematic Chinese medicine that also accommodated to Western medicine. In spite of their undoubted historical significance, it is outside the scope of the present discussion to describe these struggles in detail.

95 Qin Bowei 秦伯未 et al. 1973. Qin Bowei was, of course, one of the leading proponents of an independent Chinese medical tradition firmly anchored in its own
practices.

96 Famous physicians arguing for the importance of "disease differentiation" (*bianbing*) in Chinese medicine included Yue Meizhong 岳美中 (2000a), Pu Fuzhou
蒲辅周 (Zhonguo zhongyi yanjiuyuan 中国中医研究院 1979), and Jiang Chunhua.
See also the reply by the Beijing Chinese Medicine Research Institute (Beijing
zhongyi yanjiusuo 北京中医研究所 1962) to the article by Sun Shizhong 孙世重
(1962). For a summary of such debates, see Lü Guangrong 吕光荣 1980. Qin Shoushan 金寿山 (1978) provides one of the most convincing arguments for the clinical
usage and, indeed, necessity of Chinese medical disease differentiation in medical practice. Zhao Hongjun 赵洪钧 (1989: 213-19), who describes and analyses the
polemic regarding the unification of disease names in Chinese medicine in the
1930s, sees Yang Zemin as having carried the day in the long run. For Zhao this
"was the inevitable [outcome] of the development of academic thought" (*shi xueshu fazhan de biran* 是学术发展的必然 1989: 219). I see it as the outcome of a
historically specific alignment of infrastructures. After all, the chief actors from
within the discipline of Chinese medicine were more or less the same in the 1930s
as they were in the 1950s. What had changed were the other actors (human and nonhuman) to which they were aligned and the field of practice in which they operated.
These changed alignments may be read as stimulating a "development of academic
thought" in these actors, though there is nothing inevitable about it. The fact that
the discourse on *bianzheng lunzhi* was produced in Maoist China and not in Taiwan, Hong Kong, or San Francisco, where many eminent scholar-physicians of the
Republican Period had emigrated after 1949, is proof if any is needed.

97 Ren Yingqiu 任应秋 1966, 1980. See also Ren Yingqiu 1954 for an earlier seminal
contribution.

98 Yue Meizhong 岳美中 and Chen Keji 陈可冀 1962. Chen Keji is one of the most
prominent physicians of Chinese medicine in contemporary China. For a biography and bibliography, see Zhongguo kexue jishu xiehui 中国科学技术协会 1999:
406-25. Thematically the discussion narrated in this paragraph recapitulates the
debate of the 1930s initiated by Shi Jinmo outlined earlier in this chapter. Even
some of its participants are the same. What has changed is the knowledge participants have of Western medicine and the new framework of pattern diagnosis that
constitutes a stable background accepted by all participants.

99 Pertinent examples are Fang Yaozhong 方药中 1979; Ren Yingqiu 任应秋 1984b;
and Yue Meizhong 岳美中 1984a, 1984b.

100 A series of articles outlining these efforts was published in the *Shanghai Journal of
Chinese Medicine* from 1962 onward under the title "Linzheng bianzheng shizhi
gaiyao" 临证辨证施治概要 (Outline of clinical pattern differentiation and treatment
application).

101 Shanghai zhongyi xueyuan 上海中医学院 1964.

102 Beijing zhongyiyuan geming weiyuanhui 北京中医院革命委员会 1971. This book claims to be the second edition of a text compiled at the hospital in 1961 that I have been unable to trace. My thanks to Nathan Sivin for guiding me to this text. Shanghai zhongyi xueyuan 上海中医学院 1972. For a critical evaluation of this text from a contemporary Chinese perspective, see also Zhang Weiyao 张维耀 1994: 355.

103 Qin Bowei 秦伯未 1983a, 1983b; Ren Yingqiu 任应秋 1984b.

104 Zhao Shaoqin 赵绍琴 et al. 1982, cited in chapter 6 as a nonofficial textbook for the teaching of *wenbing* in Beijing, is one example of a later text that retains *bian-zheng shizhi*. The persistence of various designations and their subtle differences of meaning is additional evidence, of course, for the essential plurality of Chinese medicine.

105 "Zhang Zhongjing zai yixueshang de chengjiu" 张仲景在医学上的成就 (Zhang Zhongjing's achievements in medicine), reprinted in Zhu Liangchun 2000: 9–19.

106 The development of Zhang Cigong's thought is much more complex than can be discussed here. It reflects not only issues regarding the scientific status of Chinese medicine but assimilates multiple strands of debate and discourse that conjoin—to mention just a few—Japanese influences on Chinese medicine, Indian philosophy, Western medicine, nationalism, long-standing disputes within the Chinese medical community, and considerable clinical experience.

107 Shanghai zhongyi xueyuan 上海中医学院 1972: 182.

108 Zhang Xichun 张锡纯, *Yixue zhongzhong canxi lu*; Zhonguo zhongyi yanjiuyuan 1979; Zhu Chenyu 祝谌予 1982. The explicit discussions provided by modern physicians are themselves a modern reformulation of the case history genre that previously relied on implicit insinuations and tacit knowledge as discussed by Andrews (1996: chapter 7) and Shao (1998).

109 Chen Ziyin 沈白尹 1973.

110 For a biography, see Shi Yuguang 史宇广 1991: 17.

111 Yue Meizhong 岳美中 1981b: 7. Historically, this discussion may be linked to those of the previous two decades regarding the relation of patterns to diseases and interpreted as efforts by an important group of Chinese medicine physicians to assert the independence of their tradition from excessive encroachment and redefinition through Western medicine. I refuse to label these physicians, of whom Yue Meizhong is a representative, "traditional" or "conservative" because they never closed themselves to the development and transformation of Chinese medicine. They did, however, insist on a Chinese medicine that assimilated Western medicine rather than being entirely changed by it.

112 Other contributions to this debate, which was conducted in *Shangdong yixue* 山东医学 (*Shangdong Medicine*) 1980 (6) and *Shanghai zhongyiyao zazhi* 上海中医药杂志 (*Shanghai Journal of Chinese Medicine and Pharmacology*) 1981 (12), were made by Zhang Qiwen 张奇文, Zhu Hongming 朱鸿铭, Xiao Jun 消骏, Gao Dixiu 高迪旭, and Wang Zhicheng 王志成.

113 The quotes in this paragraph are taken from Yue Meizhong 岳美中 2000b. This article was not written as a contribution to the debate on type differentiation but helps us to understand why Yue should think of type differentiation as the use of "dead formulas"—a phrase that I think Yue did not use casually. In Maoist discourse (and Yue was a self-professed Maoist) duanlian 锻炼 refers to steeling body and mind through exercise and training. It evokes repetition and struggle. Furthermore, transformation and continual change are explicitly defined by Mao Zedong (1968) as characteristic aspects of living things that can only be grasped by means of the dialectical method and that must be responded to by an equally flexible and changing practice. Anyone familiar with the history of Chinese medicine will find multiple layers of reference in this analogy: from the *qi* transformations of Chinese physiology to the rejection of old formulas for the treatment of contemporary diseases that have been a recurrent topic of Chinese medical discourse since the Jin-Yuan (Ding Guangdi 丁光迪 1999). Yue's critique of type differentiation can thus be read as a failure of modernizers to adhere not merely to fundamental tenets of Chinese medicine but also to Maoist dialectics. In many ways, the shift from pattern to type differentiation therefore represents a shift from Maoist modernization in Chinese medicine under the adage "using the ancient in modern ways, using the Western in Chinese ways" (*gu wei jin yong, yang wei zhong yong* 古为今用, 洋为中用; cited in Beijing zhongyi xueyuan geming weiyuanhui 北京中医院革命委员会 1971: 2) to a post-Maoist one insisting on its integration into global markets and technoscientific networks (see chapter 9).

114 Exemplary textbooks are Li Anmin 李安民 and Long Yurong 尤玉荣 1993 and Wang Zude 王祖德 et al. 1992. Biographies of Jiang Chunhua can be found in Dong Jianhua 董建华 1990, 2: 90, Zhongguo kexue jishu xiehui 中国科学技术协会 1999: 183–96 and Zhou Fengwu 周风梧 et al. 1981, 1: 45–61.

115 Chen Ziyin himself is of the opinion that his research has initiated an entirely new vista on understanding and treating kidney disorders in Chinese medicine. See, for instance, Chen Ziyin 沈自尹 and Wang Wenjian 王文健 1988. More conservative-minded physicians think that Chen did much to promote himself and little to benefit Chinese medicine. For an overview of Chen's research, see Ma Boying 马伯英 1994: 584–86, 595–96.

116 Liang Maoxin 梁茂新 et al. 1998 is a particularly valuable example. See also the overviews in Cai Jingfeng 蔡景峰 2000: 287–89; and Meng Qingyun 孟庆云 2000: 72–92.

117 This statement is based on an extensive review of articles published in Chinese medical journals since 1984 on the topic of *bianzheng lunzhi*. For a flavor of the nature of these debates, see Fang Yaozhong 1993a; Wang Yuxi 王玉玺 1985; and Nan Zheng 南征 1986. Hu Xin 胡欣 and Ge Xiumei 葛秀梅 1994; and Ke Xuefan 柯雪帆 1987 are typical examples of the systematized orthodoxy that characterizes state-sponsored *bianzheng lunzhi* discourse in the 1990s.

118 A typical example is *Zhongyi xitonglun* 中医系统论 (*Chinese Medicine Systems*

Theory), by Zhu Jiene 祝世讷 and Sun Guilian 孙桂莲, published in 1990 as a contribution to *Dangdai zhongyi congshu* 当代中医丛书 (Contemporary Chinese Medicine Series). The series was edited by Dong Jianhua 董建华, one of the best-known and most respected Chinese medicine physicians in Beijing and a CCP member. The books in this series analyze Chinese medicine and pattern differentiation (the two are by now almost interchangeable) from various modern scientific perspectives. Systems theory, cybernetics, and informatics are recurrent topics.

119 For a useful overview of relevant research and its associated problems, see Yang Weiyi 杨维益 1997; and Meng Qingyun 孟庆云 2000: 125–43.

120 The most exemplary encyclopedias in the domain of pattern differentiation have been produced by the Academy of Chinese Medicine (Zhongguo zhongyi yanjiuyuan 中国中医研究院 1984 and 1987).

121 Zhongyi bingming zhenduan guifan ketizu 中医病名诊断规范课题组 1987.

122 Guojia jishu jianduju 国家技术鉴督局 1994, 1995, 1997a, 1997b, 1997c. See also Xinhua News Agency, 11 October 1994.

123 *Guojia jishu jianduju* 国家技术鉴督局 1995: 72.

124 Yue Meizhong 岳美中 1981b: 13.

125 That there is indeed a sense among many senior practitioners of Chinese medicine that not all is well with the direction in which their medicine is developing can be gleaned from many of the contributions to a collection of articles recently published by Cui Yueli 崔月梨 (1997), formerly minister of health.

126 As Lei (1998, 1999) shows, the discourse on the role of experience in relation to Chinese medicine has a long history. It came to twentieth-century China via Japan and Kanpo medicine, and was used in the early part of this century as a tool to legitimize Chinese medicine independent of the theories of the classical medical literature. Although modern usage is contingent on this earlier discourse, it is also significantly different in terms both of what it addresses and what it seeks to achieve.

127 I shall give just one example of the different effects of this process. In 1976, Yue Meizhong organized the First National Chinese Medicine Research Student Class in Beijing. This brought together renowned *laozhongyi* from all over China who shared their personal experiences with younger physicians who had graduated since the early 1960s. Although the participants greatly valued the experience, Yue's first class was also the last. By the late 1970s it was already impossible, according to several informants, to bring several luminaries together for another such project.

128 "Lü Bingkui cong yi 60 nian wenji" weiyuanhui 吕炳奎从医６０年文集编辑委员会 1993: 13–14, 141.

129 Liu Yue 刘越 1998a, 1999.

130 The development and transformation of the case note genre in Chinese medicine is explored in Hsu forthcoming: section 5. Andrews (1996: chapter 7) shows that

the rewriting and re-presentation of case notes of one physician by another in order to "modernize" Chinese medicine was a strategy already employed during the Nationalist period.

131 Liu Yue 刘越 1998b, 1998c. Liu adduces several pieces of supportive evidence, such as the fact that Chinese prepared medicines (chengyao 成药) can be divided into those that treat patterns and those that treat diseases.

132 Liu Yue 刘越 1999. Appendix 2 compares in detail Zhang Xichun's own presentation of a case with that of its re-presentation by Liu Yue. It is interesting that Farquhar (1994a) also repeatedly uses a diagram to represent the time line of the process of pattern differentiation.

133 A typical example is the use of the formula *Gan mai dazao tang* 甘麦大枣汤 (Liquorice, Wheat, and Jujube Decoction). This well-known formula from the *Jingui yaolue* 金匮要略 is indicated for a pattern known as "visceral agitation" (*zangzao* 脏躁) thought to occur predominantly in women. The formula is indicated for symptoms such as disorientation, frequent attacks of melancholy or crying, and inability to control oneself. Up to the present date there is little agreement among commentators as to what disease mechanism the formula actually treats or how the formula works. A contemporary textbook for teachers notes laconically that "there has existed quite considerable disagreement among physicians throughout the history [of Chinese medicine] regarding the disease location of visceral agitation" and that "regarding the problem of the formula's primary drug, not all historical formula discussions are in agreement." See Xu Jiqun 许济群 and Wang Mianzhi 王绵之 1995: 314–16. Despite such theoretical disagreements physicians have little problem diagnosing visceral agitation in practice. This is precisely because it is the formula and its memorized indications that define the pattern and lead to the diagnosis, and not the pattern (defined as a disease mechanism) that leads to the formula.

134 Ke Xuefan 柯雪帆 (1987: 31–39), for instance, lists ten different methods of pattern differentiation including differentiation of types and via formulas. Chen Keji 陈可冀 and Shi Zaixiang 史载祥 (1999) is a typical example of a modern hybrid of pattern and type differentiation that discusses treatment of various conditions under the heading of "Chinese medicine pattern differentiation and type determination" (*zhongyi bianzheng fenxing* 中医辨证分型).

135 See, for instance, the article by Li Zhizhong 李致重 from the Chinese Association of Chinese Medicine and Pharmacology 中国中医药学会 (1997a).

8. Creating Knowledge

1 Channels and collaterals (*jingluo* 经络) is the more precise term for what is commonly known in the West as "meridians."

2 See Zhang Xichun 张锡纯, *Yixue zhongzhong canxi lu*, 1: 306–37 for an overview of the treatment of wind stroke in Chinese medicine and also for the early influence

of Western medicine on the formulation of new therapeutic approaches. Porkert (1978: 162–63) describes and analyzes the status of the brain in classical anatomy and physiology.

3   An inscription device, according to Latour (1987: 68), is "any set-up . . . that provides a visual display of any sort in a scientific text." Ethnographers of laboratory life such as Knorr-Cetina (1981), Latour and Woolgar (1986: 64), and Traweek (1988: 72) provide ample evidence of the constructive role technological apparatuses play in producing the artificial realities of technoscience.

4   Taylor (2000) argues convincingly that the development of Chinese medicine since the 1950s, including the formulation of the term "traditional Chinese medicine" as the official English-language translation of the native *zhongyi*, was influenced by the desire to project a particular view of China to the outside world. Although this desire has thus been a constant for half a century, its concrete synthesis is constantly changing.

5   Chinese universities provide accommodation for students but not their families. Lack of affordable accommodation and the uncertainty of finding a job in Beijing after graduation were the main reasons why Dr. Lin did not move his family to Beijing for the time of his graduate studies. After graduation he succeeded in obtaining a position at a Beijing hospital and thereby a residence permit. His family now lives in Beijing.

6   Du Ruzhu 杜如竹 1994.

7   Dr. Lin does, however, discuss the polysemic history of the nosological category *zhongfeng* in his dissertation.

8   Gao Surong 高素荣 1993: 265–80.

9   Edwards and Bouchier 1991: 821–22.

10 It would be enlightening for the study of the synthetic emergence in contemporary China to compare in detail Dr. Lin's efforts with that of his classical ancestors. Sun Simiao's discussions of the various presentations of *fengyi* 风懿 and *fengfei* 风痱 (1993: 132–36)—to give but one example—while not showing the definitional rigor of Dr. Lin's project, are much more detailed in their portrayal of the different patterns described. Compare, for instance, this vivid description of the *Qinjiao san* 秦艽散 (*Gentianae macrophyllae Radix Powder*) pattern—one of Sun's shorter descriptions—with Dr. Lin's analyses outlined in table 5 and figure 37: "*Gentianae macrophyllae Radix Powder* is a formula for the treatment of hemiplegia, deranged speech, [periods of] alternating elation and sorrow, arched back rigidity, and wind itch of the skin."

11 Classical texts such as the *Yixue xinwu* 医学心悟 (*The Awakening of the Mind in Medical Studies*)—cited to me by Dr. Lin as one of his main inspirations and itself inspired by earlier texts such as the *Suwen* and *Lingshu* chapters cited above—discuss the nature and treatment of these pathologies in terms of the penetration of pathogenic *qi* (*xieqi* 邪气) into particular areas of the body such as the channels or visceral systems.

12 The liver visceral system of function is involved in all patterns because wind pathologies in Chinese medicine implicitly involve the liver.

13 Although this cannot be discussed here (due both to lack of space and to my intention not to violate my informants' confidence) those physicians like Dr. Lin whom I came to know quite well and with whom I discussed such issues in detail were all personally transformed in the process of transforming Chinese medicine.

14 Latour (1993) accomplishes the critical task of detailing the shortcomings of other Enlightenment critiques.

15 One of the particular advantages of my model is that it can be connected to a large research tradition that explores situated learning: for example, Lave 1993 and Lave and Wenger 1991. The work of the Russian psychologist Vygotsky and its development into "activity theory" and a theory of "mediated action" by various Russian and Western scholars is particularly noteworthy and has greatly influenced my own thinking. An introductory collection of Vygotsky's works is in Kozulin 1990; and van der Veer and Elsiner 1994. The most prominent and influential representative of Vygotskyian psychology in the West is Wertsch. For an introduction, see Wertsch 1985, 1991; and Wertsch et al. 1995. Wertsch's focus on tool-mediated action as a primary unit of analysis is drawn from the work of Vladimir Zinchenko, son of Peter Zinchenko, a collaborator of Vygotsky and member of the activity-oriented Kharkov school. Kozulin (1986) provides a brief intellectual history of activity theory. See also Bakehurst 1990: 208; and Wertsch 1985: 196–98, 205–8.

16 See Latour 1987, 1988 on "trials of strength" as that which establishes networks; and Brown and Lee 1994 on the Nietzschean character of the model. See once again Pickering 1995: 209–12, which extends a similar argument into the perspective that the present is continually breaking up into the future.

17 Benjamin 1982: 83, translated after Buck-Morss 1991: 8.

18 Nader 1996: 11.

19 See Kleinman 1995: 31 for a perspective from medical anthropology; and Valussi 1997 for an examination from the perspective of medical practice.

9. The Future of Chinese Medicine

1 My model obviously constitutes an outline rather than a fully developed theory of social practice. Processes such as the formation and control of boundaries between fields of practice, the mutual interpenetration of various levels of analysis and those of production and reproduction remain sketchy. Others, such as distinctions between different types of synthesis, have hardly been touched on. These are important lacunae that demand to be filled in. I have no excuses for these shortcomings other than that the formulation of social theory was never my primary goal but emerged in the course of writing an ethnography of plurality.

2 The titles of the articles I refer to in the text are: "My View of the 'River Chart'

and 'Luo Writing'" (*Wo kan "hetu luoshu"* 我看 "河图洛书"), "Textual Research concerning an Original Passage of the 'Jingmai' Chapter of the 'Lingshu'" ("*Lingshu: jingmai bufen yuanwen kaoding*" 灵枢: 经脉部分原文考订), "An Introduction to the Academic Tenets and Clinical Experiences of Professor Kong Guangyi" (*Kong Guangyi jiaoshou xueshu sixiang he linchuang jingyan jianjie* 孔光一教授学术思想和临床经验简介), "The Effects of Harmonising the Liver and Aiding the Spleen Drink on Body Weight and Gastric Mucosal Change in 'Spleen Depletion' CCl_4 Liver Damaged Rats" (*He gan zhu pi yin dui "pixu"* CCl_4 *gan sunshang dashu tizhong he weichang nianmo bianhua de yingxiang* 和肝助脾饮对 "脾虚" CCl_4损伤大鼠体重和胃肠粘膜变化的影响), and "The Treatment of 190 Cases of Cervical Erosion by Chinese Medicine" (*Zhongyiyao zhiliao zigongjing kuilan 190 an* 中医药治疗子宫颈溃烂 190 案).

3   Taylor (2000: 55) shows clearly that the CCP's policies regarding Chinese medicine emerged in the course of interpretations of the thought of party leaders, especially Mao Zedong, by a middle layer of "policy translators and implementers."

4   Ren Jixue 任继学 1997: 9. The differences between "awakening the mind" so as to "just know" and explicate knowing based on post-Enlightenment models of the world are discussed by Hsü 1999.

5   The original *Guang wenre lun* 广瘟热论 (*Expanded Discussion of Warm [Pathogen Epidemic] Heat [Disorders]*) by Dai Tianzhang 戴天章 dates from 1722. It was edited by Lu Jiuzhi 陆九芝 and published under the new name *Guang wen re lun* 广温热论 (*Expanded Discussion of Warm [Pathogen] Heat [Disorders]*) in 1866. It was finally reedited by He Lianchen 何廉臣 and published as *Zhongding guang wenre lun* 重订广温热论 (*Newly Revised Expanded Discussion of Warm [Pathogen] Heat [Disorders]*) in 1909. See the editor's preface to the 1960 edition.

6   All quotes are from Ren Jixue 任继学 1997: 116–17.

7   Fu Youfeng's 符有丰 (1999). *Buzhong yiqi tang* is discussed in *Neiwaishang bianhuo lun* 内外伤辨惑论 (*Clarifying Doubts about Inquiries from Internal and External Causes*, 1.1 (1993 [1247]: 15–20).

8   During my study of warm [pathogen] disorders (*wenbing* 温病) at Beijing University of Chinese Medicine, for instance, I was instructed about the importance and effectiveness of carrying out a correct pattern differentiation through the vivid recollection of emergency cases treated by my teacher and his teachers. My teacher indicated also that, in his opinion, many young doctors lacked the experience to make a correct differentiation. Note that he does not blame lack of knowledge but lack of practice.

9   In fact, it is representative only of certain dominant modes of such innovation. Other kinds of innovation follow more closely classical models of knowledge extension. A very good example is Lu Zheng's 陆拯 (1997) innovative system of treating toxicity patterns, which is modeled on Ye Tianshi's 叶天士 (1667–1746) system of treating warm pathogen diseases, yet succeeds in breaking entirely new ground.

10 I employ "global" here both in the popular sense as referring to the world as a whole and in its anthropological or social scientific sense as an instantiation of nature-culture that is opposed to local forms of nature-culture.

11 Scott 1999.

12 These center on notions such as *shi* 势 (propensity) or *yi* 意 (intention). See Jullien 1995, 1999; Liao Yujun 廖育群 1999; and Kuang Cuizhang 匡萃璋 1997.

13 The citation is from Stephen E. Straus, M.D., the director of the National Institute of Health in Bethesda, Maryland, and as such representative of biomedical physicians most immediately involved with alternative medicines. See Goldsmith 1999: 2287. One might wish to comment on the author's skillful rhetoric that succeeds in describing a standardized and routinized medical practice that has become so homogeneous that it no longer knows of alternatives as a "healing art."

Notes to Appendix A

1 Nanjing College of Chinese Medicine 南京中医学院, eds., *Zhongyixue gailun* 中医学概论 (*Outline of Chinese Medicine*). Beijing: Renmin weisheng chubanshe, 1958.

2 Chongqing Research Class of Physicians of Western Medicine Seconded from Work to Study Chinese Medicine (Chongqingshi xiyi lizhi xuexi zhongyi yanjiuban 重庆市西医离职学习中医研究班), *Zhongyi bianzheng shuyu de shentao* 中医辨证术语的深讨 (*An In-Depth Discussion of Chinese Medicine Pattern Terminology*) (Chongqing: Chongqing renmin chubanshe, 1959).

3 Qin Bowei 秦伯未 et al., *Shisi gangyao bianzheng* 十四纲要辨证 (The Fourteen Principal Rubrics of Pattern Differentiation), *Zhongyi zazhi* 中医杂志 1 (1961):5–9, 2:38–46, 3:35–41.

4 Fang Yaozhong 方药中, *Bianzheng lunzhi yanjiu ji jiang* 辨证论治研究七讲 (*Seven Lectures on Pattern Differentiation and Treatment Determination Research* (Beijing: Renmin weisheng chubanshe, 1979), 101–76.

5 *Beijing zhongyi xueyuan* 北京中医学院 1990.

6 The reasons for transferring the commission to Nanjing are complex. It appears that the institutional structure at the school was very well developed. The school had been set up in the early 1950s under Lü Bingkui, who by now was heading the Chinese Medicine Bureau at the MOH. Furthermore, the Nanjing College of Chinese Medicine is widely considered to have been the leading Chinese medicine college in the country at the time.

7 See, for instance, the comments of Lü Bingkui, in overall charge of the production of the *Outline*, cited in chapter 7.

8 These include Ding Guangdi 丁光迪, Ren Yingqiu 任应秋, Xu Jiqun 许济群, Wang Mianzhi 王绵之, and Yan Zhenghua 颜正华.

9 See Yin Huihe 印会河 1999: foreword.

10 *Chongqingshi xiyi lizhi xuexi zhongyi yanjiuban* 重庆市西医离职学习中医研究班 1959: 1.

11 These are external, internal, and miscellaneous causes. External causes generally refer to climatic factors; internal causes generally refer to emotions; miscellaneous causes include trauma and inappropriate lifestyle. The locus classicus for this threefold differentiation is the *San yin ji yi bingyuan luncui* 三因极一病源论粹 (*The Three Causes Epitomized and Verified: The Quintessence of Doctrine on the Origins of Medical Disorders*) by Chen Yan 陈言 ca. 1174, as cited for instance in the *Outline* (*Nanjing zhongyi xueyuan* 1958: 121).

12 These are translated by Farquhar (1994a: 86) as "illness factors."

13 Zhang Weiyao 1994: 352 states that the *Outline* model is not comprehensive enough.

14 See Sivin 1987: 112, which identifies a simplification of classical practices in the emphasis contemporary Chinese medicine places on visceral manifestation pattern determination.

15 See Hsu 1999: 198–206; Sivin 1987: 208–12.

BIBLIOGRAPHY OF PREMODERN CHINESE MEDICAL TEXTS

Texts in this section are identified by name rather than author. Only texts specifically consulted (i.e., not those cited merely from secondary sources) have been included. The modern editions used are specified after the listing of title, author, and date. References to the original text are by *juan*, chapter, and/or section, as appropriate (i.e., 2.1 can mean *juan* 2, chapter 1, or chapter 2, section 1). Page number references are to the modern editions consulted.

Bianzheng lu 辨证录 (*A Record of Differentiating Patterns*). Attributed to Chen Shiduo 陈士铎. 1687. Edition used is Wang Yongqian 王永谦 et al., eds. 1989. Beijing: Renmin weisheng chubanshe.

Ding Ganren yi'an 丁甘仁医案 (*Ding Ganren's Case Records*). Edited by Ding Jiwan 丁济万. 1927. Edition used is 1960. Shanghai: Shanghai kexue chubanshe.

Feng Zhaozhang miannang milu zazheng daxiao hecan 冯兆张绵囊秘录杂证大小合参 (*Feng Zhaozhang's Secret Records of the Cotton Bag: Complete Consultation of Major and Minor Miscellaneous Patterns*). Feng Zhaozhang. 1702. Edition used is Tian Sisheng 田思胜, ed., *Feng Zhaozhang yixue quanshu* 冯兆张医学全书 (*The Complete Medical Works of Feng Zhaozhang*). Beijing: Zhongguo zhongyiyao chubanshe.

Huangdi neijing 黄蒂内经 (*The Inner Classic of the Yellow Lord*). Anonymous [probably Warring States and Han]. Editions used are Ren Yingqiu, ed. 1986. *Huangdi neijing zhangju suoyin* 黄蒂内经章句索引 (*A Concordance of The Inner Classic of the Yellow Lord*). Beijing: Renmin weisheng chubanshe. Guo Aichun 郭霭春, ed. 1989. *Huangdi neijing lingshu jiaozhu yuyi* 黄蒂内经灵枢校注语译 (*The Inner Classic of the Yellow Lord Spiritual Pivot with Annotations and Translation into Modern Chinese*). Tianjin: Tianjin kexue jishu chubanshe. Guo Aichun 郭霭春, ed. 1992. *Huangdi neijing suwen jiaozhu* 黄蒂内经素问校注 (*The Inner Classic of the Yellow Lord Simple Questions with Annotations*). Beijing: Renmin weisheng chubanshe.

Jingyue quanshu 景岳全书 (*Collected Treatises of [Zhang] Jingyue*). Zhang Jiebin 张介宾. 1624. Edition used by Xiao Lixun 逍立勋, ed. 1991. Beijing: Renmin weisheng chubanshe.

Leizheng zhicai 类证治裁 (*Tailored Treatments According to Patterns*) Beijing: Renmin weisheng chubanshe. Lin Peiqin 林佩琴. 1851. Edition used is Liu Jinwen 刘荩文, ed. 1988. Beijing: Renmin weisheng chubanshe.

Linzheng zhinan yi'an 临证指南医案 (*A Case Record Compass of Clinical Patterns*). Ye Tianshi 叶天士, compiled and edited by Hua Xiuyun 华岫云. 1766. Edition used is Gao Huiyun 高慧筠 et al., eds. 1995. Beijing: Huaxia chubanshe.

Lenglu yihua 冷庐医话 (*Medical Stories from Cold Cottage*). Lu Yitian 陆以恬. Foreword 1857. Edition used is Zhu Weichang 朱伟常, ed. 1993. *Lenglu yihua kaozheng* 冷庐医话考注 (*Annotated Medical Stories from Cold Cottage*). Shanghai: Shanghai zhongyi xueyuan.

Maijing 脉经 (*Pulse Classic*). Wang Shuhe 王叔和. ca. A.D. 280. Edition used is Chen Yannan 沈炎南, ed. 1993. *Maijing yuyi* 脉经语译 (*The Pulse Classic with Translation into Modern Chinese*). Beijing: Renmin weisheng chubanshe.

Nanjing 难经 (*Classic of Difficult Issues*). Attributed to Qin Yue 秦越. Warring States. Edition used is *Nanjing benyi* 难经本义 (*Original Meaning of the Classic of Difficult Issues*). Hua Shou 滑寿. 1361. Chen Hong 陈虹 and Ni Qinyi 倪秦一, eds. 1994. Chongqing: Xinan shiyuan daxue chubanshe.

Neiwaishang bianhuo lun 内外伤辨惑论 (*Clarifying Doubts about Inquiries from Internal and External Causes*). Li Gao 李杲. 1247. Edition used is Ding Guangdi 丁光迪 and Wang Kui 王魁, eds. 1993. *Dongyuan yiji.* 东垣医集 (*The Collected Medical Works of [Li] Dongyuan*). Beijing: Renmin weisheng chubanshe.

Qianjin yaofang 千金要方 (*Important Formulas Worth a Thousand*). Sun Simiao 孙思藐. 650–659. Edition used is Liu Gengsheng 刘更生 and Zhang Ruixian 张瑞贤, eds. 1993. Beijing: Huaxia chubanshe.

Shanghan zabing lun 伤寒杂病论 (*Discussion of Cold Damage and Various Disorders*). Zhang Zhongjing 张仲景. Eastern Han. Contemporary versions are usually based on the edition of Wang Shuhe 王叔和. Song, 1065. Editions used are Li Peisheng 李培生 and Liu Duzhou 刘渡舟, eds. 1987. *Shanghan lun* 伤寒论 (*Discussion of Cold Damage*). Beijing: Renmin weisheng chubanshe. Li Keguang 李克光, ed. 1989. *Jingui yaolue* 金匮要略 (*Essentials of the Golden Casket*). Beijing: Renmin weisheng chubanshe.

Taiping huimin hejiju fang 太平惠民和剂局方 (*Prescriptions of the Public Pharmacy of the Era of Great Peace and of the Bureau of Medicines*). 1078. Edition used is Liu Jingyuan 刘景源, ed. 1985. Beijing: Renmin weisheng chubanshe.

Waitai biyao 外台秘要 (*Arcane Essentials from the Imperial Library*). Wang Tao 王焘. 752. Edition used is Gao Wenzhu 高文铸, ed. *Waitai biyao fang* 外台秘要方 (*Arcane Essentials from the Imperial Library Formulary*). 1993. Beijing: Huaxia chubanshe.

Wanbing huichun 万病回春 (*Restoration of Health from the Myriad Diseases*). Gong Tingxian 龚廷贤. 1588. Edition used is Li Shihua 李世华 and Wang Yuxue 王育学, eds. *Gong Tingxian yixue quanshu* 龚廷贤医学全书 (*The Collected Medical Works of Gong Tingxian*). 1999. Beijing: Zhongguo zhongyiyao chubanshe.

Wenbing tiaobian 温病条辨 (*Systematic Differentiation of Warm [Pathogen] Disorders*).

Wu Jutong 吳鞠通. 1798. Edition used is Li Liukun 李刘坤, ed. *Wu Jutong yixue quanshu* 吳鞠通医学全书 (*The Collected Medical Works of Wu Jutong*). 1999. Beijing: Zhongguo zhongyiyao chubanshe.

Xuezheng lun 血证论 (*Discussion of Blood Patterns*). Tang Rongchuan 唐容川. 1884. Edition used is Wang Mimi 王咪咪 and Li Lin 李林, eds. *Tang Rongchuan yixue quanshu* 唐容川医学全书 (*The Collected Medical Works of Tang Rongchuan*). 1999. Beijing: Zhongguo zhongyiyao chubanshe.

Yifang jijie 医方集解 (*Medical Formulas Collected and Analyzed*). Wang Ang 汪昂. 1682. Edition used is 1957. Shanghai: Shanghai weisheng chubanshe.

Yilin gaicuo 医林改错 (*Correction of Errors among Physicians*). Wang Qingren 王清任. 1830. Edition used is Shanxisheng zhongyi yanjiuyuan 陕西省中医研究院, eds. 1976. *Yilin gaicuo pingzhu* 医林改错评注 (*Correction of Errors among Physicians with Notes and Annotations*). Beijing: Renmin weisheng chubanshe.

Yimen falü 医门法律 (*Laws for Physicians*). Yu Chang 喻昌. 1658. Siku yixue congshu 四库医学丛书. Reprinted 1991. Shanghai: Shanghai guji chubanshe.

Yizong bidu 医宗必读 (*Essential Readings from the Medical Ancestors*). Li Zhongzi 李中梓. 1637. Edition used is Bao Laifa 包来发, ed. *Li Zhongzi yixue quanshu* 李中梓医学全书 (*The Collected Medical Works of Li Zhongzi*). 1999. Beijing: Zhongguo zhongyiyao chubanshe.

Yixue xinwu 医学心悟 (*The Awakening of the Mind in Medical Studies*). Cheng Guopeng 程国彭. 1732. Reprinted 1991. *Zhongguo yixue dacheng* 中国医学大成 (*Great Compendium of Chinese Medicine*), vol. 46. Shanghai: Shanghai kexue jishu chubanshe.

Yixue yuanliu lun 医学源流论 (*Discussions on the Origin and Development of Medicine*). Xu Dachun 徐大椿. 1757. Edition used is *Xu Dachun yishu quanji* 徐大椿医书全集 (*Complete Collected Medical Books of Xu Dachun*). 1988. Beijing: Renmin weisheng chubanshe.

Yixue zhongzhong canxi lu 医学衷中参西录 (*Records of the Assimilation of the Western to Chinese in Medicine*). 1900–34. Zhang Xichun 张锡纯. Edition used is Wang Yunkai 王云凯, Yang Yiya 杨医亚, and Li Binzhi 李彬之, eds. 1991. Shijiazhuang: Hebei kexue jishu chubanshe.

Zhengzhi zhunsheng 证治准绳 (*Indispensable Tools for Pattern Treatment*). Wang Kentung 王肯堂 1602–8. Edition used is Ni Hexian 倪和宪, ed. 1991. Beijing: Renmin weisheng chubanshe.

Zhongding guang wen re lun 重订广温热论 (*Newly Revised Expanded Discussion of Warm [Pathogen] Heat [Disorders]*). He Lianchen 何廉臣. 1909. Reprinted 1960. Beijing: Renmin weisheng chubanshe.

Zhongxi huitong yijing jingyi 中西汇通医经经义 (*The Essential Meaning of the Medical Classics from the Perspective of the Convergence of Chinese and Western Medicine*). Tang Rongchuan 唐容川. 1892. Edition used is Wang Mimi 王咪咪 and Li Lin 李林, eds. *Tang Rongchuan yixue quanshu* 唐容川医学全书 (*The Collected Medical Works of Tang Rongchuan*). 1999. Beijing: Zhongguo zhongyiyao chubanshe.

Zhubing yuan hou lun 诸病源候论 (*On the Origins and Symptoms of All Disorders*). Chao Yuanfang 巢元方. Completed 610. Edition used is Ding Guangdi 丁光迪 ed. 1992. *Zhubing yuan hou lun jiaozhu* 诸病源候论校注 (*On the Origins and Symptoms of All Disorders. Corrected and Annotated Edition*). Beijing: Renmin weisheng chubanshe.

BIBLIOGRAPHY OF MODERN CHINESE
AND WESTERN SOURCES

Abu-Lughod, Lila. 1990. "The Romance of Resistance—Tracing Transformations of Power through Bedouin Women." *American Ethnologist* 17: 41–55.

Ågren, Hans. 1974. "Patterns of Tradition and Modernization in Contemporary Chinese Medicine." In *Medicine in Chinese Cultures: Comparative Studies in Chinese and Other Cultures*, edited by Arthur Kleinman, Peter Kunstadter, E. Russell Alexander, and James L. Gale, 37–59. Washington: U.S. Dept. of Health, Education, and Welfare Public Health Service.

——. 1986. "Chinese Traditional Medicine: Temporal Order and Synchronous Events." In *Time, Science, and Society in China and the West*, edited by J. T. Fraser, N. Lawrence, and F. C. Haber, 211–18. Amherst: University of Massachusetts Press.

Ahmed, Akbar S., and Chris N. Shore, eds. 1995. *The Future of Anthropology: Its Relevance to the Contemporary World*. London: Athlone Press.

Ames, Roger T. 1984. "The Meaning of Body in Classical Chinese Thought." *International Philosophical Quarterly* 24, no. 1: 39–54.

——. 1994. "The Focus-Field Self in Classical Confucianism." In *Self as Person in Asian Theory and Practice*, edited by Roger T. Ames, Wimal Dissanayake, and Thomas P. Kasulis, 187–212. Albany: SUNY Press.

Amsterdamska, O. 1990. "Surely You Are Joking Monsieur Latour!" *Science, Technology, and Human Values* 15: 495–504.

Andrews, Bridie J. 1996. "The Making of Modern Chinese Medicine, 1895–1937." Ph.D. diss., University of Cambridge.

——. 1997a. "TB and the Assimilation of Germ Theory in China, 1895–1937." *Journal of the History of Medicine and Allied Sciences* 52, no. 1: 114–57.

——. 1997b. "Another Kind of Miracle: Medical Achievements of Pre-revolutionary China." *Times Literary Supplement*, no. 4925: 26–27.

Anonymous. 1992. *Beijing ge yiyuan zhuanjia zhuanke menzhen zhinan* 北京各医院专家专门诊指南 (*A Guide to Specialists and Specialist Outpatient Departments in Beijing*). Beijing: Neibu ziliao 内部资料.

Appadurai, Arjun. 1986. "Theory in Anthropology: Center and Periphery." *Comparative Studies in Society and History* 28: 356–61.

——. 1990. "Disjuncture and Difference in the Global Cultural Economy." *Public Culture* 2: 1–24.

——. 1995. "The Production of Locality." In *Counterworks: Managing the Diversity of Knowledge*, edited by Richard Fardon, 204–25. London: Routledge.

Archer, Margaret S. 1996. *Culture and Agency: The Place of Culture in Social Theory*. Rev. ed. Cambridge: Cambridge University Press.

Asad, Talal. 1973. *Anthropology and the Colonial Encounter*. London: Ithaca.

——. 2000. "Agency and Pain: An Exploration." *Culture and Religion* 1, no. 1. <http://www.stir.ac.uk/Departments/Arts/ReligiousStudies/C&R/cr/asad.html>.

Baer, Hans A., Merrill Singer, and Ida Susser. 1997. *Medical Anthropology and the World System: A Critical Perspective*. Westport: Bergin and Garvey.

Baer, Hans A., Cindy Jen, Lucia M. Tanassi, Christopher Tsia, and Helen Wahbeh. 1998. "The Drive for Professionalization in Acupuncture: A Preliminary View from the San Francisco Bay Area." *Social Science and Medicine* 46, nos. 4–5: 533–37.

Bailey, Paul J. 1990. *Reform the People: Changing Attitudes towards Popular Education in Early Twentieth-Century China*. Edinburgh: Edinburgh University Press.

Bakehurst, David. 1990. "Social Memory in Soviet Thought." In *Collective Remembering*, edited by D. Middleton and D. Edwards, 203–26. London: Sage.

Barnes, Linda L. 1998. "The Psychologizing of Chinese Healing Practices in the United States." *Culture, Medicine and Psychiatry* 22: 413–43.

Baum, John Alan. 1979. *Montesquieu and Social Theory*. Oxford: Pergamon.

Baum, Richard. 1982. "Science and Culture in Contemporary China." *Asian Survey*, December, 1170.

Beijing zhongyi xueyuan 北京中医学院 (Beijing College of Chinese Medicine). 1980. *Essentials of Chinese Acupuncture*. Beijing: Foreign Languages Press.

——. 1986. *Zhongyi jichu lilun* 中医基础理论 (*Basic Theory of Chinese Medicine*). Beijing: Zhongyi guji chubanshe.

Beijing zhongyi yanjiusuo 北京中医研究所 (Beijing Academy of Chinese Medicine). 1962. "Guanyu 'Bianzheng lunzhi he jiti fanyingxing wenti' yi wen shi yijian" 关于 "辨证论治和机体反应性问题" 一文时意见 (Objections to "A Pattern differentiation and treatment determination and the problem of organismic reaction" based on classical and contemporary sources). *Zhongyi zazhi*, no. 4: 14–15.

Beijing zhongyiyuan geming weiyuanhui 北京中医院革命委员会 (Beijing Hospital of Chinese Medicine Revolutionary Committee). 1971. *Bianzheng shizhi gangyao* 辨症施治纲要 (*Differentiating Symptoms and Applying Treatment: An Outline*). Beijing: Renmin weisheng chubanshe.

Benjamin, Walter. 1982. *Gesammelte Schriften*. Vol. 5: *Das Passagenwerk*. Edited by Rolf Tiedeman and Hermann Schweppenhäuser. 6 vols. Frankfurt am Main: Suhrkamp.

Bensky, Dan. 1996. "Dialogues on the Processes of Life: Selected Translations from the Huangdi Neijing." M.A. thesis, University of Washington.

——. 1998. *Eastland Press Draft Glossary of Chinese Medical Terminology*. Seattle: Eastland Press.

Bensky, Dan, and Randy Barolet. 1990. *Chinese Herbal Medicine: Formulas and Strategies.* Seattle: Eastland Press.

Bensky, Dan, and Andrew Gamble.1993. *Chinese Herbal Medicine: Materia Medica.* Rev. ed. Seattle: Eastland Press.

Berg, Marc, and Annemarie Mol, eds. 1998. *Differences in Medicine: Unraveling Practices, Techniques, and Bodies.* Durham: Duke University Press.

Berger, Peter L., and Thomas Luckmann. 1967. *The Social Construction of Reality: A Treatise in the Sociology of Knowledge.* London: Pelican Books.

Berman, Marshall. 1982. *All That Is Solid Melts into Air: The Experience of Modernity.* New York: Penguin.

Bermingham, Ann, and John Brewer, eds. 1995. *The Consumption of Culture, 1600–1800: Image, Object, Text.* London: Routledge.

Billig, Michael, Susan Condor, Derek Edwards, Mike Gane, David Middleton, and Alan Radley. 1988. *Ideological Dilemmas.* London: Sage.

Bloch, Maurice. 1985. "From Cognition to Ideology." In *Power and Knowledge: Anthropological and Sociological Approaches,* edited by Richard Fardon, 21–48. Edinburgh: Scottish Academic Press.

Bloom, Gerald, and Gu Xingyuan. 1997. "Health Sector Reform: Lessons from China." *Social Science and Medicine* 45, no. 3: 351–60.

Bloor, David. 1976. *Knowledge and Social Imagery.* London: Routledge and Kegan Paul.

———. 1999. "Anti-Latour." *Studies in History and Philosophy of Science* 30, no. 1: 81–112.

Bodenschatz, Christine. "Medizin als neokonfuzianische Praxis." Ph.D. diss., Ludwig-Maximillian Universität Munich, forthcoming.

Boltz, William G. 1994. *The Origin and Early Development of the Chinese Writing System.* New Haven: American Oriental Society.

Bourdieu, P. 1993. *The Field of Cultural Production: Essays on Art and Literature.* Edited and introduced by Randal Johnson. New York: Columbia University Press.

Bray, Francesca. 1993. "Chinese Medicine." In *Companion Encyclopedia of the History of Medicine,* edited by W. F. Bynum and Roy Porter, 728–54. London: Routledge.

Brodwin, Paul. 1996. *Medicine and Morality in Haiti: The Contest for Healing Power.* Cambridge: Cambridge University Press.

Brown, Steve, and Nick Lee. 1994. "Otherness and the Actor-Network: The Undiscovered Continent." *American Behavioral Scientist* 36: 772–90.

Buck-Morss, Susan. 1991. *The Dialectics of Seeing: Walter Benjamin and the Arcades Project.* Cambridge: MIT Press.

Cai Jingfeng 蔡景峰, Li Qinghua 李庆华, and Zhang Binghuan 张冰浣, eds. 2000. *Zhongguo yixue tongshi: xiandai juan* 中国医学通史: 现代卷 (*History of Medicine in China: The Contemporary Period*). Beijing: Renmin weisheng chubanshe.

Cai Jinggao 蔡景高. 1962. "Bianzheng yu bianbing de jiehe" 辩证与辨病的结合 (The integration of pattern differentiation and disease differentiation). *Zhongyi zazhi,* no. 9: 31–33.

Chao, Yuan-Ling. 1995. "Medicine and Society in Late Imperial China: A Study of Physicians in Suzhou." Ph.D. diss., University of California at Los Angeles.

Chen Baoming 陈宝明 and Zhao Jinxi 赵进喜. 1994. *Gu fang miao yong* 古方妙用 (*Ancient Formulas That Are Wonderfully Useful*). Beijing: Kexue tongji chubanshi.

Chen, C. C. 1989. *Medicine in Rural China: A Personal Account.* Berkeley: University of California Press.

Chen, Haifeng, ed. 1984. *Modern Chinese Medicine.* Vol. 3: *Chinese Health Care.* Lancaster: MTP Press, in association with Renmin weisheng chubanshe, Beijing.

Chen Jiaxu 陈家旭. 1992. "Ganqixu zheng zhenduan tanxi" 肝气虚证诊断探析 (An exploratory analysis regarding the diagnosis of liver *qi* depletion patterns). *Beijing zhongyi xueyuan xuebao* 15, no. 6: 6–8.

——. 1993. "Qixu yu yangxu zhi luan, mouguo yu gan" 气虚与阳虚之乱, 莫过于肝 (Confusions about *qi* and *yang* depletion pertain particularly to the liver). *Zhongyi zazhi* 34, no. 3: 183–85.

——. 1994a. "Ganqixu zheng de linzhuang zhenduan ji bianzheng guilü yanjiu" 肝气虚临床证诊及辨证规律研究 (Research regarding regularities in the clinical diagnosis and pattern differentiation of liver *qi* depletion). *Zhongguo yiyao xuebao* 9, no. 1: 12–14.

——. 1994b. "Hushi ganqixu zheng ruogan yuanyin de tantao" 忽视肝气虚证若干原因的探讨 (A reminder not to overlook the varied causes of liver *qi* depletion). *Zhongyi yanjiu* 7, no. 3: 6–8.

Chen, Jirui. 1988. *Acupuncture Case Histories from China.* Translated by Nissi Wang. Seattle: Eastland Press.

Chen Kezheng 陈克正, ed. 1992. *Gu jin zhenjiu zhiyan qinghua* 古今针灸治验精华 (*The Essence of the Clinical Experience of Classical and Contemporary Acumoxa Practitioners*). Beijing: Zhongguo zhongyiyao chubanshe.

Chen Li 陈 离, ed. 1991. *Zhongguo yixue shi* 中国医学 史 (*History of Medicine in China*). Hunan: Hunan kexue jishu chubanshe.

Chen Keji 陈可冀 and Shi Zaixiang 史载祥, eds. 1999. *Shiyong xueyuzhengxue* 实用血瘀证学 (*A Practical [Approach] to Blood Stasis Patterns*). Beijing: Renmin weisheng chubanshe.

Chen Minzhang 陈敏章, ed. 1997. *Zhongguo weisheng nianjian* 中国卫生年签 (*Year Book of Health in the People's Republic of China*). Beijing: Renmin weisheng chubanshe.

Chen, William Y. 1961. "Medicine and Public Health." In *Sciences in Communist China*, edited by Sidney H. Gould, 383–408. Westport, Conn.: Greenwood Press.

Chen Xiaoye 陈小野. 1997. "Lun zhongyi binglixue zheng, bing gainian de tongyi" 论中医病理学证, 病概念的同意 (On the sameness of pattern and disease concepts in Chinese medicine pathology). *Zhongyi zazhi* 38, no. 8: 499–501.

Chen Youbang 陈佑邦 and Deng Liangming 邓良明, eds. 1987. *Dangdai zhongguo zhenjiu linzheng jingyao* 当代中国针灸临证精要 (*Essentials of Contemporary Chinese Acupuncturists' Clinical Experiences*). Tianjin: Tianjin kexue jishu chubanshe.

Chen Yuanpeng 陈元朋. 1997. *Liang Song de 'shangyi shiren' yu 'ruyi': jianlun qi zai Jin Yuan de liubian* 两宋的'尚医士人' 与 '儒医': 兼论其在金元的流变 ("Elites Who Esteemed Medicine" and "Literati Physicians" in the Northern and Southern Song

Dynasties: With a Discussion of Their Spread and Transformation During the Jin and Yuan Dynasties]. Taibei: Guoli Taiwan daxue chubanshe.

Chen Ziyin 沈自尹. 1973. "Neike zhongxiyi jiehe de chubu tantao" 内科领城里中西医结合的初步探讨 (A First Outline of the Integration of Chinese and Western Medicine within Internal Medicine). *Xinyiyao zazhi* 新医药杂志, no. 4: 2.

Chen Ziyin 沈自尹 and Wang Wenjian 王文健. 1988. "Achievements in the Investigation of the Kidney in TCM." *Zhongxiyi jiehe zazhi* Special Issue 2: 96–99.

Cheng Menxue 程门雪. 1986. *Jingui bianjie* 金匮篇解 (*Explanations on the [Essentials of the] Golden Casket*). Beijing: Renmin weisheng chubanshe.

Cheng Shao'en 程绍恩, Xu Baofeng 徐宝丰, Mei Guohui 美国辉, and Xia Yuehui 夏月辉. 1990. *Zhongyao xinfa* 中药心法 (*The Essence of the Chinese Materia Medica*). Beijing: Beijing kexue jishu chubanshe.

Cheng Shide 程士德, ed. 1987. *Neijing* 内经 (*The Inner Classic*). Teaching Reference Works for Tertiary-Level Chinese Medicine. Beijing: Renmin weisheng chubanshe.

Chi, C., J. L. Lee, J. S. Lai, et al. 1996. "The Practice of Chinese Medicine in Taiwan." *Social Science and Medicine* 43: 1329–41.

Chiu, Martha Li. 1986. "Mind, Body, and Illness in a Chinese Medical Tradition." Ph.D. diss., Harvard University.

Chongqingshi xiyi lizhi xuexi zhongyi yanjiuban 重庆市西医离职学习中医研究班 (Chongqing Research Class of Western Medicine Physicians Seconded from Work to Study Chinese Medicine). 1959. *Zhongyi bianzheng shuyu de shentao* 中医辨证术语的深讨 (*An In-Depth Discussion of Chinese Medicine Pattern Terminology*). Chongqing: Chongqing renmin chubanshe.

Clarke, J. J. 1997. *Oriental Enlightenment: The Encounters Between Asian and Western Thought*. London: Routledge.

Clifford, James. 1988. *The Predicament of Culture: Twentieth-Century Ethnography, Literature, and Art*. Cambridge: Harvard University Press.

Collins, Harry, and Trevor Pinch. 1982. *Frames of Meaning*. London: Routledge.

Comaroff, Jean. 1983. "The Defectiveness of Symbols or the Symbols of Defectiveness? On the Cultural Analysis of Medical Systems." *Culture, Medicine and Psychiatry* 7: 3–20.

———. 1985. *Body of Power, Spirit of Resistance: The Culture and History of a South African People*. Chicago: University of Chicago Press.

Cooper, William C., and Nathan Sivin. 1973. "Man as Medicine: Pharmacological and Ritual Aspects of Traditional Therapy Using Drugs Derived from the Human Body." In *Chinese Science: Explorations of an Ancient Tradition*, edited by Shigeru Nakayama and Nathan Sivin, 203–72. Cambridge: MIT Press.

Croizier, Ralph C. 1968. *Traditional Medicine in Modern China*. Cambridge: Harvard University Press.

———. 1976. "The Ideology of Medical Revivalism in Modern China." In *Asian Medical Systems: A Comparative Study*, edited by Charles Leslie, 341–55. Berkeley: University of California Press.

Cui Yueli 崔月梨. 1980. "Jicheng fazhan zuguo yiyaoxue, jiakuai zhongxiyi jiehe bufa, wei sihua jianshe zuochu geng dade gongxian" 继承发展祖国医药学, 加快中西医结合步伐, 为四化建设作出更大的贡献 (Developing the medical and pharmacological inheritance of our motherland and stepping up the pace of integration of Chinese and Western medicine is yet another great achievement of carrying out the four modernizations). Beijing: Quanguo zhongyi he zhongxiyi jiehe gongzuohui.

——. 1990. Foreword to Dong Jianhua 董建华 1990.

——, ed. 1997. *Zhongyi chensi lu* 中医沉思录 (*Pondering Core Issues of Chinese Medicine*). Beijing: Zhongyi guji chubanshe.

Cussins, Charis M. 1998. "Ontological Choreography: Agency for Women Patients in an Infertility Clinic." In M. Berg and A. Mol, 184–222. Durham: Duke University Press.

de Certeau, Michel. 1988 [1984]. *The Practice of Everyday Life*. Translated by Steven Rendall. Berkeley: University of California Press.

Deadman, Peter, and Mazin Al-Khafaji. 1995. "The Treatment of Psycho-emotional Disturbance by Acupuncture with Particular Reference to the Du Mai." *Journal of Chinese Medicine* 47: 30–34.

Deleuze, Gilles, and Félix Guattari. 1983. *Anti-Oedipus: Capitalism and Schizophrenia*. Translated by Robert Hurley. Minneapolis: University of Minnesota Press.

Deng Tietao 邓铁涛, ed. 1984. *Zhongyi zhenduanxue* 中医诊断学 (*Chinese Medical Diagnosis*). Teaching Materials for Tertiary Medical and Pharmaceutical Schools and Colleges. Shanghai: Shanghai kexue jishu chubanshe.

——, ed. 1987. *Zhongyi zhenduanxue* 中医诊断学 (*Chinese Medical Diagnosis*). Teaching Reference Works for Tertiary-Level Chinese Medicine. Beijing: Renmin weisheng chubanshe.

——, ed. 1999. *Zhongyi jindai shi* 中医近代史 (*A History of Chinese Medicine in the Modern Era*). Guangzhou: Guangdong gaodeng jiaoyu chubanshe.

DeWoskin, Kenneth J. 1983. *Doctors, Diviners, and Magicians of Ancient China: Biographies of Fang-shih*. New York: Columbia University Press.

Ding Guangdi 丁光迪, ed. 1999. *Jin Yuan yixue pingxi* 金元医学评析 (*A Critical Analysis of Jin-Yuan Medicine*). Beijing: Renmin weisheng chubanshe.

Dissanayake, Wimal, ed. 1996. *Narratives of Agency: Self-Making in China, India, and Japan*. Minneapolis and London: University of Minnesota Press.

Dodds, E. A. 1973. *The Greeks and the Irrational*. Berkeley: University of California Press.

Dong Hanliang 董汉良. 1986. "Yang Zemin shengping shilue yu qi dui zhongyi tongyi bingming de jianjie" 扬则民生平事略与其对中医统一病名的见解 (A short biographical account of Yang Zemin's life and his views on the unification of Chinese medical disease names). *Zhonghua yishi zazhi* 16, no. 1: 35–37.

Dong Hanliang 董汉良 and Chen Tianxiang 陈天详. 1981a. "Yang Zemin xiansheng ji qi xueshu sixiang" 扬则民先生及其学术思想 (Mr. Yang Zemin and his scholarly thought). *Zhejiang zhongyiyao zazhi*, no. 7: 293–294.

———. 1981b. "Yang Zemin xiansheng yanjiu 'Neijing' xueshu sixiang jianjie" 扬则民先生研究《内经》学术思想间介 (A brief introduction to Mr. Yang Zemin's scholarly thought regarding research into the "Neijing"). *Zhejiang zhongyi xueyuan xuebao*, no. 4: 23–24.

Dong Jianhua 董建华, ed. 1990. *Zhongguo xiandai mingzhongyi yi'an jinghua* 中国现代名中医医案精华 (*Essential Case Histories of Famous Contemporary Physicians of Chinese Medicine*). 3 vols. Beijing: Beijing chubanshe.

Douglas, Mary. 1966. *Purity and Danger.* London: Routledge and Kegan Paul.

Downey, Gary Lee, and Joseph Dumit, eds. 1997. *Cyborgs and Citadels: Anthropological Interventions in Emerging Sciences and Technologies.* Santa Fe: School of American Research Press.

Du Ruzhu 杜如竹. 1994. "Zhongyiyao 'ba wu' kezhi zheng guan xinxi" 中医药'八五'科技政关信息 (Information on TCM research programs in the Eighth Five-Year Plan). *Zhongguo zhongyiyao xinxi zazhi* 1, no. 1: 35–36.

Dunn, Fred L. 1976. "Traditional Asian Medicine and Cosmopolitan Medicine as Adaptive Systems." In *Asian Medical Systems: A Comparative Study*, edited by Charles Leslie, 133–58. Berkeley: University of California Press.

Dutton, Michael. 1998. *Streetlife China.* Cambridge: Cambridge University Press.

Eastman, Lloyd E. 1988. *Family, Fields, and Ancestors: Constancy and Change in China's Social and Economic History, 1550-1949.* Oxford: Oxford University Press.

Eberhardt, Wolfram. 1971. *Moral and Social Values of the Chinese: Collected Essays.* Taipei: Chinese Materials and Resource Centre.

Edwards, C. R. W., and I. A. D. Bouchier, eds. 1991. *Davidson's Principles and Practice of Medicine.* 16th ed. Edinburgh: Churchill Livingstone.

Eisenberg, Leon. 1977. "Disease and Illness." *Culture, Medicine and Psychiatry* 1: 9–23.

EIU (Economist Intelligence Unit). 1998. *Healthcare in China into the Twenty-first Century.* London: Economist Intelligence Unit, 17 July.

Epler, Deane C. Jr. 1977. "The Concept of Disease in Two Third Century Chinese Medical Texts." Ph.D. diss., University of Washington.

Fabrega, H., and D. B. Silver. 1973. *Illness and Shamanistic Curing in Zinacantan.* Stanford: Stanford University Press.

Fang Yaozhong 方药中. 1955. "Guanyu xuexi Shanghan lun yu Jingui yaolue jidian jiben gainian" 关于学习伤寒论与金匮要略的几点基本概念 (Some basic concepts concerning the study of the *Shanghan lun* and the *Jinkui yaolue*). *Jiangxi zhongyiyao* 5, no. 6.

———. 1979. *Bianzheng lunzhi yanjiu ji jiang* 辨证论治研究七讲 (*Seven Lectures on Pattern Differentiation and Treatment Determination Research*). Beijing: Renmin weisheng chubanshe.

———. 1983. "Xue yi sishi nian de huigu" 学医四十年的回顾 (Reviewing forty years of studying medicine). In Zhou Fengwu 周风梧 et al., 1981–85, 1: 172–89.

———. 1993a [1977]. "Tan bianzheng lunzhi de qiben jingshen ji qi zai linzhuang yunyong zhong de buzhou he fangfa" 谈辨证论治的基本精神及其在临床运用中的步骤和方法

(On the basic spirit of pattern differentiation and treatment determination and procedures and methods regarding its clinical application). In 1993b, 203–8.

——. 1993b. *Yixue chengqi ji* 医学承启集 (*Collected Writings concerning Continuation and Innovation in Medicine*). Beijing: Zhongyi guji chubanshe.

Fardon, Richard. 1995. "Latticed Knowledge: Eradication and Medical Dispersal of the Unpalatable in Islam, Medicine and Anthropological Theory." In *Counterworks: Managing the Diversity of Knowledge,* edited by Richard Fardon, 143–63. London: Routledge.

Farquhar, Judith. 1986. "Knowledge and Practice in Chinese Medicine." Ph.D. diss., University of Chicago.

——. 1987. "Problems of Knowledge in Contemporary Chinese Medical Discourse." *Social Science and Medicine* 24: 1013–21.

——. 1992a. "Objects, Processes and Female Infertility in Chinese Medicine." *Medical Anthropology Quarterly* 14: 370–99.

——. 1992b. "Time and Text: Approaching Chinese Medical Practice through Analysis of a Published Case." In Charles Leslie and Allan Young 1992, 62–71.

——. 1994a. *Knowing Practice: The Clinical Encounter in Chinese Medicine.* Boulder: Westview Press.

——. 1994b. "Multiplicity, Point of View, and Responsibility in Traditional Chinese Healing." In Angela Zito and Tani E. Barlow 1994a, 78–99.

——. 1996a. "Market Magic: Getting Rich and Getting Personal in Medicine after Mao." *American Ethnologist* 23, no. 2: 239–57.

——. 1996b. "'Medicine and the Changes are One': An Essay in Divination Healing with Commentary." *Chinese Science* 16: 107–34.

——. *Appetites: Food and Sex in Post-socialist China.* Durham: Duke University Press, forthcoming.

Farquhar, Judith, and James L. Hevia. 1993. "Culture and Postwar American Historiography of China." *positions* 1, no. 2: 486–525.

Featherstone, Mike. 1990. *Global Culture, Nationalism, Globalisation, and Modernity.* London: Sage.

Fei Xiaotong. 1992. *From the Soil: The Foundations of Chinese Society. A Translation of Fei Xiaotong's Xiangtu zhongguo with an introduction and epilogue by Gary Hamilton and Wang Zheng.* Berkeley: University of California Press.

Feuchtwang, Stephen. 1992. *The Imperial Metaphor.* London: Routledge.

Flaws, Bob. 1992. "Thoughts on Acupuncture, Internal Medicine and TCM in the West." *Journal of Chinese Medicine* 38: 1–7.

Foucault, Michel. 1979. *Discipline and Punish: The Birth of the Prison.* Harmondsworth: Penguin.

——. 1980. *Power/Knowledge: Selected Interviews and Other Writings, 1972–1977.* Edited and translated by C. Gordon. Brighton: Harvester Press.

——. 1990 [1976]. *The History of Sexuality.* Vol. 1: *An Introduction.* Harmondsworth: Penguin.

Frankel, Stephen, and Gilbert Lewis, eds. 1989. *A Continuing Trial of Treatment: Medical Pluralism in Papua New Guinea*. Dordrecht: Kluwer.

Franklin, Sarah. 1995. "Science as Culture, Cultures of Science." *Annual Review of Anthropology* 24: 163–84.

Fu Youfeng 符有丰. 1999. "Dongyuan 'piwei neishangbing' jinhuan kao" 东垣 "脾胃内伤病" 急缓考 (Investigating the acute or chronic nature of Dongyuan's "spleen stomach internal damage disorder"). *Yiguwen zhishi*, no. 3: 28–29.

Fuller, Steve. 2000. *Thomas Kuhn: A Philosophical History for Our Times*. Chicago: University of Chicago Press.

Fung, Yu-lan. 1953. *A History of Chinese Philosophy: The Period of Classical Learning*. Translated by Derk Bodde. 2 vols. Princeton: Princeton University Press.

Furth, Charlotte. 1988. "Androgynous Males and Deficient Females: Biology and Gender Boundaries in Sixteenth Century China." *Late Imperial China* 9, no. 2: 1–31.

———. 1999. *A Flourishing Yin: Gender in China's Medical History, 960–1665*. Berkeley: University of California Press.

Galison, Peter, and David J. Stump, eds. 1996. *The Disunity of Science: Boundaries, Contexts, and Power*. Stanford: Stanford University Press.

Gao Dixiu 高迪旭. 1981. "Shitan fenxing lunzhi baobian wojian" 试谈分型论治褒贬我见 (A personal appraisal of type discrimination and treatment determination). *Shanghai zhongyiyao zazhi*, no. 12: 4–6.

Gao Huiyuan 高辉远. 1983. "Xiansheng Pu Fuzhou de zhixue jingshen yu yixue chengjiu" 先生蒲辅周的治学精神与医学成就 (The dynamism of Mr. Pu Fuzhou's clinical studies and his medical achievements). *Shangdong zhongyi zazhi*, no. 1: 40–42.

Gao Luwen 高渌纹. 1993. *Shiyong youdu zhongyao linchuang shouce* 实用有毒中药临床手册 (*Clinical Handbook of Practically Applied Poisonous Chinese Medical Drugs*). Beijing: Xueyuan chubanshe.

Gao Surong 高素荣. 1993. *Shiyuzheng* 失语症 (*Aphasia*). Beijing: Zhongguo xiehe yike daxue lianhe chubanshe.

Gasché, Rodolphe. 1986. *The Tain of the Mirror: Derrida and the Philosophy of Reflection*. Cambridge: Harvard University Press.

Gauld, Robin D. C. 1998. "A Survey of the Hong Kong Health Sector: Past, Present and Future." *Social Science and Medicine* 47, no. 7: 927–39.

Geertz, Clifford. 1977. "On the Notion of Anthropological Understanding." In *Annual Editions in Anthropology*. Guildford, Conn.: Dushkin.

Gergen, Kenneth J. 1989. "Social Psychology and the Wrong Revolution." *European Journal of Social Psychology* 19: 463–84.

———. 1990. "Social Understanding and the Inscription of Self." In *Cultural Psychology: Essays on Comparative Human Development*, edited by James W. Stigler, Richard A. Shweder, and Gilbert Herdt, 569–606. Cambridge: Cambridge University Press.

Giddens, Anthony. 1990. *Modernity and Self Identity*. Cambridge: Polity Press.

———. 1991. *The Consequences of Modernity*. Cambridge: Polity Press.

Gieryn, Thomas F. 1995. "Boundaries of Science." In *Handbook of Science and Tech-

nology Studies, edited by Sheila Jasanoff, Gerald E. Markle, James C. Petersen, and Trevor Pinch, 393–443. London: Sage.

——. 1999. *Cultural Boundaries of Science: Credibility on the Line.* Chicago: University of Chicago Press.

Gingras, Yves. 1995. "Following Scientists through Society? Yes, but at Arms' Length!" In *Scientific Practice*, edited by Z. Buchwald, 123–48. Chicago: University of Chicago Press.

——. 1997. "The New Dialectics of Nature." *Social Studies of Science* 27, no. 2: 317–34.

Goldsmith, Marsha S. 1999. "2020 Vision: NIH Heads Foresee the Future." *Journal of the American Medical Association* 282: 2287–90.

Golinski, Jan. 1998. *Making Natural Knowledge: Constructivism and the History of Science.* Cambridge: Cambridge University Press.

Good, Byron J. 1977. "The Heart of What's the Matter: The Semantics of Illness in Iran." *Culture, Medicine and Psychiatry* 1: 25–28.

——. 1994. *Medicine, Rationality, and Experience: An Anthropological Perspective.* Lewis Henry Morgan Lecture Series. Cambridge: Cambridge University Press.

Greenwood, Bernard. 1992. "Cold or Spirits? Ambiguity and Syncretism in Moroccan Therapeutics." In *The Social Basis of Health and Healing in Africa*, edited by Steven Feierman and John M. Janzen, 285–314. Berkeley: University of California Press.

Gu Zhishan 顾植山. 1982. "Ye tan zhongyi gejia xueshuo de yanjiu fanchou ji liupai wenti" 也谈中医各家学说的研究范畴级流派问题 (A further discussion of the scope of research in doctrines of schools of Chinese medicine: Regarding the problem of [medical] streams). *Zhongyi zazhi*, no. 3: 10–13.

Guo Mingxin 郭铭信. 1980. "Sanjiao gainian de yantao ji qi linchuang de yingyong" 三焦概念的研讨及其临床的应用 (A discussion of the concept of the *sanjiao* and its clinical applications). *Zhongyi zazhi*, no. 8: 567.

Guojia jishu jianduju 国家技术鉴督局 (State Bureau of Technical Supervision). 1994. *Zhongyi bing zheng zhenduan liaoxiao biaozhun* 中医病证诊断疗效标准 (*Standards of Diagnosis and Therapeutic Effect for Diseases and Patterns in Chinese Medicine*). Zhonghua renmin gongheguo guojia biaozhun 中华民共和国国家标准 (National Standards of the People's Republic of China). ZY/T001-94. Beijing: Zhongguo bioazhun chubanshe.

——. 1995. *Zhongyi bing zheng fenlei yu daima* 中医病证分类与代码 (*Classification and Codes for Diseases and Patterns in Chinese Medicine*). Zhonghua renmin gongheguo guojia biaozhun 中华人民共和国国家标准 (National Standards of the People's Republic of China). GB/T15657-1995. Beijing: Zhongguo bioazhun chubanshe.

——. 1997a. *Zhongyi linchuang zhenliao shuyu jibing bufen* 中医临床诊疗术语疾病部分 (*Clinical Terminology of Chinese Medical Diagnosis and Treatment—Diseases*). Zhonghua renmin gongheguo guojia biaozhun 中华人民共和国国家标准 (National Standards of the People's Republic of China). GB/T16751.1-1997. Beijing: Zhongguo bioazhun chubanshe.

——. 1997b. *Zhongyi linchuang zhenliao shuyu zhenghou bufen* 中医临床诊疗术语证

候部分 (*Clinical Terminology of Chinese Medical Diagnosis and Treatment—Patterns*). Zhonghua renmin gongheguo guojia biaozhun 中华人民共和国国家标准 (National Standards of the People's Republic of China). GB/T16751.2-1997. Beijing: Zhongguo bioazhun chubanshe.

———. 1997c. *Zhongyi linchuang zhenliao shuyu zhifa bufen* 中医临床诊疗术语治发部分 (*Clinical Terminology of Chinese Medical Diagnosis and Treatment—Therapeutic Methods*). Zhonghua renmin gongheguo guojia biaozhun 中华人民共和国国家标准 (National Standards of the People's Republic of China). GB/T16751.3-1997. Beijing: Zhongguo bioazhun chubanshe.

Guojia zhongyiyao guanliju 国家中医药管理局 (State Administration of Chinese Medicine and Pharmacology). 1997 [1992]. "Jianshe zhongguo teyoude zhongyiyao guanli tizhi" 建设中国特有的中医药管理体制 (Constructing a regulatory system of Chinese medicine and pharmacology with Chinese characteristics). In Cui Yueli 崔月梨 1997a, 213–26.

Guojia zhongyiyao guanliju yizhengsi 国家中医药管理局医政司 (State Administration of Chinese Medicine and Pharmacology, Bureau of Medical Administration). 1991. *Zhongyi bing'an shuxie guifan* 中医病案书写规范 (*Standards for Writing Up Chinese Medicine Case Histories*). Beijing: Guojia zhongyiyao guanliju yizhengsi.

Guojia zhongyiyao guanliju zhengce faguisi 国家中医药局管理局政策发规司 (State Administration of Chinese Medicine and Pharmacology, Bureau of Policy and Laws). 1992. *Zhonghua renmin gongheguo xianxing zhongyiyao fagui huibian 1949–1991* 中华人民共和国现行中医药发规汇编 *1949–1991* (*Edited Collection of Currently Effective Laws on Chinese Medicine and Pharmacology of the People's Republic of China 1949–1991*). Beijing: Zhongguo zhongyiyao chubanshe.

Gusterson, Hugh. 1996. *Nuclear Rites: An Anthropologist among Weapon Scientists.* Berkeley: University of California Press.

Habermas, Jürgen. 1987. *The Philosophical Discourse of Modernity.* Oxford: Polity Press.

Hacking, Ian. 1996. "Matter over Mind." *Times Literary Supplement,* 10 May, 15.

Hahn, Robert A., and Arthur Kleinman. 1983. "Biomedical Practice and Anthropological Theory: Frameworks and Directions." *Annual Review of Anthropology* 12: 305–33.

Hammer, Leon. 1991. "Duelling Needles: Reflections on the Politics of Medical Models." *American Journal of Acupuncture* 19, no. 3.

Hammes, Michael, and Thomas Ots. 1994. *33 Fallbeispiele zur Akupunktur aus der VR China: Ein klinisches Kompendium.* Stuttgart: Hippokrates Verlag.

Han Zhirong 韩智荣 and Liu Jinsheng 刘金声. 1990. "Zhang Xichun wenbu ganqi sixiang chutan" 张锡纯温补肝气思想初探 (An introduction to Zhang Xichun's theories on the warming and supplementing of liver *qi*). *Hebei zhongyi zazhi* 12, no. 1: 5.

Hannerz, Ulf. 1992. *Cultural Complexity: Studies in the Social Organization of Meaning.* New York: Columbia University Press.

Hanson, Marta E. 1997. "Inventing a Tradition in Chinese Medicine: From Universal

Canon to Local Medical Knowledge in South China, the Seventeenth to the Nineteenth Century." Ph.D. diss., University of Pennsylvania.

Haraway, Donna. 1989. *Primate Visions: Gender, Race, and Nature in the World of Modern Science.* New York: Routledge.

——. 1991. "A Cyborg Manifesto: Science, Technology and Socialist Feminism in the Late Twentieth Century." In *Simians, Cyborgs, and Women: The Reinvention of Nature*, 149–81. London: Free Association Books.

——. 1993. "The Biopolitics of Postmodern Bodies: Determinations of Self in Immune Systems Discourse." In *Knowledge, Power and Practice: The Anthropology of Medicine and Everyday Life*, edited by Shirley Lindenbaum and Margaret Lock, 364–410. Berkeley: University of California Press.

Hare, Martha L. 1993. "The Emergence of an Urban U.S. Chinese Medicine." *Medical Anthropology Quarterly* 7, no. 1: 30–49.

Harré, Rom, ed. 1986. *The Social Construction of Emotions.* Oxford: Basil Blackwell.

Hay, John. 1983a. "The Human Body as a Microcosmic Source of Macrocosmic Values in Calligraphy." In *Theories of the Arts in China*, edited by Susan Bush and Christian Murck, 74–102. Princeton: Princeton University Press.

——. 1983b. "Values and History in Chinese Painting (I)." *Res* 6: 72–111.

——. 1983c. "Values and History in Chinese Painting (II)." *Res* 7–8: 102–36.

——. 1994. "The Body Invisible in Chinese Art?" In Angela Zito and Tani E. Barlow 1994a, 42–77.

He Puren 贺普仁, ed. 1989. *Zhen ju zhen fa* 针具针法 (*Acupuncture Tools and Methods*). Beijing: Kexue jishu wenzai chubanshe.

He Shixi 何时希. 1991. "Menghe Dingshi sandai mingyi" 孟河丁氏三代名医 (Three Generations of Famous Physicians in the Menghe Ding Family). In *Haishang yilin* 海上医林 (*Physicians of Shanghai*), edited by Shanghaishi wenshi ziliaohui 上海市文史资料会 (Shanghai Literary and Historical Materials Committee), 1–11. Shanghai: Shanghai renmin chubanshe.

——. 1997. *Jindai yilin yishi* 近代医林轶事 (*Anecdotes from the World of Medicine in the Modern Era*). Shanghai: Shanghai zhongyiyao daxue chubanshe.

He Yumin 何裕民. 1987. *Zhongyixue daolun* 中医学导论 (*Guide to Chinese Medicine*). Shanghai: Shanghai zhongyi xueyuan chubanshe.

Henderson, Gail. 1993. "Public Health in China." In *China Briefing, 1992*, edited by William A. Joseph, 103–24. Boulder: Westview Press.

Henderson, Gail, et al. 1994. "Equity and the Utilization of Health Services: Report of an Eight Province Survey in China." *Social Science and Medicine* 39, no. 5: 687–700.

Henriques, J., W. Hollway, C. Urwin, C. Venn, and V. Walkerdine. 1984. *Changing the Subject: Psychology, Social Regulation and Subjectivity.* London: Methuen.

Hess, David J. 1997a. *Science Studies: An Advanced Introduction.* New York: New York University Press.

——. 1997b. "If You're Thinking of Living in STS: A Guide for the Perplexed." In Gary Lee Downey and Joseph Dumit 1997, 143–64.

Hillier, Sheila M., and J. A. Jewell. 1983. *Health Care and Traditional Medicine in China, 1800-1982.* London: Routledge and Kegan Paul.

Hinrichs, T. J. 1995. "Official Responses to Epidemics in the Song and the Medical Civilising of the South." Paper presented at the Liu-Gweidjen Memorial Workshop. Cambridge: Needham Research Institute.

———. 1998. "New Geographies of Chinese Medicine." *Osiris* 13: 287–325.

Ho, D. Y. F. 1975. "On the Concept of Face." *American Journal of Sociology* 81: 867–84.

Hoizey, Dominique, and Marie-Joseph Hoizey. 1993. *A History of Chinese Medicine.* Edinburgh: Edinburgh University Press.

Horton, Richard. 1967. "African Traditional Thought and Western Science." *Africa* 38: 50–71, 155–87.

Hsu, Elisabeth. 1991. "The Reception of Western Medicine in China: Examples from Yunnan." In *Science and Empires,* edited by P. Petitjean et al., 89–101. Amsterdam: Kluwer.

———. 1995. "The Manikin in Man: Culture Crossing and Creativity." In *Syncretism and the Commerce of Symbols,* edited by Goran Aijmer. Goteborg: Institute for Advanced Studies in Social Anthropology.

———. 1996. "Innovations in Acumoxa: Analgesia, Scalp and Ear Acupuncture in the People's Republic of China." *Social Science and Medicine* 42, no. 3: 421–30.

———. 1999. *The Transmission of Chinese Medicine.* Cambridge: Cambridge University Press, 1999.

———. 2001. *Innovation in Chinese Medicine.* Cambridge: Cambridge University Press.

Hsu, Francis L. 1971. "Psychological Homeostasis and *Jen:* Conceptual Tools for Advancing Psychological Anthropology." *American Anthropologist* 73: 23–44.

Hu, Hsien-chin. 1944. "The Chinese Concept of Face." *American Anthropologist* 46: 45–64.

Hu Xin 胡欣 and Ge Xiumei 葛秀梅. 1994. *Zhongyi bianzheng lunzhi jiaocheng* 中医辨证论治教程 (*A Course in Chinese Medical Pattern Differentiation and Treatment Determination*). Beijing: Huayi chubanshe.

Hu Yulun 胡玉伦. 1986. "Guanyu gan yang (qi) xu de jige wenti" 关于肝阳（气）虚的几个问题 (Some questions concerning liver *yang* and *qi* depletion). *Xin zhongyi* 18, no. 5: 51–54.

Hua, Shiping. 1995. *Scientism and Humanism: Two Cultures in Post-Mao China.* Albany: SUNY Press.

Huang, Shumin. 1988. "Transforming China's Collective Health Care System: A Village Study." *Social Science and Medicine* 27, no. 9: 879–88.

Huang Xingyuan 黄星垣. 1985. *Zhongyi neike jizheng zhengzhi* 中医内科急症证治 (*Pattern Treatment of Akute Symptoms in Internal Chinese Medicine*). Beijing: Renmin weisheng chubanshe.

Huang Zili 黄自立. 1988. *Zhongyi baijia yilun huicui* 中医百家医论荟萃 (*A Collection of Medical Writings from Diverse Medical Schools*). Chongqing: Chongqing chubanshe.

Hui, Wang. 1997 [1995]. "The fate of 'Mr. Science' in China: The Concept of Science and Its Application in Modern Chinese Thought." In *Formations of Colonial Modernity in East Asia*, edited by Tani E. Barlow, 21–81. Durham: Duke University Press.

Hwang, Kwang-Kuo. 1987. "Face and Favour: The Chinese Power Game." *American Journal of Sociology* 92, no. 4: 944–74.

Hymes, Robert P. 1987. "Not Quite Gentlemen? Doctors in Song and Yuan." *Chinese Science* 8: 9–76.

Ilg, Renate. 2001. "Famous Contemporary Chinese Physicians: Professor Li Zhongyu." *Journal of Chinese Medicine* 66: 51–54.

Jacobs, J. Bruce. 1979. "A Preliminary Model of Particularistic Ties in Chinese Political Alliance: *Kan-ch'ing* and *Kuan-hsi* in a Rural Taiwanese Township." *China Quarterly* 78: 237–73.

Janes, Craig R. 1995. "The Transformations of Tibetan Medicine." *Medical Anthropology Quarterly* 9: 6–12.

——. 1999. "The Health Transition, Global Modernity and the Crisis of Traditional Medicine: The Tibetan Case." *Social Science and Medicine* 48: 1803–20.

Jia Dedao 贾得道. 1993. *Zhongguo yixueshi lue* 中国医学史略 (*A Synopsis of The History of Medicine in China*). Taiyuan: Shanxi kexue jishu chubanshe.

Jia, Huanguang. 1997. "Chinese Medicine in Post-Mao China: Standardization and the Context of Modern Science." Ph.D. diss., University of North Carolina.

Jiang Keming 江克明 and Bao Mingzhong 包明蕙, eds. 1989. *Jianming fangji cidian* 简明方剂辞典 (*Concise Dictionary of Formulas*). Shanghai: Shanghai kexue jishu chubanshe.

Jiangsu xinyi xueyuan 江苏新医学院, eds. 1977. *Zhongyao dacidian* 中药大辞典 (*Great Encyclopedia of Chinese Drugs*). Shanghai: Shanghai kexue jishu chubanshe.

Jiao Shude 焦树德. 1982. *Cong bingli tan bianzheng lunzhi* 从病例谈辨证论治 (*A Discussion of Pattern Discrimination and Treatment Determination on the Basis of Case Studies*). Beijing: Renmin weisheng chubanshe.

Jullien, François. 1995. *The Propensity of Things: Toward a History of Efficacy in China*. Translated by Janet Lloyd. New York: Zone Books.

——. 1999. *Über die Wirksamkeit*. Translated by Gabriele Rick and Ronald Voullié. Berlin: Merve Verlag.

Kaptchuk, Ted. 1983. *Chinese Medicine: The Web That Has No Weaver*. London: Rider.

——. 1996. Preface to MacPherson and Kaptchuk 1966, xii–xxi.

Ke Xuefan 柯雪帆, ed. 1987. *Zhongyi bianzhengxue* 中医辨证学 (*Chinese Medical Pattern Differentiation*). Shanghai: Shanghai zhongyi xueyuan chubanshe.

King, Ambrose Yeo-chi. 1994. "Kuan-hsi and Network Building: A Sociological Interpretation." In *The Living Tree: The Changing Meaning of Being Chinese Today*, edited by Tu Wei-ming, 109–26. Stanford: Stanford University Press.

Kipnis, Andrew. 1997. *Producing Guanxi: Sentiment, Self, and Subculture in a North China Village*. Durham: Duke University Press.

Kleinman, Arthur. 1980. *Patients and Healers in the Context of Culture, Comparative*

Studies of Health Systems and Medical Care. Berkeley: University of California Press.

——. 1986. *Social Origins of Distress and Disease.* New Haven and London: Yale University Press.

——. 1995. *Writing at the Margin: Discourse between Anthropology and Medicine.* Berkeley: University of California Press.

Knorr-Cetina, Karin. 1981. *The Manufacture of Knowledge: An Essay on the Constructivist and Contextual Nature of Science.* Oxford: Pergamon.

Kou Huaxing 寇华胜. 1990. *Zhongyi shengjiangxue* 中医生升降学 (*A Study of Ascending and Directing Downward in Chinese Medicine*). Nanchang: Jiangxi kexue jishu chubanshe.

Kozulin, Alex. 1986. "The Concept of Activity in Soviet Psychology: Vygotsky, His Disciples and Critics." *American Psychologist* 41, no. 3: 264–74.

——. 1990. *Vygotsky's Psychology: A Biography of Ideas.* London: Harvester.

Kuang Cuizhang 匡萃璋. 1997 [1995]. "Xiandai kezhi zhishi beijingxia de zhongyixue" 现代科技知识背景下的中医学 (Chinese medicine against the background of contemporary knowledge in science and technology). In Cui Yueli 崔月梨 1997, 89–97.

Kubny, Manfred. 1995. *Qi Lebenskraftkonzepte in China: Definition, Theorien und Grundlagen.* Heidelberg: K. F. Haug.

Kunstadter, Peter. 1976a. "The Comparative Medical Anthropological Study of Medical Systems in Society." In *Medicine in Chinese Cultures: Comparative Studies in Chinese and Other Cultures,* edited by Arthur Kleinman, Peter Kunstadter, E. Russell Alexander, and James L. Gale, 683–96. Washington: U.S. Dept. of Health, Education, and Welfare, Public Health Service.

——. 1976b. "Do Cultural Differences Make Any Difference? Choice Points in Medical Systems Available in Northwestern Thailand." In *Medicine in Chinese Cultures,* 351–84.

Kuper, Adam. 1999. *Culture: The Anthropologist's Account.* Cambridge: Harvard University Press.

Kuriyama, Shigehisa. 1986. "Varieties of Haptic Experience: A Comparative Study of Greek and Chinese Pulse Diagnosis." Ph.D. diss., Harvard University.

Kwok, Daniel W. Y. 1965. *Scientism in Chinese Thought 1900–1950.* New Haven and London: Yale University Press.

Laderman, Carol, and Marina Roseman, eds. 1996. *The Performance of Healing.* London: Routledge.

Lampton, David L. 1977. *The Politics of Medicine in China: The Policy Process 1949–1977.* Folkestone: Dawson.

Last, Murray. 1992. "The Importance of Knowing about Not Knowing: Observations from Hausaland." In *The Social Basis of Health and Healing in Africa,* edited by Steven Feierman and John M. Janzen, 393–406. Berkeley: University of California Press.

Latané, B., and S. Wolf. 1981. "The Social Impact of Majorities and Minorities." *Psychological Review* 88: 438–53.

Latour, Bruno. 1987. *Science in Action.* Cambridge: Harvard University Press.

———. 1988. *The Pasteurization of France.* Translated by Alan Sheridan and John Law. Cambridge: Harvard University Press.

———. 1990. "Postmodern? No Simply Amodern. Steps toward an Anthropology of Science." *Studies in the History and Philosophy of Science* 21, no. 1: 145–71.

———. 1993. *We Have Never Been Modern.* Translated by Catherine Porter. Cambridge: Harvard University Press.

———. 1997. "A Few Steps towards an Anthropology of the Iconoclastic Gesture." *Science in Context* 10, no. 1: 63–83.

Latour, Bruno, and S. Woolgar. 1986. *Laboratory Life: The Construction of Scientific Knowledge.* 2d ed. Princeton: Princeton University Press.

Lave, Jean. 1993. "The Practice of Learning." In *Understanding Practice: Perspectives on Activity and Context,* edited by Seth Chaiklin and Jean Lave, 3–32. Cambridge: Cambridge University Press.

Lave, Jean, and Etienne Wenger. 1991. *Situated Learning: Legitimate Peripheral Participation.* Cambridge: Cambridge University Press.

Leach, Edmund R. 1964 [1954]. *Political Systems of Highland Burma: A Study of Kachin Social Structure.* Edited by James Woodburn. London: Athlone Press.

Lee, Rance P. L. 1980. "Perceptions and Uses of Chinese Medicine among the Chinese in Hongkong." *Culture, Medicine and Psychiatry* 4, no. 4: 345–75.

Lee, Sing. 1999. "Diagnosis Postponed: Shenjing Shuairuo and the Transformation of Psychiatry in Post-Mao China." *Social Science and Medicine* 23: 349–80.

Lei, Sean Hsianglin. 1998. "When Chinese Medicine Encountered the State: 1910–1949." Ph.D. diss., University of Chicago.

———. 1999. "From *Changshan* to a New Anti-malarial Drug: Re-networking Chinese Drugs and Excluding Chinese Doctors." *Social Studies of Science* 29, no. 3: 323–58.

Leslie, Charles. 1976a. Introduction to *Asian Medical Systems: A Comparative Study,* edited by Charles Leslie, 1–17. Berkeley: University of California Press.

———. 1976b. "The Ambiguities of Medical Revivalism in Modern India." In *Asian Medical Systems: A Comparative Study,* edited by Charles Leslie, 356–67. Berkeley: University of California Press.

———. 1980. "Medical Pluralism in World Perspective." *Social Science and Medicine* 14B: 191–99.

Leslie, Charles, and Allan Young, eds. 1992. *Paths to Asian Medical Knowledge.* Comparative Studies of Health Systems and Medical Care, edited by John M. Janzen. Berkeley: University of California Press.

Lewis, Gilbert. 1975. *Concepts of Health and Illness in a Sepik Society.* London: Athlone Press.

Li Anmin 李安民 and Long Yurong 尤玉荣. 1993. *Zhongxi canzhao neike bingzheng zhiliaoxue* 中西参照内科病证治疗学 (*A Cross-Reference Manual of Chinese and Western Internal Medicine Diseases and Patterns and Their Treatment*). Tianjin: Tianjin keji fanyi chubanshe.

Li, Jianmin. 1997. "Jinfang: The Transmission of Secret Techniques in Ancient China." *Bulletin of the Institute of History and Philology Academia Sinica* 68, no. 1: 117–66.

Li Jingwei 李经纬, ed. 1988. *Zhongyi renwu cidian* 中医人物词典 (*Biographical Dictionary of Chinese Medicine*). Shanghai: Shanghai cishu chubanshe.

Li Keguang 李克光, ed. 1989. *Jingui yaolue* 金匮要略 (*Essentials of the Golden Casket*). Teaching Reference Works for Tertiary-Level Chinese Medicine. Beijing: Renmin weisheng chubanshe.

Li Jingwei 李经纬, Deng Tietao 邓铁涛, et al., eds. 1995. *Zhongyi dacidian* 中医大辞典 (*Encyclopedia of Chinese Medicine*). Beijing: Renmin weisheng chubanshe.

Li Xiaohai 李晓海. 1988. "Lun qingdai de ganbing sangang bianzhi xueshuo" 论清代的肝病三纲辨治学说 (A discussion of Qing dynasty doctrines regarding the three rubrics for differentiating and treating liver disorders). *Beijing zhongyi xueyuan xuebao* 11, no. 5: 40–41.

Li Yun 李云, ed. 1988. *Zhongyi renming cidian* 中医人名词典 (*Biographical Dictionary of Chinese Medicine*). Beijing: Guoji wenhua chuban gongsi.

Li Zhizhong 李致重. 1997a [1996]. "Zheng, zheng, zheng, hou de yange he zhenghou dingyi de yanjiu" 證, 证, 症, 侯的沿革和证候定义的研究 (Researching the evolution of the concepts evidence, pattern, symptom and sign, and the definition of patterns). In Cui Yueli 崔月梨 1997, 177–89. Beijing: Zhongyi guji chubanshe.

Li Zhizhong 李致重. 1997b [1996]. "Cong wenhua yu kexue de jiaodu lun 'zhong xi yi jiche'" 从文化与科学角度论 "中西医结合 (Discussing the "Integration of Chinese and Western medicine" from the perspectives of culture and science). In Cui Yueli 崔月梨 1997, 153–63.

Liang Maoxin 梁茂新, Liu Jin 刘进, Hong Zhiping 洪治平, and Xu Yueying 徐月英. 1998. *Zhongyi zheng yanjiu de kungan he duice* 中医证研究的困惑与对策 (*The Encumberment of Research on Chinese Medicine Patterns and What to Do about It*). Beijing: Renmin weisheng chubanshe.

Liao Yujun 廖育群. 1999. "Guanyu zhongguo chuantong yixue de yige chuantong guannian" 关于中国传统医学的一个传统观念——医者意也 (On a traditional concept of traditional Chinese medicine—medicine is intention). Paper presented at the Chinese Academy of Social Sciences, Beijing, 30 June.

Lin Ganliang 林乾良. 1960. "Lun zhongyi de bianzheng lunzhi" 论中医的辨证论治 (On pattern differentiation and treatment determination in Chinese medicine). *Jiangsu zhongyi*, no. 5: 59–61.

Lincoln, Bruce. 1989. *Discourse and the Construction of Society: Comparative Studies of Myth, Ritual and Classification.* New York and Oxford: Oxford University Press.

Liscomb, Kathleen M. 1993. *Learning from Mt. Hua: A Chinese Physician's Illustrated Travel Record and Painting Theory.* Cambridge: Cambridge University Press.

Liu Duzhou 刘渡舟. 1983. "Xuexi zhongyi de diandi tihui" 学习中医的点滴体会 (Studying Chinese medicine as a process of gradual realization). In Zhou Fengwu 周风梧 et al. 1981–85, 1: 102–13. Jinan: Shandong kexue jishu chubanshe.

Liu, G., X. Liu, and Q. Meng. 1994. "Privatization of the Medical Market in Socialist China: A Historical Approach." *Health Policy* 27: 157–73.

Liu, Inmao. 1986. "Chinese Cognition." In *The Psychology of the Chinese People*, edited by Michael Harris Bond, 73–105. Hong Kong: Oxford University Press.

Liu Ruchen 刘汝琛, ed. 1983. *Zhongyixue bianzhengfa gailun* 中医学辩证法概论 (*Outline of Chinese Medical Dialectics*). Guangzhou: Guangdong keji chubanshe.

Liu, X., and W. Hsiao. 1995. "The Cost Escalation of Social Health Insurance Plans in China: Its Implications for Public Policy." *Social Science and Medicine* 41, no. 8: 1095–1101.

Liu Yue 刘越. 1998a. *Liu Yue yi'an yilun ji* 刘越医案医论集 (*Liu Yue's Collected Case Histories and Medical Essays*). Beijing: Xueyuan chubanshe.

——. 1998b. "'Sheng jiang' yu 'shi gang bianzheng' lun '升降' 于 '十纲辨证' 论 (A discussion of "Ascending and Directing Downward" and the "Ten Rubrics for Differentiating Patterns"). In 1998a, 386–94.

——. 1998c. "Zhongyi bianzheng yu bianbing de jicheng yu fazhan" 中医辨证于辨病的继承于发展 (Inheriting and developing pattern and disease differentiation in Chinese medicine). In 1998a, 394–98.

——, ed. 1999. *Zhang Xichun yi'an* 张锡纯医案 (*Zhang Xichun's Case Histories*). Beijing: Xueyuan chubanshe.

Lock, Margaret. 1980. *East Asian Medicine in Urban Japan: Varieties of Medical Experience*. Berkeley: University of California Press.

——. 1990. "Rationalization of Japanese Herbal Medicine: The Hegemony of Orchestrated Pluralism." *Human Organization* 49, no. 1: 41–47.

——. 1993a. *Encounters with Aging: Mythologies of Menopause in Japan and North America*. Berkeley: University of California Press.

——. 1993b. "Cultivating the Body: Anthropologies and Epistemologies of Bodily Practice and Knowledge." *Annual Review of Anthropology* 22: 133–55.

Lock, Margaret, and Deborah Gordon, eds. 1988. *Biomedicine Examined*. Dordrecht: Kluwer.

Lou Shaolai 楼绍来 and Ren Tianluo 任天洛. 1998. "Zhou Enlai dui zhongyi shiye de jiechu gongxian" 周恩来对中医事业的杰出贡献 (Zhou Enlai's outstanding contribution to the cause of Chinese Medicine). *Shanghai zhongyiyao daxue Shanghaishi zhongyiyao yanjiuyuan xuebao* 12, no. 1: 4–6.

"Lü Bingkui cong yi 60 nian wenji" weiyuanhui 吕炳奎从医６０年文集编辑委员会 (Editorial Committee for the "Festschrift for Lü Bingkui's 60th Anniversary as Physician"), ed. 1993. *Lü Bingkui cong yi 60 nian wenji* 吕炳奎从医６０年文集 (*Festschrift for Lü Bingkui's 60th Anniversary as Physician*). Beijing: Huajia chubanshe.

Lu Ganfu 陆干甫 and Xie Yongxin 谢永新. 1986. *Zhongyixue bianzhengfa yuanli* 中医学辩证法原理 (*Principles of Chinese Medical Dialectics*). Beijing: Zhongyi guj chubanshe.

Lü Guangrong 吕光荣. 1980. "Xiandai zhongyi xueshu zhengming wenti" 现实中医学术争鸣问题 (Academic debates and problems in modern Chinese medicine). *Yunnan zhongyi xueyuan xuebao*, no. 1: 19–25.

Lu Gwei-Djen and Joseph Needham. 1980. *Celestial Lancets: A History and Rationale of Acupuncture and Moxa*. Cambridge: Cambridge University Press.

———. 2000. *Science and Civilization in China*. vol. 6, part 6, edited by Nathan Sivin. Cambridge: Cambridge University Press.

Lü Jingshan 吕景山. 1982. *Shi Jinmo duiyao linchuang jingnian ji* 施今墨对药临床经验集 (*Shi Jinmo's Collected Clinical Experience in the Use of Synergistic Drugs*). Beijing: Renmin weisheng chubanshe.

Lu Zheng 陆拯. 1997. *Duzheng lun* 毒证论 (*Discussion of Toxicity Patterns*). Beijing: Renmin weisheng chubanshe.

Lu Zhongyue 陆中岳 and Hong Shenglin 洪胜林. 1998. "'Zhongyi fukexue' (wuban jiao-cai) quefan piyin lunzhi quyi" 中医妇科学（五版教材）缺乏脾阴论治刍议 (A modest proposal regarding the lack of discussion on the treatment of spleen *yin* depletion in the fifth edition teaching material "Chinese Medical Gynecology"). *Shanghai zhongyiyao daxue shanghaishi zhongyi yanjiuyuan xuebao*, no. 12: 26–28.

Luhmann, Niklas. 1995. *Social Systems*. Translated by John Bednarz Jr. and Dirk Baecker. Stanford: Stanford University Press.

Lutz, Catherine. 1988. *Unnatural Emotions: Everyday Sentiments on a Micronesian Atoll and Their Challenge to Western Theory*. Chicago: University of Chicago Press.

Lynch, Michael. 1996. "Review of 'The Mangle of Practice.'" *Contemporary Sociology* 25: 809–11.

Ma Boying 马伯英. 1993. *Zhongguo yixue wenhua shi* 中国医学文化史 (*A History of Chinese Medicine in Chinese Culture*). Shanghai: Shanghai People's Publishing House.

Ma Boying 马伯英, Gao Xi 高晞, and Hong Zhongli 洪中立. 1994. *Zhong wai yixue wenhua jiaoliu shi* 中外医学文化交流史 (*A History of Intercultural Exchange in Medicine between China and Other Countries*). Shanghai: Wenhui chubanshi.

Ma Zhongxue 麻仲学, ed. 1991. *Zhongguo yixue zhenfa daquan* 中国医学诊法大全 (*Compendium of Chinese Medical Diagnostic Methods*). Jinan: Shandong kexue jishu chubanshe.

MacIntyre, Alasdair C. *After Virtue: A Study in Moral Theory*. 2d ed. London: Duckworth.

Maciocia, Giovanni. 1989. *The Foundations of Chinese Medicine*. Edinburgh: Churchill Livingstone.

———. 1996. Foreword. In MacPherson and Kaptchuk 1996, ix–xi.

MacPherson, Hugh, and Ted Kaptchuk, eds. 1996. *Acupuncture in Practice: Case History Insights from the West*. Edinburgh: Churchill Livingstone.

Mao Zedong 毛泽东. *Mao zhuxi yulu* 毛主席语录 (*Sayings by Chairman Mao*). N.p., n.d.

———. 1968. *Maodun lun* 矛盾论 (*On Practice*). In *Mao Zedong xuanji* 毛泽东选集 (*Selected Works by Mao Zedong*), 274–312. Beijing: Renmin chubanshe.

Marcus, George E. 1995. "Ethnography in/of the World: The Emergence of Multi-sited Ethnography." *Annual Review of Anthropology* 24: 95–117.

Marcus, George E., and Michael M. J. Fischer. 1986. *Anthropology as Cultural Critique: An Experimental Moment in the Human Sciences*. Chicago: University of Chicago Press.

Martin, Emily. 1987. *The Woman in the Body: A Cultural Analysis of Reproduction.* Milton Keynes: Open University Press.

McLennan, Gregor. 1995. *Pluralism.* Buckingham: Open University Press.

Mencius. *Mengzi.* 1970. Translated by D. C. Lau. Harmondsworth: Penguin.

Meng Jingchun 孟景春 and Zhou Zhongying 周仲瑛, eds. 1994. *Zhongyixue gailun: xiudingben* 中医学概论: 修订本 (*Outline of Chinese Medicine.* Rev. ed.). Beijing: Renmin weisheng chubanshe.

Meng Qingyun 孟庆云, ed. 2000. *Zhongguo zhongyiyao fazhan 50 nian: 1949-1999* 中国中医药发展五十年: 1949-1999 (*Fifty Years of Development of Chinese Medicine and Pharmacology in China: 1949-1999*). Zhengzhou: Henan yike daxue chubanshe.

Meng Shujiang 孟澍江, ed. 1985. *Wenbingxue* 温病学 (*Warm [Pathogen] Disorders*). Shanghai: Shanghai kexue jishu chubanshe.

"Mingyi yaolan" bianshen weiyuanhui 名医摇篮编审委员会 (Editorial Committee of "Cradle of Famous Physicians"). *Mingyi yaolan* 名医摇篮 (*Cradle of Famous Physicians*). Shanghai: Shanghai zhongyiyao chubanshe.

Miyashita, Saburo. 1986. "A Historical Analysis of Chinese Formularies and Prescriptions: Three Examples." In *History of Traditional Medicine: Proceedings of the 1st and 2nd International Symposia on the Comparative History of Medicine—East and West,* edited by Teizo Ogawa, 101-16. Tokyo: Taniguchi Foundation.

Mol, Annemarie, and John Law. 1994. "Regions, Networks, and Fluids: Anaemia and Social Topology." *Social Studies of Science* 24: 641-71.

Moore, M. 1992. "Competition and Pluralism in Public Bureaucracies." *IDS Bulletin* 23, no. 4: 65-77.

Nader, Laura. 1996. "Anthropological Inquiry into Boundaries, Power, and Knowledge." In *Naked Science: Anthropological Inquiry into Boundaries, Power, and Knowledge,* edited by Laura Nader, 1-25. New York and London: Routledge.

Nan Zheng 南征. 1986. "Bianzheng lunzhi de qiantan" 辨证论治的浅谈 (A brief discussion of pattern differentiation and treatment determination). *Jilin zhongyiyao,* no. 4: 44-45.

Nandy, Ashis, ed. 1998. *Science, Hegemony and Violence: A Requiem for Modernity.* Delhi: Oxford University Press.

Nanjing College of TCM. 1990. *Acupuncture Treatment of Common Diseases Based upon Differentiation of Syndromes.* Beijing: People's Medical Publishing House.

Nanjing zhongyi xueyuan 南京中医学院 (Nanjing College of Chinese Medicine), ed. 1958. *Zhongyixue gailun* 中医学概论 (*Outline of Chinese Medicine*). Beijing: Renmin weisheng chubanshe.

———. 1997. *Zhongyi fangji dacidian* 中医方剂大辞典 (*Great Encyclopaedia of Chinese Medicine Formulas*). 11 vols. Beijing: Renmin weisheng chubanshe.

Nathan, Andrew J. 1993. "Is Chinese Culture Distinctive? A Review Article." *Journal of Asian Studies* 4: 923-36.

Needham, Joseph, ed. 1956. *Science and Civilisation in China: History of Scientific Thought.* Vol. 2: *Science and Civilisation in China.* Cambridge: Cambridge University Press.

Needham, Joseph, and Gwei-djen Lu. 1975. "Problems of Translation and Modernisation of Ancient Chinese Technical Terms: Manfred Porkert's Interpretations of Terms in Ancient and Medieval Chinese Natural and Medical Philosophy." *Annals of Science* 32, no. 5: 491–502.

Obeyesekere, Gananath. 1992. "Science, Experimentation, and Clinical Practice in Ayurveda." In Leslie and Young 1992, 160–76. Berkeley: University of California Press.

Ogden, Suzanne. 1992. *China's Unresolved Issues: Politics, Development and Culture.* Englewood Cliffs, N.J.: Prentice-Hall.

Oi, Jean C. 1989. *State and Peasant in Contemporary China: The Political Economy of Village Government.* Berkeley: University of California Press.

Ong, Aihwa. 1987. *Spirits of Resistance and Capitalist Discipline: Factory Women in Malaysia.* Albany: SUNY Press.

———. 1995. "Anthropology, China and Modernities." In *The Future of Anthropological Knowledge*, edited by Henrietta L. Moore, 60–92. London: Routledge.

———. 1997. "Chinese Modernities: Narratives of Nation and of Capitalism." In *Underground Empires: The Cultural Politics of Modern Chinese Transnationalism*, edited by Aihwa Ong and D. Nonini, 171–202. London: Routledge.

Ots, Thomas. 1990a. *Medizin und Heilung in China.* 2d ed. Berlin: Dietrich Reimer Verlag.

———. 1990b. "The Angry Liver, the Anxious Heart and the Melancholy Spleen: The Phenomenology of Perceptions in Chinese Culture." *Culture, Medicine and Psychiatry* 14: 25–58.

Ouyang Qi 欧阳琦. 1993. *Zheng bing jiehe yongyao shi* 证病结合用药式 (*A Method for Using Drugs [Based on] Integrated Pattern and Disease Differentiation*). Chansha: Hunan kexue jishu chubanshe.

Parsons, Talcott. 1968 [1937]. *The Structure of Social Action.* New York: Free Press.

Pei Xueyi 裴学义 and Kong Xiangqi 孔祥琦. 1981. "Xian shi Kong Bohua xiansheng xue-shu guankui" 先师孔伯化先生学术管窥 (A humble description of the learning of our former teacher, Mr. Kong Bohua). In Zhou Fengwu 周风梧 et al. 1981–85, 3: 99–112. Jinan: Shandong kexue jishu chubanshe.

Pelto Perrti, J., and Gretel H. Pelto. 1990. "Field Methods in Medical Anthropology." In *Medical Anthropology: Contemporary Theory and Method*, edited by Thomas M. Johnson and Carolyn F. Sargent, 269–97. New York: Praeger.

———. 1975. "Intracultural Diversity: Some Theoretical Issues." *American Ethnologist* 2: 1–18.

Pickering, Andrew. 1995. *The Mangle of Practice: Time, Agency, and Science.* Chicago: University of Chicago Press.

———. 1997. "Concepts and the Mangle of Practice: Constructing Quaternions." In *Mathematics, Science, and Postclassical Theory*, edited by Barbara Herrnstein-Smith and Arkady Plonitsky, 40–82. Durham: Duke University Press, 1997.

Pinch, Trevor. 1999. "Mangled Up in Blue." *Studies in History and Philosophy of Science* 30, no. 1: 139–47.

Polanyi, Michael. 1958. *Personal Knowledge*. Chicago: University of Chicago Press.

Porkert, Manfred. 1978. *The Theoretical Foundations of Chinese Medicine: Systems of Correspondence*. Cambridge: MIT Press.

——. 1983. *The Essentials of Chinese Diagnostics*. Zurich: Acta Medicinae Sinensis.

——. 1998. "Die chinesische Medizin verkürzt und verbilligt." *Chinesische Medizin* 13, no. 3: 80–85.

Prakash, Gyan. 1990. "Writing Post-orientalist Histories of the Third World: Perspectives from Indian Historiography." *Comparative Studies in Society and History* 32, no. 2: 383–408.

Pu Zhixiao 蒲志孝. 1985. "Pu Fuzhou yishi" 蒲辅周轶事 (Anecdotes about Pu Fuzhou). *Shandong zhongyi zazhi*, no. 2: 29–31.

Qian Zifen 钱自奋, Zhang Yuxuan 张育轩, and Guo Saishan 郭赛珊, eds. 1993. *Zhu Chenyu linchuang jingyan ji* 祝谌予临床泾验集 (*The Collected Clinical Experience of Zhu Chengyu*). Beijing: Beijing yike daxue with Zhongguo banhe yike daxue.

Qin Bowei 秦伯未. 1929. *Jiaowu baogao* 教务报告 (*Report by the Dean*). *Zhongguo yixueyuan kan* 1, Appendix: 6–7.

——, ed. 1959 [1928]. *Qingdai mingyi yi'an jinghua* 清代名医医案精华 (*Essential Case Histories of Famous Qing Dynasty Physicians*). Shanghai: Shanghai zhongyi shuju; reprinted, Shanghai kexue jishu chubanshe.

——. 1983a [1957]. "Qian tan 'bianzheng lunzhi'" 浅谈 "辨证论治" (A preliminary talk on pattern differentiation and treatment determination). Reprinted in Qin Bowei 秦伯未 1983e, 27–37.

——. 1983b [1962]. "Mantan chufang yongyao" 漫谈处方用药 (An informal discussion of the use of drugs in writing a prescription). Reprinted in Qin Bowei 秦伯未 1983e, 267–84.

——. 1983c [1963]. "Wenbing yide" 温病一得 (What I have learned about warm [pathogen] disorders). Reprinted in Qin Bowei 秦伯未 1983e, 390–414.

——. 1983d [1964]. "Ruhe zhiliao xiyi zhenduan de jibing" 如何治疗西医诊断的疾病 (How to treat illnesses having been diagnosed by Western medicine). Reprinted in Qin Bowei 秦伯未 1983e, 443–68.

——. 1983e. *Qin Bowei yiwen ji* 秦伯未医文集 (*A Collection of Qin Bowei's Writings on Medicine*). Edited by Wu Dazhen 吴大真 and Wang Fengqi 王凤岐. Changsha: Hunan kexue jishu chubanshe.

Qin Bowei 秦伯未, Li Yan 李岩, Zhang Tianren 张田仁, and Wei Zhizhen 魏执真. 1973 [1963]. "Bianzheng lunzhi qianshuo" 辨证论治浅说 (An elementary introduction to pattern differentiation and treatment determination). In *Zhongyi linchuang lueyao* 中医临床备要 (*Essential Reference for the Clinical Practice of Chinese Medicine*), 239–57. Beijing: Renmin weisheng chubanshe.

Qin Bowei 秦伯未, Li Yinglin 李英麟, Yin Fengli 殷凤礼, Jiao Shude 焦树德, Kang Tingpei 康廷培, Wu Zemin 武泽民, Geng Fusi 耿富思, and Liao Jiamo 廖家模. 1961. "Zhongyi bianzheng lunzhi gangyao" 中医辨证论治纲要 (Outline of Chinese medical pattern differentiation and treatment determination). *Zhongyi zazhi*, no. 1: 5–9, no. 2: 38–46, no. 3: 35–41.

Qin Shoushan 金寿山. 1978. "Tantan bian zhongyi de bing" 谈谈辨中医的病 (Chats concerning the differentiation of diseases in Chinese medicine). *Xinyi yaoxue zazhi*, no. 9: 5–8.

Qiu Peiran 裘沛然. 1995. *Jianfenglou shi chao* 剑风楼诗抄 (*Sable Wind Tower Poems Copied*). Shanghai: Shanghai zhongyiyao daxue chubanshe.

Qiu Peiran 裘沛然 and Ding Guangdi 丁光迪, eds. 1992. *Zhongyi ge jia xueshuo* 中医各家学说 (*Doctrines of Schools of Chinese Medicine*). Teaching Reference Works for Tertiary-Level Chinese Medicine. Beijing: Renmin weisheng chubanshe.

Quanguo gaodeng jiaoyu zixue kaoshi zhidao weiyuanhui 全国高等教育自学考试指导委员会 (National Tertiary-Level Self-Study Examination Guides Committee). 1986. *Zhongyi zhuanye kaoshi jihua* 中医专业考试计划 (*Chinese Medicine Professional Examination [Self-Study] Program*). Shanghai: Shanghai zhongyi xueyuan chubanshe.

Rabinow, Paul. 1996 [1992]. "Artificiality and Enlightenment: From Sociobiology to Biosociality." In *Essays on the Anthropology of Reason*, 91–111. Princeton: Princeton University Press.

Rapp, Rayna. 1997. "Real-Time Fetus: The Role of the Sonogram in the Age of Monitored Reproduction." In Gary Lee Downey and Joseph Dumit eds., 1997, 31–48.

Ren Jixue 任继学, ed. 1997. *Zhongyi jizhenxue* 中医急诊学 (*Chinese Emergency Medicine*). Shanghai: Shanghai kexue jishu chubanshe.

Ren Yingqiu 任应秋. 1954. "Zhongyi bianzheng lunzhi tixi" 中医辨证论治体系 (The system of Chinese medicine pattern differentiation and treatment determination). *Zhongyi zazhi*, no. 4: 19

——. 1966. "Bianzheng lunzhi zhong de jige wenti" 辨证论治中的几个问题 (Some questions concerning pattern differentiation and treatment determination). Reprinted in Ren Yingqiu 1984a, 99–113.

——. 1980. "Lue tan bianzheng yu bianbing" 略谈辨证与辨病 (A synopsis of pattern differentiation and disease differentiation). Reprinted in Ren Yingqiu 1984a, 138–40.

——. 1981. "Yixue liupai suhui lun" 医学流派溯洄论 (Tracing medical streams back to their source). *Beijing zhongyi xueyuan xuebao*, no. 1: 1–6.

——. 1984a. *Ren Yingqiu lunyi ji* 任应秋论医集 (*Ren Yingjiu's Collected Writings on Medicine*). Beijing: Renmin weisheng chubanshe.

——. 1984b. "Zhongyixue jichu lilun liu jiang" 中医学基础理论六讲 (Six lectures on the basic theories of Chinese medicine). In Ren Yingqiu 1984a, 168–208.

Rheinberger, Hans-Jörg. 1999. "Reenacting History." *Studies in History and Philosophy of Science* 30, no. 1: 163–66.

Rhodes, Lorna Amarasingham. 1990. "Studying Biomedicine as a Cultural System." In *Medical Anthropology: Contemporary Theory and Method*, edited by Thomas M. Johnson and Carolyn F. Sargent, 159–73. New York: Praeger.

Rofel, Lisa. 1992. "Rethinking Modernity: Space and Factory Discipline in China." *Cultural Anthropology* 1, no. 1: 93–114.

——. 1999. *Other Modernities: Gendered Yearnings in China after Socialism*. Berkeley: University of California Press.

Rosaldo, Renato. 1995. Introduction to *Hybrid Cultures: Strategies for Entering and Leaving Modernity*, edited by Nestor Garcia Canclini, xi–xvii. Minneapolis: University of Minnesota Press.

Rosenberg, Charles. 1992. *Explaining Epidemics and Other Studies in the History of Medicine*. Cambridge: Cambridge University Press.

Rouse, Joseph. 1992. "What Are Cultural Studies of Scientific Knowledge." *Configurations* 1, no. 1: 1–22.

——. 1996. *Engaging Science: How to Understand Its Practices Philosophically*. Ithaca: Cornell University Press.

Rubel, Arthur J., and Michael Hass. 1990. "Ethnomedicine." In *Medical Anthropology: Contemporary Theory and Method*, edited by Thomas M. Johnson and Carolyn F. Sargent, 115–31. New York: Praeger.

Sahlins, Marshall. 1993. "Goodbye to Tristes Tropes: Ethnography in the Context of Modern World History." *Journal of Modern History* 65: 1–25.

Said, Edward W. 1985. *Orientalism*. Harmondsworth: Penguin.

Schatzki, Theodore. 1999. "To Mangle: Emergent, Unconstrained, Posthumanist?" *Studies in History and Philosophy of Science* 30, no. 1: 157–61.

Scheid, Volker. 1995a. "The Great *Qi:* Zhang Xichun's Reflections on the Nature, Pathology and Treatment of the *Daqi.*" *Journal of Chinese Medicine* 49: 5–16.

——. 1995b. "Essay Review of 'Chinese Acupuncture' by Georges Soulié de Morant." *China Review International* 3, no. 1: 59–61.

——. 2001. "Shaping Chinese Medicine: Two Case Studies from Contemporary China." In *Chinese Medicine: Innovation, Convention, and Controversy*, edited by Elisabeth Hsu, 370–404. Cambridge: Cambridge University Press.

Scheper-Hughes, Nancy. 1992. *Death without Weeping: The Violence of Everyday Life in Brazil*. Berkeley: University of California Press.

Scheper-Hughes, Nancy, and Margaret Lock. 1987. "The Mindful Body: A Prolegomenon to Future Work in Medical Anthropology." *Medical Anthropology Quarterly* 1: 6–41.

Schleifer, Ronald, Robert Con Davis, and Nancy Mergler. 1992. *Culture and Cognition: The Boundaries of Literary and Scientific Inquiry*. Ithaca: Cornell University Press.

Schoenhals, Martin. 1993. *The Paradox of Power in a People's Republic of China Middle School*. Armonk, N.Y.: M. E. Sharpe.

Schwartz, Benjamin. 1985. *The World of Thought in Ancient China*. Cambridge: Belknap Press of Harvard University Press.

Scott, Colin. 1996. "Science for the West, Myth for the Rest? The Case of James Bay Creek Knowledge Construction." In *Naked Science: Anthropological Inquiry into Boundaries, Power, and Knowledge*, edited by Laura Nader, 69–86. London: Routledge.

Scott, James C. 1998. *Seeing like a State: How Certain Schemes to Improve the Human Condition Have Failed*. New Haven: Yale University Press.

Seltzer, Mark. 1992. *Bodies and Machines*. New York: Routledge.

Serres, Michel, and Bruno Latour. 1995. *Conversations on Science, Culture and Time.* Translated by Roxanne Papidus. Ann Arbor: University of Michigan Press.

Shaffer, Simon. 1991. "The Eighteenth Brumaire of Bruno Latour." *Studies in History and Philosophy of Science* 22: 174–92.

Shanghai zhongyi xueyuan 上海中医学院 (Shanghai College of Chinese Medicine), ed. 1964. *Zhongyi neikexue jiangyi* 中医内科学讲义 (*Lecture Notes on Chinese Internal Medicine*). Shanghai: Shanghai kexue jishu chubanshe.

——. 1972. *Bianzheng shizhi* 辨症施治 (*Differentiating Symptoms and Applying Treatment*). Shanghai: Shanghai renmin chubanshe.

Shao, Jing. 1998. "Reifying Embodiment: Writing Case-Records in a Contemporary Hospital of Chinese Medicine." Paper presented at the conference "The Case History in Chinese Medicine: History, Science, and Narrative," University of California, Los Angeles, 24 January. Published at <www.isop.ucla.edu/ccs/seminar.htm>.

——. 1999. "'Hospitalizing' Traditional Chinese Medicine: Identity, Knowledge, and Reification." Ph.D. diss., University of Chicago.

Shaw, R., and C. Stewart. 1994. Introduction to *Syncretism/Anti-Syncretism: The Politics of Religious Synthesis*, edited by C. Stewart and R. Shaw, 1–26. London: Routledge.

Shi Lanhua 史兰化. 1992. *Zhongguo chuantong yixue shi* 中国传统医学史 (*A History of Traditional Medicine in China*). Beijing: Kexue chubanshi.

Shi Qi 施杞 and Xiao Mincai 萧敏材. 1993. *Zhongyi bing'an xue* 中医病案学 (*The Study of Chinese Medical Case Records*). Shanghai: Zhongguo dabaike quanshu chubanshe (Shanghai fenshe).

Shi Yuguang 史宇广, ed. 1989. *Zhongguo zhongyi jigou zhi* 中国中医机构志 (*The Organization of Chinese Medicine in China*). Beijing: Zhongyi guji chubanshe.

——, ed. 1991. *Zhongguo zhongyi renming cidian* 中国中医人名辞典 (*Biographical Dictionary of Chinese Medicine*). Beijing: Zhongyi guji chubanshe.

Shi Yuguang 史宇广 and Shan Shujian 单书健, eds. 1992. *Dangdai mingyi linzheng jinghua* 当代名医临证精华 (*The Essence of Clinical Pattern Diagnosis of Famous Contemporary Physicians*). 21 vols. Beijing: Zhongyi guji chubanshe.

Shore, Bradd. 1982. *Sala'ilula: A Samoan Mystery.* New York: Columbia University Press.

Shweder, Richard A., and Edmund J. Bourne. 1982. "Does the Concept of the Person Vary Cross-Culturally?" In *Cultural Conceptions of Mental Health and Therapy*, edited by Anthony J. Marsella and Geoffrey M. White, 97–137. Dordrecht: Kluwer.

Sidel, Victor W., and Ruth Sidel. 1974. *Serve the People: Observations on Medicine in the People's Republic of China.* Boston: Beacon Press.

Sivin, Nathan. 1968. *Chinese Alchemy: Preliminary Studies.* Cambridge: Harvard University Press.

——. 1987. *Traditional Medicine in Contemporary China.* Ann Arbor: Center for Chinese Studies, University of Michigan.

——. 1990. "Reflections on the Situation in the People's Republic of China, 1987." *American Journal of Acupuncture* 18, no. 4: 341–43.

——. 1995. "Text and Experience in Classical Chinese Medicine." In *Knowledge and the Scholarly Medical Traditions*, edited by Don Bates, 177–204. Cambridge: Cambridge University Press.

——. 1997. "Translating Chinese Medicine: Not Just Philology." Paper presented at the conference "New Directions in the History of Chinese Science," UCLA Center for Chinese Studies, 24 May.

Smith, Richard J. 1983. *China's Cultural Heritage: The Ch'ing Dynasty 1644–1912*. Boulder: Westview Press.

Son, Annette H. K. 1999. "Modernization of Medical Care in Korea (1876–1990)." *Social Science and Medicine* 49: 543–50.

Soulié de Morant, Georges. 1994 [1972]. *Chinese Acupuncture*. Translated by Lawrence Grinell, Claudy Jeanmougin, and Maurice Leveque. Brookline, Mass.: Paradigm.

Spivak, Gayatri Chakravorty, and Sara Harasym. 1990. *The Post-colonial Critique: Interviews, Strategies, Dialogues*. New York: Routledge.

Strathern, Marylin. 1991. *Partial Connections*. Savage, Md.: Rowman and Littlefield.

——. 1992a. *After Nature: English Kinship in the Late Twentieth Century*. Cambridge: Cambridge University Press.

——. 1992b. *Reproducing the Future: Anthropology, Kinship and the New Reproductive Technologies*. London: Routledge.

——. 1995a. "Afterword: Relocations." In *Shifting Contexts: Transformations in Anthropological Knowledge*, edited by Marilyn Strathern, 177–85. London: Routledge.

——. 1995b. "The Nice Thing about Culture Is That Everyone Has It." In *Shifting Contexts*, 153–76.

Sun Shizhong 孙世重. 1962. "Bianzheng lunzhi he jiti fanyingxing wenti" 辨证论治和机体反应性问题 (Pattern differentiation and treatment determination and the problem of organismic reaction). *Zhongyi zazhi*, no. 1: 2–5.

Swartz, Marc J., Victor Turner, and Arthur Tuden, eds. 1966. *Political Anthropology*. Chicago: University of Chicago Press.

Tanford, S., and S. Penrod. 1984. "Social Influence Model: A Formal Integration of Research on Majority and Minority Influence Processes." *Psychological Bulletin* 95: 189–225.

Tang Shenglan, Gerald Bloom, Xushen Feng, Henry Lucas, Xingyuan Gu, and Malcolm Segall, with Gail Singleton and Polly Payne. 1994. "Financing Health Services in China: Adapting to Economic Reform." Brighton: Institute for Development Studies.

Taussig, Michael T. 1980. "Reification and the Consciousness of the Patient." *Social Science and Medicine* 14B: 3–13.

Taylor, Charles. 1989. *Sources of the Self. The Making of Modern Identity*. Cambridge: Cambridge University Press.

Taylor, Kim. 1999. "Paving the Way for TCM Textbooks: The Chinese Medical Improvement Schools." Paper presented at the Ninth International Conference on the History of Science in East Asia, the East Asian Institute, National University of Singapore, 23–27 August.

——. 2000. "Medicine of Revolution: Chinese Medicine in Early Communist China 1945–1963." Ph.D. diss., University of Cambridge.

Toulmin, Stephen. 1990. *Cosmopolis: The Hidden Agenda of Modernity.* Chicago: University of Chicago Press.

Traweek, Sharon. 1988. *Beamtimes and Lifetimes.* Cambridge: Harvard University Press.

——. 1993. "An Introduction to Cultural, Gender, and Social Studies of Sciences and Technologies." *Culture, Medicine and Psychiatry* (special issue: *Biopolitics: The Anthropology of the New Genetics and Immunology*) 17: 3–25.

Tu, Weiming. 1994. "Embodying the Universe: A Note on Confucian Self-Realization." In *Self as Person in Asian Theory and Practice,* edited by Roger T. Ames, Wimal Dissanayake, and Thoma P. Kasulis, 177–86. Albany: SUNY Press.

Turner, Stephen. 1994. *The Social Theory of Practices: Tradition, Tacit Knowledge and Presuppositions.* Cambridge: Polity Press.

——. 1999. "Practice in Real Time." *Studies in History and Philosophy of Science* 30, no. 1: 149–56.

Twitchett, Denis Crispin, John King Fairbank, and Kwang-Ching Liu. 1978. *The Cambridge History of China.* Cambridge: Cambridge University Press.

Unschuld, Paul U. 1973. *Die Praxis des traditionellen chinesischen Heilsystems. Unter Einschluss der Pharmazie dargestellt an der heutigen Situation auf Taiwan.* Edited by Wolfgang Bauer and Hubert Franke. Wiesbaden: Franz Steiner Verlag.

——. 1975. "Medico-Cultural Conflicts in Asian Settings: An Explanatory Theory." *Social Science and Medicine* 9: 303–12.

——. 1976. "The Social Organization of Medical Practice in Taiwan." In *Asian Medical Systems,* edited by Charles Leslie, 300–316. Berkeley: University of California Press.

——. 1979. *Medical Ethics in Imperial China: A Study in Historical Anthropology.* Berkeley: University of California Press.

——. 1985. *Medicine in China: A History of Ideas.* Berkeley: University of California Press.

——. 1986a. *Medicine in China: A History of Pharmaceutics.* Berkeley: University of California Press.

——. 1986b. *Nan Ching: The Classic of Difficult Issues.* Berkeley: University of California Press.

——, ed. 1989. *Approaches to Traditional Chinese Medical Literature: Proceedings of an International Symposium on Translation Methodologies and Terminologies.* Boston: Kluwer.

——. 1990. "Gedanken zur kognitiven Ästhetik Europas und Ostasiens." *Geschichte in Wisenschaft und Unterricht* 12: 735–44.

——. 1992. "Epistemological Issues and Changing Legitimation: Traditional Chinese Medicine in the Twentieth Century." In *Paths to Asian Medical Knowledge,* edited by Charles Leslie and Allan Young, 44–63. Berkeley: University of California Press.

——. 1994. "Der chinesische 'Arzneikönig' Sun Simiao. Geschichte—Legende—Ikono-graphie. Zur Plausibilität naturkundlicher und übernatürlicher Erklärungsmo-delle." *Monumenta Sinica* 42: 217–57.

——. 1997. *Chinesische Medizin*. Munich: C. H. Beck.

Valussi, Marco. 1997. "What Does 'Alternative Medicine' Really Mean?" *European Journal of Herbal Medicine* 3, no. 1: 38–44.

van der Veer, René, and Jaan Valsiner, eds. 1994. *The Vygotsky Reader*. Oxford: Blackwell.

Varela, Francisco, Evan Thompson, and Eleanor Rosch. 1995. *The Embodied Mind: Cognitive Science and Human Experience*. Cambridge: MIT Press.

Wakeman, Frederic, Jr. 1995. *Policing Shanghai: 1927–37*. Berkeley: University of California Press.

Walder, Andrew. 1986. *Communist Neo-traditionalism: Work and Authority in Chinese Industry*. Berkeley: University of California Press.

Wang Huaimei 王怀美, Chen Jing 陈静, and Wu Xifang 吴翠芳. 1998. "'Bagang bianzheng' yuanliu xiaokao" '八纲辨证' 源流小考 (A brief examination of the origins of "eight rubric pattern differentiation"). *Anhui zhongyi linzhuang zazhi* 10, no. 6: 188.

Wang, Jing. 1996. *High Culture Fever: Politics, Aesthetics, and Ideology in Deng's China*. Berkeley: University of California Press.

Wang Ji 王琦. 1993. "21 shiji—zhongyiyao de shiji" 二十一 世纪—中医药的世纪 (The 21st century—the century of Chinese medicine). *Chuantong wenhua yu xiandaihua*, 64–67.

Wang Miqu 王米渠, Wang Keqin 王克勤, Zhu Wenfeng 朱文锋, and Zhang Liutong 张六通. 1986. *Zhongyi xinlixue* 中医心理学 (*Chinese Medical Psychology*). Huanggang: Hubei kexue jishu chubanshe.

Wang Qiaochu 王翘楚. 1998. *Yilin chunqiu—Shanghai zhongyi zhongxiyi jiehe fazhan shi* 医林春秋－上海中医中西医结合发展史 (*Spring and Autumn of the Medical World: A History of the Development of Chinese and Integrated Chinese and Western Medicine in Shanghai*). Shanghai: Wenhui chubanshe.

Wang Songbao 汪松葆, ed. 1987. *Gaodeng zhongyi jiaoyu yu guanli* 篙等中医教育与管理 (*Chinese Medical Further Education and Administration*). Zhangsha: Hunan kexue jishu chubanshe.

Wang Xinhua 王新华, ed. 1983. *Zhongyi lidai yilun xuan* 中医历代医论选 (*Selected Medical Essays by Traditional Chinese Doctors of Past Generations*). Nanjing: Jiangsu kexue jishu chubanshe.

Wang Xudong 王旭东. 1989. *Zhongyi meixue* 中医美学 (*Aesthetics of Chinese Medicine*). Nanjing: Dongnan daxue chubanshe.

Wang Yuxi 王玉玺. 1985. "Bianbing xiaoyi" 辨病小议 (A brief discussion of disease differentiation). *Jilin zhongyiyao*, no. 4: 7–8.

Wang Zhicheng 王志成. 1981. "Ye tan fenxing lunzhi yu bianzheng lunzhi" 也谈分型论治与辨证论治 (Contributing to discussing type discrimination and treatment determination and pattern discrimination and treatment determination). *Shanghai zhongyiyao zazhi*, no. 12: 7.

Wang Zhipu 王致谱 and Cai Jingfeng 蔡景峰, eds. 1999. *Zhongguo zhongyiyao 50 nian* 中国中医药50年 (*Fifty Years of Chinese Medicine and Pharmacology in China*). Fuzhou: Fujian kexue jishu chubanshe.

Wang Ziqiang 王自强. 1994. *Nei Nan jing sanshi lun* 内难经三十论 (*Thirty Essays on the Neijing and Nanjing*). Beijing: Zhongyi zhongyao chubanshe.

Wang Zude 王祖德, ed. 1992. *Zhongxiyi jiehe zhenliao zhinan* 中西医结合诊疗指南 (*A Guide to Diagnosis and Treatment of Integrated Chinese and Western Medicine*). Shanghai: Tongji daxue chubanshe.

Watson, James L. 1982. "Of Flesh and Bones: The Management of Death Pollution in Cantonese Society." In *Death and the Regeneration of Life*, edited by Maurice Bloch and Jonathan Parry, 155–86. Cambridge: Cambridge University Press.

Weber, Max. 1968. *Economy and Society*. Berkeley: University of California Press.

Wertsch, James V. 1985. *Vygotsky and the Social Formation of Mind*. Cambridge: Harvard University Press.

——. 1991. *Voices of the Mind: A Sociocultural Approach to Mediated Action*. Cambridge: Harvard University Press.

——. 1995. "Sociocultural Research in the Copyright Age." *Culture and Psychology* 1: 81–102.

Wertsch, James V., Pablo del Rio, and Amelia Alvarez, eds. 1995. *Sociocultural Studies of Mind*. Cambridge: Cambridge University Press.

White, G. M., and J. Kirkpatrick, eds. 1985. *Person, Self and Experience: Exploring Pacific Ethnopsychologies*. Berkeley: University of California Press.

White, Sidney D. 1993. "Medical Discourses, Naxi Identities, and the State: Transformations in Socialist China." Ph.D. diss., University of California.

——. 1998. "From 'Barefoot Doctor' to 'Village Doctor' in Tiger Springs Village: A Case Study of Health Care Transformation in Socialist China." *Human Organization* 57, no. 4: 480–90.

——. 1999. "Deciphering 'Integrated Chinese and Western Medicine' in the Rural Lijiang Basin: State Policy and Local Practice(s) in Socialist China." *Social Science and Medicine* 49: 1333–47.

WHO Regional Committee for the Western Pacific. 1994. "Guidelines for Clinical Research on Acupuncture." Draft report in the private collection of the author.

Wiseman, Nigel. 1995. *Ying-han, han-ying zhongyi cidian* 英汉汉英词典 (*English-Chinese, Chinese-English Dictionary of Chinese Medicine*). Zhangsha: Hunan kexue jishu chubanshe.

Woolgar, Steve. 1988. *Science: The Very Idea*. Chichester: Ellis Horwood and Tavistock.

Woolgar, Steve, and Malcolm Ashley. 1988. "Introduction to the Reflexive Project." In *Knowledge and Reflexivity*, edited by Steve Woolgar. London: Sage.

World Bank. 1996. *China: Issues and Options in Health Financing*. Report no. 15278 CHA. Washington, D.C.: World Bank.

Worsley, Peter. 1982. "Non-Western Medical Systems." *Annual Review of Anthropology* 11: 315–48.

Wu Boping 吴伯平. 1985. "Yi Qin Bowei laoshi de zhixue jingshen" 忆秦伯未老师的治学精神 (A recollection of the spirit in which teacher Qin Bowei carried out his studies). In Zhou Fengwu 周风梧 et al. 1981–85, 3: 339–50.

Wu Dazhen 吴大真 and Wang Fengqi 王凤岐. 1984. "Yi Qinlao" 忆秦老 (Remembering Elder Qin). In Qin Bowei 1983e, 1–10.

Wu, Yi-Li. 1998. "Transmitted Secrets: The Doctors of the Lower Yangzi Region and Popular Gynecology in Late Imperial China." Ph.D. diss., Yale University.

Wu, Yiyi. 1993–94. "A Medical Line of Many Masters: A Prosopographical Study of Liu Wansu and His Disciples from the Jin to the Early Ming." *Chinese Science* 11: 36–65.

Wujinxian weishengju bianshi xiuzhi lingdao xiaozu 武进县卫生局编史修志史修志领导小组 (Wujin County Department of Health Leadership Group for the Editing of Historical Material and the Compilation of the Gazeteer). 1985. *Wujin weishengzhi: 1879–1983* 武进卫生志: 1879–1983 (*Health Gazeteer of Wujin County: 1879–1983*). Wujn: Wujinxian weishengju (neibu ziliao).

Xiao Jun 消骏. 1981. "Women dui fenxing lunzhi de kanfa" 我们对分型论治的看法 (Our view of type discrimination and treatment determination). *Shanghai zhongyiyao zazhi*, no. 12: 2–3.

Xie Guan 谢观. 1935. *Zhongguo yixue yuanliu lun* 中国医学源流论 (*On the Origins and Development of Medicine in China*). Shanghai: Shanghai zhongyi shuju.

Xinhua News Agency. 1993 [1992]. "Die chinesische Medizin passt sich der modernen Welt an." In *ChinaMed*, 2–11 November, 20.

Xu Jiqun 许济群. 1985. *Fangjixue* 方济学 (*Formulas*). Shanghai: Shanghai kexue jishu chubanshe.

Xu Jiqun 许济群 and Wang Mianzhi, eds. 王绵之 1995. *Fangjixue* 方济学 (*Formulas*). Teaching Reference Works for Tertiary-Level Chinese Medicine. Beijing: Renmin weisheng chubanshe.

Xu, Liangying, and Dainian Fan. 1980. *Science and Socialist Construction in China.* Translated by C. S. Hsu. Armonk, N.Y.: M. E. Sharpe.

Xu Ping 许平. 1990. *Kuizeng lisu* 馈赠礼俗 (*The Etiquette and Customs Attached to the Presentation of Gifts*). Beijing: Huaqiao chubanshe.

Xu, Xiaqun. 1997. "'National Essence' versus 'Science': Chinese Native Physicians' Fight for Legitimacy 1912-32." *Modern Asian Studies* 31, no. 4: 847–78.

Yan, Yunxiang. 1996. *The Flow of Gifts: Reciprocity and Social Networks in a Chinese Village.* Stanford: Stanford University Press.

Yan Zhenghua 颜正华, ed. 1991. *Zhongyaoxue* 中药学 (*Chinese Materia Medica*). Teaching Reference Works for Tertiary-Level Chinese Medicine. Beijing: Renmin weisheng chubanshe.

Yang, C. K. 1961. *Religion in Chinese Society: A Study of Contemporary Social Functions of Religion and Some of Their Historical Factors.* Berkeley: University of California Press.

Yang, Mayfair Mei-hui. 1988. "The Modernity of Power in the Chinese Socialist Order." *Cultural Anthropology* 3: 408–27.

——. 1994. *Gifts, Favours, and Banquets: The Art of Social Relationships in China.* Wilder House Series in Politics, History, and Culture. Ithaca: Cornell University Press.

——. 1995. "Travelling Theory and Modernity in China." In *The Future of Anthropological Knowledge,* edited by Henrietta L. Moore, 93–114. London: Routledge.

Yang Weiyi 杨维益, ed. 1988. *Zhongyi zhenduanxue* 中医诊断学 (*Chinese Medical Diagnosis*). Huabei diqu gaodeng zhongyiyao yuanxiao jiaocai 华北地区高等中医药院校教材. Teaching Materials for Tertiary-Level Chinese Medicine and Pharmacology Colleges and Schools in North China. Beijing: Zhongyi guji chubanshe.

——. 1997 [1994]. "Zhong ti xi yong yu 'zheng' de dongwu moxing" 中体西用于 "证" 的动物模型 (Chinese in essence Western in application and animal models of "patterns"). In Cui Yueli 崔月梨 1997, 131–40.

Yang Xinglin 扬杏林 and Tang Xiaohong 唐晓红, eds. 1991. *Shanghai zhongguo xixueyuan yuanshi* 上海中国医学院院史 (*History of the Shanghai China Medicine College*). Shanghai: Shanghai kexue jishu wenxian chubanshe.

Yang Yiya 杨医亚, ed. 1994. *Fangjixue* 方济学 (*Formulas*). Shijiazhuang: Hebei kexue jishu chubanshe.

Yang Zemin 扬则民. 1985. *Qianguang yihua* 潜广医话 (*Medical Essays by Qianguang*). Edited by Dong Hanliang 董汉良 and Chen Tianxiang 陈天详. Beijing: Renmin weisheng chubanshe.

Yin Huihe 印会河. 1999. *Zhongyi neike xinlun* 中医内科新论 (*A Fresh Discussion of Chinese Internal Medicine*). Taiyuan: Shanxi kexue jishu chubanshe.

Young, Allan. 1980. "The Discourse on Stress and the Re-production of Conventional Knowledge." *Social Science and Medicine* 14B: 133–46.

——. 1981. "When Rational Men Fall Sick: An Inquiry into Some Assumptions Made by Medical Anthropologists." *Culture, Medicine and Psychiatry* 5: 317–35.

——. 1990. "Moral Conflicts in a Psychiatric Hospital Treating Combat-Related Posttraumatic Stress Disorder." In *Social Science Perspectives on Medical Ethics,* edited by G. Weisz, 65–82. Dordrecht: Kluwer.

——. 1995. *The Harmony of Illusions: An Ethnographic Account of Posttraumatic Stress Disorder.* Princeton: Princeton University Press.

Yu Shenchu 俞慎初. 1983. *Zhongguo yixue jianshi* 中国医学简史 (*Short History of Medicine in China*). Fuzhou: Fujian kexue zhishu chubanshe.

Yu Yunxiu 余云岫. 1954. *Gudai jibing minghou shuyi* 古代疾病名侯疏志义 (*Explanations Regarding the Meaning of Ancient Disease Names*). Renmin weisheng chubanshe.

Yue Meizhong 岳美中. 1981a. "Shitan fenxing lunzhi de juxianxing" 试谈分型论治的局限性 (An examination of the limitations of type discrimination and treatment determination). *Shanghai zhongyiyao zazhi*, no. 1: 6–7.

——. 1981b. "Wu heng nanyi zuo yisheng" 无恒难以做医生 (Without persevering it is difficult to become a physician). In Zhou Fengwu 周风梧 et al. 1981–88, 1: 1–19.

——. 1984a. "Bianzheng lunzhi de fangfa gangyao" 辨证论治的方法纲要 (An outline of the method of pattern differentiation and treatment determination). In Yue Mei-zhong 1984c, 43–45.

———. 1984b. "Xu tan bianzheng lunzhi" 续谈辨证论治 (A further chat on pattern differ-entiation and treatment determination). In Yue Meizhong 1984c, 45–50.

———. 1984c. *Yue Meizhong yihua ji* 岳美中医话集 (*A Collection of Yue Meizhong's Talks on Medicine*), edited by Zhongyi yanjiuyuan Xiyuan yiyuan 中医研究院西苑医院 (Academy of Chinese Medicine Xiyuan Hospital). Beijing: Zhongyi guji chubanshe.

———. 2000a. "Bianzheng lunzhi de tantao" 辨证论治的探讨 (An exploration of pattern differentiation and treatment determination). Reprinted in Yue Meizhong 2000c, 3–15.

———. 2000b. "Lun zhongyi jibengong de duanlian" 论中医基本功的锻炼 (On mastering the essential skills of Chinese medicine). Reprinted in Yue Meizhong 2000c, 26–36.

———. 2000c. *Yue Meizhong yixue wenji* 岳美中医学文集 (*A Collection of Yue Meizhong's Writings on Medicine*). Edited by Chen Keji 陈可冀. Beijing: Zhongguo zhongyiyao chubanshe.

Yue Meizhong 岳美中 and Chen Keji 陈可冀. 1962. "Bianzheng lunzhi shizhi tantao" 辨证论治实质探讨 (Exploring the essence of pattern differentiation and treatment determination). *Fujian zhongyiyao*, no. 7: 1–5.

Zang Kuntang 臧坤堂 and Wu Keqiang 吴克强, eds. 1990. *Zhongyao gu jin yingyong zhidao* 中药古今应用指导 (*A Practical Guide to Traditional and Modern Uses of Chinese Medicinal Drugs*). Guangzhou: Guangdong keji chubanshe.

Zehentmayer, Franz, and Cinzia Scorzon. 2000. "Famous Contemporary Chinese Physi-cians: Professor Li Ding." *Journal of Chinese Medicine* 64: 35–39.

Zhang Baiyu 张伯臾, Dong Jianhua 董建华, and Zhou Zhongying 周仲瑛, eds. 1988. *Zhongyi neikexue* 中医内科学 (*Chinese Internal Medicine*). Beijing: Renmin wei-sheng chubanshe.

Zhang, Dengbu. 1994. *Acupuncture Case Histories from China: A Digest of Difficult and Complicated Cases*. Edinburgh: Churchill Livingstone.

Zhang Ji 张吉, ed. 1994. *Ge jia zhenjiu yiji xuan* 各家针灸医籍选 (*A Selection of Medical Texts from the Various Acumoxa Schools*). Beijing: Zhongguo zhongyiyao chuban-she.

Zhang Mingdao 张明岛 and Shao Jieqi 邵洁奇, eds. 1998. *Shanghai weisheng zhi* 上海卫生志 (*Shanghai Health Gazetter*). Shanghai: Shanghai shehui xueyuan chubanshe.

Zhang Qiwen 张奇文. 1980. "Dui fenxing shizhi de shangque" 对分型施治的商榷 (A dis-cussion of type discrimination and treatment application). *Shandong yixue*, no. 6: 50–51.

Zhang Weiyao 张维耀. 1994. *Zhongyi de xianzai yu weilai* 中医的现在与未来 (*The Present and Future of Chinese Medicine*). Tianjin: Tianjin kexue jishu chubanshe.

Zhang Xiaoping 章笑平. 1991. *Xiandai zhongyi ge jia xueshuo* 现代中医各家学说 (*Doc-trines of Modern Schools of Chinese Medicine*). Beijing: Zhongguo zhongyiyao chu-banshe.

Zhang Yingcai 张英才. 1993. "Zhang Xichun lunzhi ganqixu chutan" 张锡纯论治肝气虚

初探 (An introduction to Zhang Xichun's differentiation and treatment of liver *qi* depletion). *Sichuan Zhongyi*, no. 2: 13–14.

Zhang Yuankai 张元凯, ed. 1985. *Menghe sijia yiji* 孟河四家医集 (*The Collected Medical Works of Four Menghe Families*). Nanjing: Jiangsu kexue jishu chubanshe.

Zhao Enjian 赵恩俭, ed. 1990. *Zhongyi maizhen xue* 中医脉诊学 (*The Study of Pulse Diagnosis in Chinese Medicine*). Tianjin: Tianjin kexue jishu chubanshi.

Zhao Hongjun 赵洪钧. 1989. *Jindai zhong xi yi lunzheng shi* 近代中西医论争史 (*History of the Polemics between Chinese and Western Medicine in Modern Times*). Hefei: Anhui kexue jishu chubanshe.

Zhao Shaoqin 赵绍琴, Hu Dingbang 胡定邦, and Liu Jingyuan 刘景源. 1982. *Wenbing zongheng* 瘟病纵横 (*Warm [Pathogen] Disorders in Detail*). Beijing: Renmin weisheng chubanshe.

Zhen Zhiya 甄志亚, ed. 1987. *Zhongguo yixue shi* 中国医学史 (*History of Medicine in China*). Nanchang: Jiangxi kexue jishu chubanshe.

Zhen Zhiya 甄志亚 and Fu Weikang 傅维康, eds. 1991. *Zhongguo yixue shi* 中国医学史 (*History of Medicine in China*). Beijing: Renmin weisheng chubanshe.

Zheng, X., and S. Hillier. 1995. "The Reforms of the Chinese Health Care System. County Level Changes: The Jiangxi Study." *Social Science and Medicine* 41, no. 8: 1057–64.

Zhongguo kexue jishu xiehui 中国科学技术协会 (China Science and Technology Association), ed. 1999. *Zhongguo kexue jishu zhuanjia chuanlu. Yixue bian. Zhongyixue, juan 1* 中国科学技术专家传略·医学编·中医学·卷 1 (*Summary Biographies of Chinese Science and Technology Experts. Medicine: Chinese Medicine, vol. 1*. Beijing: Renmin weisheng chubanshe.

Zhongguo yixuehui Shanghai fenzhi yixueshi xuehui 中国医学会上海分支医学史学会 (Medical History Association of the Shanghai Branch of the Chinese Medical Association). 1954. "Yu Yunxiu xiansheng zhuanlue he nianpu" 余云岫先生传略和年谱 (Biographical sketch and chronology of the life of Mr. Yu Yunxiu). *Zhonghua yishi zazhi*, no. 2: 81–84.

Zhonghua renmin gongheguo weishengbu zhongyisi 中华人民共和国卫生部中医司 (Chinese Medicine Bureau of the Ministry of Health of the People's Republic of China). 1985. *Zhongyi gongzuo wenjian huibian* 中医工作文件汇编 (*Collection of Documents relating to the Work [of the Ministry] on Chinese Medicine*). Beijing: Zhonghua renmin gongheguo weishengbu zhongyisi.

Zhongshan yiyuan "zhongyi fangji xuanjiang" bianxiezu 中山医院 "中医方剂选讲" 编写组 (Zhongshan Hospital "Selected Lectures on Chinese Medical Formulas" Editorial Committee), ed. 1983. *Zhongyi fangji xuanjiang* 中医方剂选讲 (*Lectures on Selected Chinese Medical Formulas*). Guangdong: Guangdong kexue chubanshe.

Zhonguo zhongyi yanjiuyuan 中国中医研究院 (Academy of Chinese Medicine). 1979. *Pu Fuzhou yiliao jingnian* 蒲辅周医疗经验 (*The Therapeutic Experience of Pu Fuzhou*). Beijing: Renmin weisheng chubanshe.

——, ed. 1984. *Zhongyi zhengzhuang bianbie zhenduanxue* 中医证状鉴别诊断学 (*Dis-*

tinguishing Signs in Chinese Medical Diagnosis). Beijing: Renmin weisheng chubanshi.

———. 1987. *Zhongyi zhenghou jianbie zhenduanxue* 中医疾病鉴别诊断学 (*The Discrimination of Patterns in Chinese Medical Diagnosis*). Beijing: Renmin weisheng chubanshe.

———. *Zhongyi jibing jianbie zhenduanxue* 中医证侯鉴别诊断学 (*The Discrimination of Diseases in Chinese Medical Diagnosis*). Beijing: Renmin weisheng chubanshe, forthcoming.

Zhongyi bingming zhenduan guifan ketizu 中医病名诊断规范课题组 (Discussion Group of Standards for Disease Names and Diagnostic Categories in Chinese Medicine). 1987. *Zhongyi bingming zhenduan guifan chugao* 中医病名诊断规范初稿 (*Standards for Disease Names and Diagnostic Categories in Chinese Medicine: A First Draft*). Hubeisheng zhongyiyao yanjiusuo.

Zhou Fengwu 周凤梧, Zhang Qiwen 张启文, and Cong Lin 丛林, eds. 1981–85. *Ming laozhongyi zhi lu* 名老中医之路 (*Paths of Renowned Senior Chinese Physicians*). 3 vols. Jinan: Shandong kexue jishu chubanshe.

Zhou Weixin 周味辛. 1954. "Lun zhongyi de zhiliao face" 论中医的治疗法则 (On the methods of Chinese medical therapeutics). *Beijing zhongyi* 10, no. 10: 14–16.

Zhu Chenyu 祝谌予. 1981. "Zhongyi xueshu yingdang fazhan tigao" 中医学术应当发展提高 (Chinese medical science should be developed and improved). In Zhou Fengwu 周凤梧 et al. 1981–85, 1: 261–74. Jinan: Shandong kexue jishu chubanshe.

———, ed. 1982. *Shi Jinmo linchuang jingnian ji* 施今墨临床经验集 (*The Collected Clinical Experience of Shi Jinmo*). Beijing: Renmin weisheng chubanshe.

———. 1985. "Yi dai ming yi-Shi Jinmo" 一代明医－施今墨 (A brilliant physician of our time: Shi Jinmo). In Zhou Fengwu 周凤梧 et al. 1981–85, 3: 71–76.

Zhu Hongming 朱鸿铭. 1980. "Yong bianzheng weiwu zhuyi zhidao zhongyi lilun yanjiu" 用辩证唯物主义指导中医理论研究 (Using dialectical materialism to guide research on Chinese medical theory). *Shandong yixue*, no. 6: 51–52.

Zhu Jiene 祝世讷 and Sun Guilian 孙桂莲. 1990. *Zhongyi xitonglun* 中医系统论 (*Chinese Medicine Systems Theory*). Chongqing: Chongqing chubanshe.

Zhu Liangchun 朱良春. 1962. "Bianzheng yu bianbing xiang jiehe de zhongyaoxing ji qi guanxi de tantao" 辨证与辨病相结合的重要性及其关系的探讨 (An Inquiry into the significance of the mutual integration of pattern differentiation and disease differentiation and their relation). *Zhongyi zazhi*, no. 4: 16.

———. 2000. *Zhang Cigong yishu jingyan ji* 章次公医术经验集 (*A Collection of Zhang Cigong's Medical Skills and Experience*). Changsha: Hunan kexue jishu chubanshe.

Zhu Wenfeng 朱文锋, ed. 1995. *Zhongyi zhenduanxue* 中医诊断学 (*Chinese Medical Diagnosis*). Standard Teaching Materials for Tertiary-Level Education in Chinese Medicine and Pharmacology Courses. Shanghai: Shanghai kexue jishu chubanshe.

Zhu Yan 朱彦. 1954. "Zhongguo gujing zhenghou zhiliao de yiban guilu 中国古典症候治疗的一般规律 (General laws regarding the treatment of symptom patterns in China's classics). *Zhonghua yishi zazhi*, no. 9: 734.

Zhu Ziqing 朱子青. 1963. "Tantan bianbing, bianzheng yu bianzheng lunzhi de fazhan" 谈谈辨病, 辨证与辨证论治的发展 (A chat about the development of disease differentiation, pattern differentiation, and pattern differentiation and treatment determination). *Jiangsu zhongyi*, no. 3: 1–3.

Zimmerman, Francis. 1978. "From Classic Texts to Learned Practice: Methodological Remarks on the Study of Indian Medicine." *Social Science and Medicine* 12: 97–103.

Zito, Angela. 1994. "Silk and Skin: Significant Boundaries." In Angela Zito and Tani E. Barlow 1994b, 103–30.

Zito, Angela, and Tani E. Barlow. 1994a. "Introduction: Body, Subject, and Power in China." In Angela Zito and Tani E. Barlow 1994b, 1–22.

——, eds. 1994b. *Body, Subject and Power in China*. Chicago: University of Chicago Press.

INDEX

ben 本/biao 标 (root and manifestations), 108, 111, 138, 160, 202

benevolence (ren 仁), 59, 139; benevolent physicians, 168; practiced benevolence, 20–21

Benjamin, Walter, 259

bianbing 辨病 (disease differentiation), 346 n.96

bianfang 辨方 (differentiation via formulas), 237, 332 n.43

bianzheng fenxi 辨症分析 (analysis of symptom differentiation), 225

bianzheng lunzhi 辨证论治, 200–204, 234, 238, 264, 267, 275, 279, 281; as continuation and development of methods and theories, 203; debates on, 281; as defining feature of Chinese medicine, 228; formation of, 219, 221; according to fourteen rubrics, 283; history of, 204; input of Western medicine physicians in the formation of, 281; in late Ming medical treatises, 206; in Maoist China, 209; in modern medical discourse, 344 n.85; role of, 219; systematization of, 288; as way of practicing medicine, 202. *See also* pattern differentiation

Bianzheng lunzhi yanjiu qi jiang 辨证论治研究七讲 (*Seven Lectures on Pattern Differentiation and Treatment Determination Research*), 275, 285

bianzheng shizhi 辨证施治 (differentiating patterns and applying treatment), 223

Bianzheng shizhi gangyao 辨症施治纲要 (*Differentiating Symptoms and Applying Treatment: An Outline*), 223, 225

bing, 病, 336 n.5. *See also* disease

biomedicine, 4, 89, 94, 137–138, 155, 163, 256; biomedical diagnoses, 137; biomedical disease categories, 267; biomedical drugs, 138; biomedical investigative techniques, 147; biomedical knowledge, employment of, 157; bio-medical signs and disease categories, 121; biomedical technology, 153, 265; biomedical treatment, side effects of, 271; as a tool to confirm Chinese medical knowledge, 157

body: anatomical body of biomedicine and functional body of Chinese medicine, 152; in Chinese medicine, 28; as represented on modern acupuncture charts, 41; as revealed by biomedical technology, 161; structure and function of, 27; of viscera and vessels, 161. See also *hsing; shen; ti*

Buzhong yiqi tang 补中益气汤 (Decoction to Supplement the Middle and Benefit *Qi*), 145, 190, 267

canonical texts, 14

Cao Xiping, 曹希平, 232

case records, 99–103, 137

case study approach, 61

Central Institute of National Medicine (*Zhongyang guoyi guan* 中央国医馆), 215

channels and collaterals (*jingluo* 经络), 41, 240

Chen Chun, 陈淳, 51

Chen Keji, 陈可冀, 222

Chen Shenwu, 陈慎吾, 75

Chen Ziyin, 沈自尹, 226–228

China-Japan Friendship Hospital, 87, 94–95, 111, 128, 192

Chinese Communist Party (CCP), 65, 68, 90, 171, 201, 264; emergence of policy on Chinese medicine, 353 n.3

Chinese drugs. See *Zhongyao dacidian* 中药

Chinese emergency medicine (*zhongyi jizhen* 中医急诊), 264

Chinese medical dialectics, 217; resonance with Maoist dialectics, 217

Chinese medical improvement schools (*zhongyi jinxiu xuexiao* 中医进修学校), 69, 214, 342 n.70

Chinese medicine, 3, 16, 295; as an

discipleship (*continued*)
ship, 182. *See also* apprenticeship;
master and disciple

disease, 206; biomedical or Western
medicine disease categories, 121, 226,
267; causes (*bingyin* 病因), 201, 280,
284; condition (*bingqing*), 病情), 280;
as diagnostic classifier, 205; differentiation (*bianbing* 辨病), 346; essential
character of (*bingxing* 病性), 201;
location (*bingwei* 病位), 201, 280;
mechanism (*bingji* 病机), 105, 158, 201,
231, 316 n.95; models, 30; names, 229–
230; patterns of, 208; standardization
of, 230. See also *bing*

distinguishing types and applying treatment (*fenxing shizhi* 分型施治), 226

diversity, 10, 12, 32; intracultural, 22

divination (*suanming* 算命), 16

doctoral supervisor (*boshi daoshi* 博士导师): status of, 242

Doctrine of the Mean (*zhongyong* 中庸),
139

Dong Jianhua, 董建华, 92

Dongzhimen Hospital of Chinese Medicine, 18, 86, 128, 136, 183, 281

drugs: adding and subtracting (*jiajian*
加减), 140; biomedical, 138; cooperation within a formula of, 156; entering
into a particular vessel, 156; synergistic
combinations (*duiyao* 对药), 141–142;
toxic, 147, 149–150

Du Zeming 杜自明, 72

Duhuo jisheng tang 独活寄生汤 (Duhuo
and Mistletoe Decoction), 146

duiyao (synergistic combinations), 141–
142

education: inheritance in, 213; political
control of, 178

efficacy, 138; attributions of, 108, 118. See
also *linghuo* 灵活

eight rubrics. See *ba gang*

Eighth Five-Year Plan, 93, 314 n.61

emergence, 52–53; Chinese medicine as
a dynamic process of, 13, 20; and disappearance, 13, 52, 56, 65; and process
of innovation, 161; and synthesis, 104,
130

Enlightenment: perceptions of knowledge, 23; subject, 165

Erchen tang 二陈汤 (Two Cured Decoction), 155–156

etheral soul (*hun* 魂), 50

ethnography, 61; as approach to Chinese medicine, 1; and fieldwork, 14,
307 n.84; interventionist, 60; in the
sociology of scientific knowledge, 298
n.63

experience (*jingyan* 经验), 231, 270, 340
n.55

face, 170, 176, 183, 335 n.89

Fang Yaozhong, 方药中, 213–214, 231,
275, 289, 341 n.66

Fangjixue 方剂学 (*Formulas*), 180

Farquhar, Judith, 50, 102, 121, 135, 139,
164, 192, 201, 212, 277

Fei Shengfu, 费绳甫, 131

Feng Zhaozhang, 冯兆张, 153

fenxing shizhi 分型施治 (distinguishing
types and applying treatment), 226

field of practice, 55, 58, 165, 198, 255, 307
n.84

filiality, 57

First and Second National Health Conferences, 67–68

five cardinal relationships (*wu lun* 五伦),
169

five phases (*wu xing* 五行), 214, 289, 342
n.68

formulas (*fangji* 方剂), 140, 180, 323
n.11; classical, 159; differentiation via
formulas (*bianfang* 辨方), 237; genealogy of, 154; merging formulas from
shanghan and *wenbing* traditions,
160; research into, 168; secret (*mifang*
秘方), 183–184; single drug formulas
(*danfang* 单方), 342 n.71; standard
additions and subtractions (*jiajian*
加减) for, 180; standardization of, 93

four modernizations, 81

Kant, Immanuel, 23

kexuehua, 科学化. *See* scientization

Kong Bohua, 孔伯化, 201

Kuang Ankun, 矿安昆, 229

laozhongyi, 老中医, 14, 142, 191–192, 214, 231, 257, 264, 285, 349 n.127; how to become a *ming laozhongyi,* 329 n.20; *ming laozhongyi,* 120, 166, 171, 183, 197

Lei, Sean, 349 n.126

Leizheng zhicai 类证治裁 (Tailored Treatments According to Patterns), 207

li 礼 (rules of correct conduct; ritualized behavior), 169, 173

Li Chongren, 李重人, 75

Li Dingming, 李鼎铭, 187

Li Gao, 141, 145, 148, 152, 190, 267

Li Zhongzi, 李中籽, 188

Lin Peiqin, 林佩琴, 207

Ling gui zhu gan tang 苓桂术甘汤 (Poria, Cinnamon, Atractylodes, and Liquorice Decoction), 162

linghuo, 灵活, 180, 331 n.42

literati physicians (*ruyi* 儒医), 169

Liu Duzhou, 刘渡舟, 232

Liu Shaoqi, 刘少奇, 71–72

Liu Yue, 刘越, 234, 236

Li zhong wan 理中丸 (Regulate the Middle Pill), 145

Lock, Margaret, 90

Lü Bingkui, 吕炳奎, 74, 79, 81–83, 179, 186, 231–232

Luhmann, Niklas, 23

Ma Yuanyi, 马元仪, 132

mangle of practice, 44, 233: Pickering's model of, 54; problems with model of, 52

Mao Zedong, 毛泽东, 67–69, 72, 75, 83, 90, 264, 311 nn.16 and 17; on practice, 229

Marcus, George E., 54

master and disciple: social relations between, 169. *See also* apprenticeship; discipleship

May Fourth Movement (*wu si yundong*), 34

medical archive, 192; formulas in, 159

medical ethics, 150, 173

medical pluralism, 11–12, 90, 128, 292 n.8

medical practice, 13; social organization of, 31

medical systems, 11–12, 21; comparison between, 109, 121; of non-Han minority cultures (*minzu yixue* 民族医学), 16

medicine and art, 139

mētis, 270

Ministry of Education (MOE, Jiaoyubu 教育部), 91–93

Ministry of Health (MOH, Weishengbu 卫生部), 68, 77, 82, 84, 91, 93, 171, 178, 202, 211, 217, 224, 229, 276–277; policy toward Chinese medicine of, 70

Ministry of Personnel (Renshibu 人事部), 171

modernity, 42, 90; definitions of, 35, 303 n.39; different modernities, 304 n.46; discourse of, 41; as locally emergent, 42; and powers of nation-state, 269; romanticist critiques of, 43

modernization, 32, 35, 40, 98, 194, 269, 272; of Chinese medicine, 17, 39, 348 n.113; and scientification, 194

Montesquieu, Charles-Louis de Secondat, 23, 53

multiplicity, 34, 58–59, 158

multisited ethnography, 53, 65

Nanjing 难经 (*Classic of Difficult Issues*), 28

Nanjing College of Chinese Medicine (Nanjing zhongyi xueyuan 南京中医学院), 135, 179, 277

national curriculum, 190

National Medicine (*guoyi* 国医), 66

National Standards for Clinical Diagnosis and Treatment Terminologies, 93

Nationwide Classes for Physicians of Western Medicine Studying Chinese

Medicine (Quanguo juban xiyi xuexi zhongyi ban 全国举办西医学习中医班), 276

needle technique (shoufa 手法), 31, 36, 40, 56, 304 n.43

Neijing, 内经. See Huangdi neijing

Neiwaishang bian huo lun 内外伤辨惑论 (Clarifying Doubt about Injury from Internal or External Causes), 141

networks, 57, 192–193, 196–198; of descent, 199; as one particular type of synthesis, 198; relational, 197; of social relations, 15

New Culture Movement (xin wenhua yundong 新文化运动), 34

new medicine (xinyi 新医), 33, 68, 76, 83, 223, 254

Ninth Five-Year Plan, 93

objective knowledge: as equated with the perceptually visible, 153

orchestrated medical pluralism, 90, 251

orientalism, 21–22, 176, 294 n.20; and modes of representation, 21; orientalist knowledge, 13

origin: image of the, 259

Ots, Thomas, 108

Outline of Chinese Medicine. See Zhongyixue gailun 中医学概论)

pai 派 (streams [in Chinese medicine]), 31, 196, 301 n.21

Pang Anshi, 庞安时, 152

pathogenic qi (xieqi 邪气), 141, 151, 159

patients, 10, 107; complexity of behavior, 128; physical bodies of, 159

patrilineal descent: classical ideologies of, 174

pattern differentiation, 30, 40, 124, 150, 187, 200–201, 212, 215, 256, 271; analysis of symptom patterns (bianzheng fenxi) 辨症分析, 225; as invention of Northern Song, 338 n.37; methods of, 344 n.90; as pivot of Chinese medical practice, 277; in relation to dialectics, 212; of symptoms and signs, 12;

systematization of, 285; and Western medical disease diagnosis, 215. See also bianzheng lunzhi

People's Health Press (Renmin weisheng chubanshe 人民卫生出版社), 92

personal relationships, 161

Ph.D. research: outline criteria, 243

phlegm (tan 痰), 152, 154, 163; phlegm-rheum (tanyin 痰饮), 143, 154; phlegm-rheum disease (tanyinbing 痰饮病), 221; tangible or formed and intangible or formless, 152; to transform (huatan 化痰), 154

physician: becoming a, 164; benevolent, 168; duty as a, 149; famous and influential physicians, 295 n.25; virtuosity of, 180

physiognomy (xiangmian 相面), 16

Pickering, Andrew, 44, 47, 52

plural health care system, 312 n.40, 316 n.96

pluralism, 322 n.45

plurality, 12, 23–4, 30, 53, 55, 59, 69, 163, 195, 197, 263; of Chinese medicine practice, 303 n.36; and cultural processes, 256; in health care, 81; as an intrinsic and irreducible aspect of Chinese medicine 13; of knowledge, 195; three constitutional aspects of, 56

polluted blood (wuxue 污血), 139

posthumanists, 47

practice, 52–54; dialectical, 213; disciplinary, 163; flexibility of, 270; mangle of, 44, 233; of writing a prescription (chufang 处方), 140. See also mangle of practice

practitioners of Chinese medicine studying Western medicine (zhongyi xuexi xiyi 中医学习西医), 137

practitioners of Western medicine studying Chinese medicine (xiyi xuexi zhongyi 西医学习中医), 218–219

prescription (chufang 处方 or fangzi 方子), 99, 102, 167; formulating a, 199; reading and writing of, 139–40; standardization of, 94; trading of, 191 principles of medicine (*yili* 医理), 210

Pu Fuzhou, 蒲辅周, 72, 179, 189, 216, 226, 343 n.82

pulse (*mai* 脉), 151; diagnosis, 30, 122–123, 143; pulse records (*mai'an* 脉案), 102–104

Pure Chinese Medicine Correspondence University (Guangming Zhongyi Hanshou Daxue 光明中医函授大学), 232

qi, 34, 48, 50, 59

Qi ju dihuang wan 杞菊地黄丸 (Lycium Berry, Chrysanthemum, and Rhemannia Decoction), 112

Qian Xinzhong, 钱信忠, 75

Qianjin yaofang 千金要方 (*Important Formulas Worth a Thousand*), 206, 265–266

Qin Bowei, 秦伯未, 72, 75, 127, 131, 179, 189, 211, 221, 224, 230, 281, 286, 288

quest for health, 118, 132

Ren Yingqiu, 任应秋, 75, 179, 206, 222, 277

renqing, 人情, 173

research: applied and clinical, 243; Chinese medicine, 94; into formulas, 168; interdisciplinary, 1

resistance, 107, 129; Foucault on, 321 n.37

resistance and accommodation, 46, 258, 322 n.45

rheum (*yin* 饮), 152, 154

righteousness (*yi* 义), 51

root (*ben* 本), 108, 111, 138, 160, 288; in Chinese medicine treatment, 108

Rouse, Joseph, 47

rubrics (*gang* 纲), 234; for the analysis of patterns, 234; eight, 188, 220, 277; fourteen, 281

Sahlins, Marshall, 19

sanjiao, 三焦, 28, 32

San ren tang 三仁汤 (Three Seed Decoction), 217

scalp acupuncture, 254–255

scholarly streams, 131

science: anthropology of, 24–25; construction of, 24–25; definition of, 98; natural and social, 20; and technology, 32, 34; universality of, 23; Western, 257

science and technology studies (STS), 13, 24, 44, 294 n.21

scientism, 43, 302 n.25

scientization, 90

Scott, James, 269

sectarianism (*zongpaizhuyi* 宗派主义), 90

Self-Strengthening movement (*yangwu yundong* 洋务运动), 34

Serres, Michel, 199

Shanghai College of Chinese Medicine (*Shanghai zhongyi xueyuan* 上海中医学院), 140, 223

shanghan 伤寒 (cold damage), 268, 284; disorders, 268; scholarly stream, 131, 159; therapeutics, 160; and *wenbing* four aspects, 225; and *wenbing* streams, 159, 219

Shanghan lun, 伤寒论, 74, 159, 170, 285; pattern of diagnosis and treatment in, 224

Shanghan zabing lun 伤寒杂病论 (*Discussion of Cold Damage and Various Disorders*), 140, 203–204, 216

Shao Jing, 104

shen 身 (lived body), 28

Sheng mai san 生脉散 (Generate the Pulse Powder), 139

Sheng xian tang 升陷汤 (Decoction to Raise What Has Sunk), 190

Shi Jinmo, 施今墨, 73, 210, 215, 220–221, 226, 230, 340 n.53, 343 n.75, 346 n.98

sifting of the national medical heritage (*zhengli zuguo yixue yichan* 整理祖国医学遗产), 21

simplification, 285; of Chinese medicine, 231

situated learning, 177, 330 n.30, 352 n.15

Sivin, Nathan, 10, 169, 171, 201, 277

social relationships, 161; connection to

medical practice, 164; construction of, 56. See also *guanxi*

social topography, 65, 165, 307 n.89

social topology, 60, 165, 197, 307 n.89

sociology of scientific knowledge (SSK), 24

standardization (*guifanhua* 规范化), 21, 230, 241, 271; of Chinese medicine, 32, 181, 222; of classical medical knowledge, 178; of teaching, practice, and bureaucratic control, 269

State, 65–66; influence on medical research, 93–94; and keeping of medical records, 93, 98, 100–101, 105; and standardization of medical practice, 93

State Administration of Chinese Medicine and Pharmacology (Guojia zhongyiyao guanliju 国家中医药管理局), 243

state education, 177; in Chinese medicine, 178; system, 198

state health care sector, 15–16

"state simplifications," 269

students (*xuesheng* 学生), of Chinese medicine, 166–168, 178; postgraduate, 183; undergraduate, 182

studentship, 177, 196; and discipleship, 182; plurality of, 195

subject formation, 23

subjectivity, 16, 165, 195

subject positionality, 165

Sun Simiao, 孙思邈, 17, 150, 247, 251, 253

surface manifestations, 138. See also *ben/biao*

syncretism, 23–24, 122–123, 158

synthesis, 13, 54–55, 58–59, 104, 107, 160, 199, 238, 252, 258–259, 271; conjunctive, 198; connective, 198; in contemporary Chinese, 238; emergent, 130; ethnography of, 54; formation, 161; instability of, 256; Kantian conception of, 53; ontology of, 258; process of, 255; as a process of simultaneous emerging and disappearing, 268; stability of, 258

systematization, 90, 271, 278–279, 281; of Chinese medical diagnostic categories, treatment methods, and measurements of therapeutic outcomes, 98; of Chinese medicine, 217; of diseases, patterns, symptoms, and signs, 207; of pattern differentiation, 285

taijiquan, 太气拳, 114

Tang Youzhi, 唐由之, 214

Tang Zonghai, 唐宗海, 189

Taylor, Kim, 67, 72

teacher-student relationships, 244; homogenization of, 181

teaching materials, 74, 178

terminology, 3; clinical, 189

testing memorized knowledge, 178

textbooks, 189; compilation of, 187

theoretical knowledge (*lilun* 理论), 17

"three paths" (*san daolu* 三道路) policy, 82

three theories (*san lun* 三论), 229

ti 体 (embodiment of any number of things, including spiritual, cosmic, and moral states), 28

Tianma gouteng yin 天麻钩藤饮 (Gastrodia and Uncaria Beverage), 157

toxic drugs, 147; side effects of, 147; use of, 149

traditional Chinese medicine (TCM), 3, 35, 43, 65, 293 n.11, 295 n.28

tradition and modernity, 98; as locally configured, 44; opposition between, 43

treatment: determination (*lunzhi*), 202; formulation of, 161; record, 166; strategy, 30, 137, 139, 156–159

types (*xing* 型), 151, 226, 325 n.43; criticism of, 151

unify Chinese and Western medicine (*zhongxiyi tuanjie* 中西医团结), 68, 214

Unschuld, Paul, 30–31, 48

visceral systems of function (*zangfu* 脏腑), 28, 188, 256, 286

Volker Scheid is Wellcome Trust Research Fellow in the Department
of History, School of Oriental and African Studies (soas), at the
University of London.

Library of Congress Cataloging-in-Publication Data
Scheid, Volker G.
Chinese medicine in contemporary China : plurality and synthesis /
Volker Scheid.
p. cm. — (Science and cultural theory)
Includes bibliographical references and index.
ISBN 0-8223-2857-7 (cloth : alk. paper) —
ISBN 0-8223-2872-0 (pbk. : alk. paper)
1. Medicine—China.   2. Medicine, Chinese—China   I. Title.   II. Series.
R601 .S355   2002   610'.951—dc21   2001056851